The Therapeutic Use of Ayahuasca

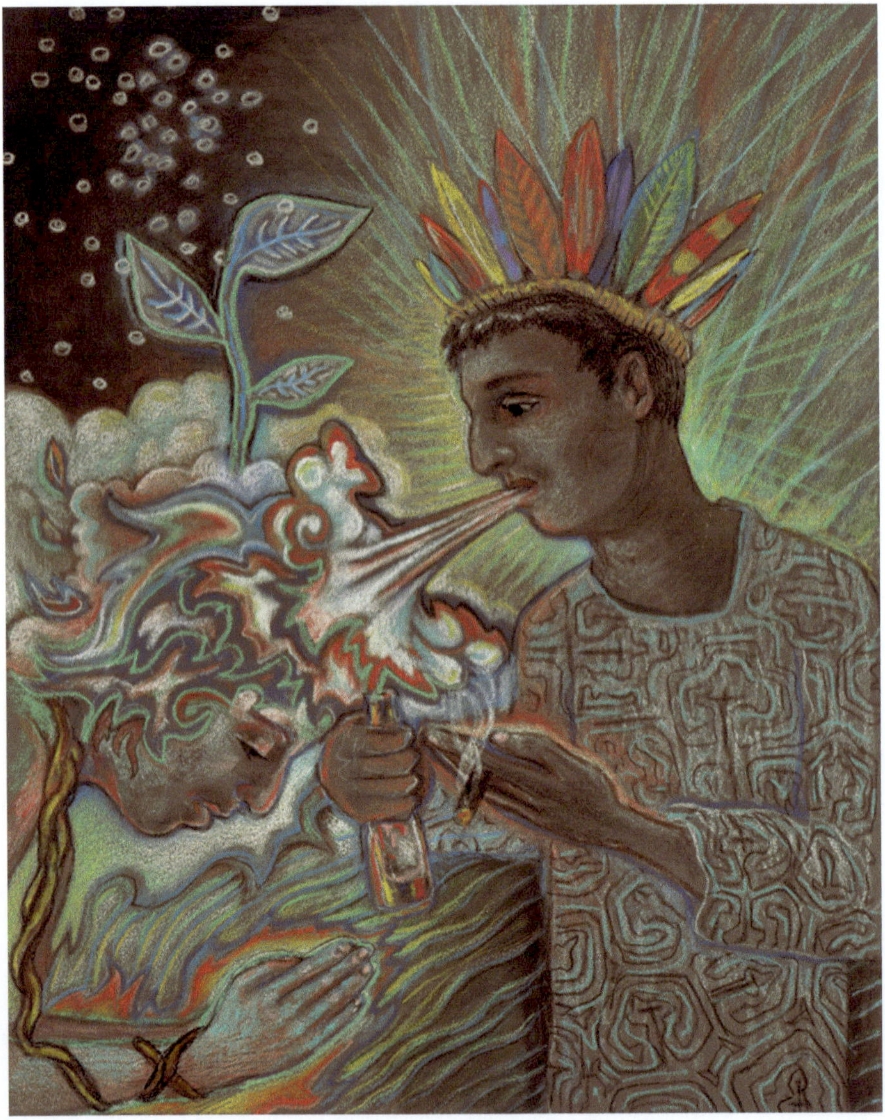

Chamán Soplando [Shaman Blowing] by Clancy Cavnar, 2012

Beatriz Caiuby Labate · Clancy Cavnar
Editors

The Therapeutic Use of Ayahuasca

Springer

Editors
Beatriz Caiuby Labate
Center for Economic Research
and Education (CIDE)
Aguascalientes, AGS, Mexico

Clancy Cavnar
Nucleus for Interdisciplinary Studies
of Psychoactives (NEIP)
San Francisco, CA, USA

ISBN 978-3-642-40425-2 ISBN 978-3-642-40426-9 (eBook)
https://doi.org/10.1007/978-3-642-40426-9

Springer Heidelberg New York Dordrecht London
Library of Congress Control Number: 2013950740

Springer is part of Springer Science+Business Media (www.springer.com)

We dedicate this book to the healing plants of the Amazon Forest

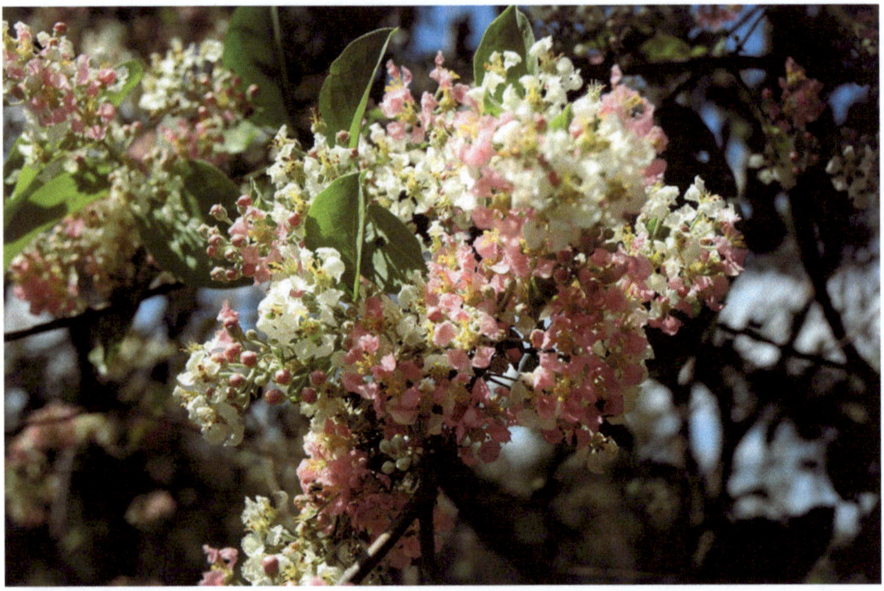

Banisteriopsis caapi flowers. © Thais Rebello

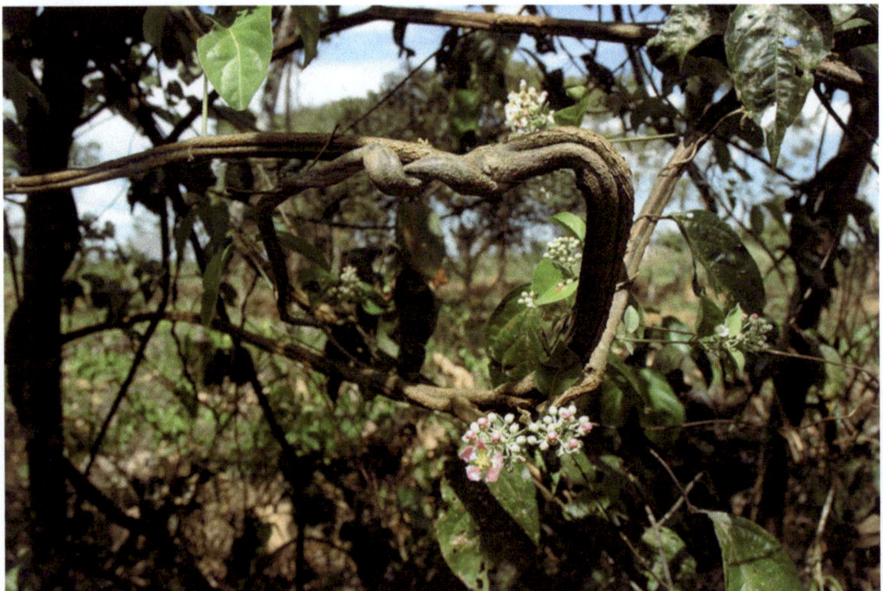

Banisteriopsis caapi vine. © Thais Rebello

Foreword

Ancient Medicine and the Modern World

Ayahuasca, the "great medicine" of the Amazon rain forest, was, for millennia, entirely unknown to Western Euro-American civilization. While first scientifically identified, catalogued, and recorded in the mid-nineteenth century by the English botanist and explorer Richard Spruce, it had earlier been the object of brutal suppression by Spanish and Portuguese invaders of the New World who attempted to violently extinguish its ceremonial use by the indigenous people of the Amazon. Employing the harshest measures of the Inquisition, in 1616, the Catholic Church formally condemned the use of plant hallucinogens by the native people of the New World with punishment by extreme tortures and death. Use of powerful plants employed by native peoples for purposes of healing, divination, and cultural cohesion was virtually eliminated and forced deeply underground and, in the case of ayahuasca, into the remote regions of the forest, far from the reach of the marauding Europeans and their descendants. While occasional reports from traders and missionaries filtered out of indigenous use of ritual plants, it was not until Spruce obtained samples of the bark of *Banisteriopsis caapi*, a woody vine and one of the central plants used in the decoction ayahuasca, that the Western world took note.

In recent years, some controversy has arisen over the antiquity of ayahuasca. Given the climactic and soil conditions in the Amazon Basin, archeological finds have been limited, and suggestions have been made that the potent plant hallucinogen decoction may have existed only for a few hundred years. While definitive evidence does not exist, it seems highly unlikely that the indigenous people who traditionally made the region their home would have been ignorant of these powerful psychoactive plants that grew throughout the geographic region they knew so intimately. Rather, it is highly likely that traditional ayahuasca use, particularly in the Upper Amazon, dates long before the arrival of the first Europeans.

Lack of awareness of the existence of plant hallucinogens around the world by Euro-American culture has itself been endemic over time. In the classic *Plants of the Gods* by Richard Evans Schultes and Albert Hofmann, the very first sentence in the book states that "the use of hallucinogenic plants has been a part of human experience for many millennia, yet modern Western societies have only recently become aware of the significance that these plants have had in shaping the history of primitive and even of advanced cultures." A telling example was the collective ignorance, until the mid-twentieth century, of the existence of hallucinogenic mushrooms. It was not until R. Gordon Wasson's "discovery" in June 1955 of indigenous Mazatec healers' use of highly potent *Psilocybe cubensis* in a remote region of the state of Oaxaca in Mexico, that Western scientists accepted such powerful psychotropic fungi as something other than the products of myth. In the case of ayahuasca, the earliest known commentary on its existence came from Jesuit missionaries in the 1600s, who spoke of "diabolical potions" made from lianas growing in the Peruvian Amazon. Throughout the New World, and particularly South of the Equator, with its lush tropics and extraordinary plant diversity, the new European overlords, in the wake of their conquest of the native peoples, harshly condemned the use of sacred plants they observed as part of aboriginal religion and ritual. Hernando Ruiz de Alarcon, an early Spanish chronicler of native customs, described his observation of how the plants "when drunk deprive of the senses, because it is very powerful, and this means they communicate with the devil, because he talks with them when they are deprived of judgment with the said drink, and deceive them with different hallucinations, and they attribute it to a god they say is inside the seed." With forced conversion to Christianity and the eradication of native cultures and traditions, the great secrets of the forest could not be tolerated openly, and, as was the case throughout Central and South America with the remarkable psychoactive plant pharmacopeia endemic to the region, the use and even knowledge of their existence faded from awareness. Not until the waning of the Inquisition and the end of forced imposition of Church decree, along with the advent of the Age of Enlightenment and the rise of Western scientific inquiry, did the very presence of these taboo plants begin to re-emerge.

In regard to ayahuasca, following isolated reports of native heresies from missionaries in remote forest outposts, the first notable subjective account of the effects of ayahuasca came from Manuel Villavicencio, an Ecuadoran geographer, who studied tribal groups in the Rio Napo area of Ecuador; he became intrigued by the use of *yagé* (another term for ayahuasca), and sought the opportunity to investigate first-hand the effects of this beverage. In a written account published in 1858, Villavicencio described how

> In a few moments, it begins to produce the most rare phenomena. Its action appears to excite the nervous system; all the senses liven up and all faculties awaken; they feel vertigo and spinning in the head, followed by a sensation of being lifted into the air and beginning an aerial journey; the possessed begins in the first moments to see the most delicious apparitions, in conformity with his ideas and knowledge; the savages [apparently the Zaparo of eastern Ecuador] say that they see gorgeous lakes, forests covered with fruit, the prettiest birds who communicate to them, the nicest and the most favorable things they want to hear, and other beautiful things relating to their savage life… As for myself I can say for a fact that when I've taken ayahuasca, I've experienced dizziness, then an aerial journey in which I recall perceiving the most gorgeous views, great cities, lofty towers,

> beautiful parks, and other extremely attractive objects; then I imagined myself to be alone in a forest and assaulted by a number of terrible beings from which I defended myself; thereafter I had the strong sensation of sleep.

By the early twentieth century, increasingly sophisticated laboratory technology allowed scientists to isolate the principle biologically active alkaloids from psychotropic plants. Working from available samples of *Banisteriopsis*, Louis Lewin, later renowned as a principle founder of the field of modern psychopharmacology, identified a compound he called banisterine, later renamed harmine (and, for a time, telepathine, after ayahuasca's reputed capacity to induce telepathic phenomena, though this term did not gain traction in the West). For several years, harmine even entered the formal medical pharmacopeia, valued as a treatment for Parkinson's disease. Only with the discovery of L-Dopa by the pharmaceutical industry, and its promotion as a "modern" treatment of Parkinson's in the 1930s, did harmine fade from medical use and interest.

Ayahuasca did not come to the attention of Western science again until the explorations of the renowned Harvard ethnobotanist, R. E. Schultes, who, during the Second World War, had been tasked by the United States government to survey the prevalence of wild rubber trees in the remote Amazon. These had become a matter of strategic concern following the Japanese Army occupation of Malaysia, the only previous substantive source of rubber, deemed essential for the Allied war effort. Schultes, who had previously studied the ritual use of peyote by the indigenous people of the Southwestern United States, learned of the use of ayahuasca by tribal groups he encountered during his solo and often hazardous trek navigating and mapping the remote Amazon. Among other observations, Schultes identified the presence of a second critical plant necessary for ayahuasca's extraordinary psychoactive potency: the leaves of the dimethyltryptamine (DMT)-rich *Psychotria viridis*. Decades later, a new generation of scientists, including ethnopharmacologist Dennis McKenna at the University of British Columbia, established the biochemical mechanism for the central nervous system activation of DMT-containing *Psychotria*, a plant that, when taken orally and alone, is entirely inactivated in the gut by the monoamine oxidase (MAO) enzyme system, but, when brewed together with *Banisteriopsis*-containing monoamine oxidase inhibiting (MAOI) harmala alkaloids, induces a far-reaching range of profound psychoactive effects. The origins of this remarkably sophisticated plant pharmacology, seemingly discovered by indigenous people throughout the Amazon long before the arrival of the European invaders, remains a mystery. Whether through methodical, reductionist, trial-and-error sampling of the various plants in the geographical region or through some form of divine or spiritual intercession, as some have proposed, the actual process of the initial discovery of ayahuasca will likely never be known.

Since the early 1990s, ayahuasca has been subjected to rigorous clinical assessment utilizing state-of-the-art research methodologies. In 1993, along with my colleagues Dennis McKenna and Jace Callaway, I had the opportunity to travel to the capital of the Brazilian state of Amazonia, the city of Manaus, a large metropolis located at the confluence of the Rio Solimoes and Rio Negro, and the origins of the Rio Amazonas. Here, we conducted a study of a randomly selected group of volunteers who were members of the syncretic religion União do Vegetal (UDV), a church that had achieved formal government sanction to use ayahuasca as a ceremonial sacrament in their religious ceremonies in the late 1980s. Beyond establishing vital safety standards and documenting that ayahuasca, when taken within the structure of the UDV, can be safely administered to well-prepared and carefully monitored subjects, we were also able to explore effects on neuropsychological function, personality characteristics, cardiovascular reactivity, and pharmacokinetic profiles of the four primary alkaloids involved in ayahuasca function (DMT, harmine, harmaline, and tetrahydroharmine), as well as apparent modulation of a primary central nervous system neurotransmitter, serotonin. Through our investigations, we were also able to discern that, when taken under optimal, culturally specific conditions, ingestion of ayahuasca had the capacity to facilitate impressive degrees of psychological healing, including mood stabilization and recovery from chronic alcoholism and other addictive behaviors.

While almost entirely unknown to mainstream Western culture until 20 years ago, beyond a few exotic and often fanciful accounts, such as the experiences of iconoclast bohemian writers Allen Ginsberg and William Burroughs during the 1950s, in recent decades, a growing movement of Brazilian syncretic churches has spread the use of ayahuasca from the Amazon to the urban centers of southern Brazil. In addition to the UDV, the Santo Daime and Barquinha churches have also established religions sanctioned to utilize ayahuasca ceremonially, though with markedly different structures and belief systems than the UDV. Legal status in Brazil through much of the twentieth century remained at issue and, in 1985, ayahuasca was formally, albeit briefly, classified as a dangerous drug of abuse. Nevertheless, legal sanction was achieved shortly thereafter, following extensive investigations by government commissions which were favorably impressed with the sincerity, ethical integrity, and psychological health of the ayahuasca religion members they interviewed. Full approval to use ayahuasca within religious contexts in Brazil was granted in 1987. This in itself was an extraordinary historical precedent. While some countries, including the United States, have allowed their indigenous populations the right to resume their tribal traditions (e.g., the use of peyote by Native Americans is protected by law), the removal of ayahuasca from legal strictures in Brazil was an important step. A further development over the last few decades has been the establishment of branches of the Brazilian ayahuasca churches in the United States and Europe. In 2006, a landmark decision was issued (unanimously) by the US Supreme Court authorizing the legal use of ayahuasca when taken within the UDV religious structure. More recently, efforts to restrict the sacramental use of ayahuasca by the Santo Daime were dismissed on the state court level in Oregon. Nevertheless, while use of ayahuasca within the context of established religion (e.g., UDV) may now be considered legal in the United States, other models and settings for its utilization remain in a legal gray area.

Traditionally, ayahuasca was used from coastal Panama and the Orinoco Basin and south of Bolivia; from coastal Brazil across the vast expanse of the Amazon Basin to the foothills of the Andes; as well as in Colombia and Ecuador. In the shamanic model, ayahuasca is seen as a magic intoxicant, which the indigenous people believe can free the soul from corporeal confinement. Above all, ayahuasca is considered a medicine: the great medicine. Practically, in today's world, the shamanic model incorporates easily-transferable features, including group structure, attention to set and setting, import of intention, and proper preparation for and integration of the experience. For both safety and efficacy, any future clinical research with these compounds will need to seriously examine these aspects of the traditional shamanic model.

Beyond Brazil, other modern forms of ayahuasca use have evolved elsewhere in the Amazon Basin. Primarily in Peru, but also in Ecuador, Bolivia, and Colombia, a tradition of mestizo healing has existed for the past century. Until recently, this was an entirely local phenomenon, known only to the generally low socio-economic status inhabitants of the region. A tradition of healing has been cultivated over time, with the avocation of ayahuasquero (facilitators of ayahuasca ceremonies) often passed down in families from generation to generation. Generally used to diagnose and treat medical, psychological, and psychosomatic disorders, this form of healing was often perceived as a culturally acceptable alternative to the ministrations of conventional physicians and surgeons. Over the past two decades, however, increasing interest in ayahuasca by North Americans and Europeans has led to an influx of westerners seeking their own healing and spiritual transformation. The emergence of positive accounts in the mainstream press has encouraged increasing numbers of such seekers, some of whom fall prey to poorly trained facilitators lacking requisite knowledge, background, and ethical orientation, unfortunately leading to cases of psychological decompensation and at least a handful of deaths, the circumstances of which have sometimes remained obscure. While highly reputable ayahuasqueros have facilitated positive and often transformative experiences for the vast majority of Euro-Americans coming to the Amazon, the risks of exploitation and injury to naïve and vulnerable seekers is starting to receive more attention. The late anthropologist Marlene Dobkin de Rios, in particular, has called attention to this dark side of ayahuasca use, both in the region of its origins in the Amazon and as it has spread to North America and Europe.

With interest growing in the potential psychospiritual healing capacity of ayahuasca, it is becoming increasingly clear that efforts need to be undertaken to further rigorously investigate its range of effects, safety parameters, and potential to be utilized to treat individuals suffering from the psychological malaise endemic to the modern world. Important foundational studies have already been established, particularly at the Autonomous University of Barcelona in Spain, where pharmacology researcher Jordi Riba and neuropsychologist José Carlos Bouso have, for the past 15 years, conducted carefully designed explorations of the neuropsychological and physiological effects of freeze dried ayahuasca (necessary in the experimental context to ensure consistency of dose and concentration of alkaloids) with normal volunteers in a laboratory setting. More recently, in established and reputable medical institutions in Brazil, a series of exciting and potentially valuable research studies have been initiated by Draulio Araujo, Jaime Hallak, and others, exploring effects of ayahuasca on brain function.

One potentially promising approach now being actively pursued, particularly in Brazil, is the ayahuasca treatment model for individuals suffering from alcoholism and other addictive disorders. Consistent with valuable, albeit long neglected, studies in the United States, Canada, and Europe, of synthetic hallucinogens for the treatment of alcohol and drug abuse in the 1950s and 1960s, which were regrettably terminated by the early 1970s because of political pressure emanating from the cultural wars of that era, the ayahuasca treatment model presents a new opportunity. Interestingly, encouraging signs of change have been in increasing evidence in recent years, particularly the authorization of clinical research of the classical hallucinogen psilocybin in the US, including a Heffter Research Institute-developed study treating alcoholics at the University of New Mexico, along with initial efforts by other investigators to conduct controlled addiction research with ayahuasca in South America. Further buttressing the growing interest and activity in this area has been a recently conducted study from northwest Canada using an ayahuasca treatment model (employing an imported traditional ayahuasquero from the Shipibo tradition of Peru) to treat long-term, refractory alcoholics of the First Nation people of Canada (indigenous tribal people of Canada) with highly promising preliminary results.

The growing use of ayahuasca for purposes of healing represents a particular challenge to mainstream medical orthodoxy. Examining traditional use of such visionary plants, it is clear that a consistent element of the experience is the awareness of alternative and unusual dimensions of consciousness, including the realm of spirits. Indeed, the translation of ayahuasca from the native Quechua language is "vine of the spirits," or "vine of the dead." Incorporating such phenomena into our consensus model of reality will test the limits of conventional thought. Nevertheless, awareness and validation of these unusual realms is integral to cultures that have used ayahuasca throughout time, up to the current awakening of interest by modernity. Reconciling such divergent belief systems and constructs of reality will certainly test the inherent cognitive flexibility of modern culture and science as we attempt to comprehend the implications of the emergence of these ancient mysteries of the forest into the modern world.

While it is essential to utilize standard and state-of-the-art scientific and medical methodologies when investigating the range of effects of ayahuasca, including its safety, efficacy, and mechanism of action, appreciation needs to also be accorded to traditional models and the knowledge and lessons accrued over time. In order to ensure safety and optimal outcome, careful attention needs to be given to structures employed by cultures remote in time and place from our own. Particular attention must be given to proper screening and preparation, whether it be for subjects in scientific and medical investigations or for those in less-structured settings seeking their own healing and personal transformation. Individual vulnerability, in regard to psychological stability and seriousness of purpose, needs to be taken into account and, when indicated, inappropriate candidates may have to be turned away. As a *mestre* (master) of the UDV told me during our research investigations in Manaus many years ago, the *vegetal* (a UDV term for ayahuasca) is for everyone, but not everyone is for the vegetal. Particularly, given the challenges of integrating the use of ayahuasca into the modern world, care must be taken to minimize the likelihood that individuals will suffer from serious adverse consequences. Potentially dangerous drug and alcohol interactions with ayahuasca need to be avoided. Attentiveness to set and setting, including preparation and scrupulous examination of intention, must be emphasized. Particular elements of preparation emphasized among the earliest practitioners of ayahuasca use, including special diets (excluding salt, sugar, processed foods, etc.) and a period of sexual abstinence, may have a role in ensuring safety and determining outcome and need to be explored, in spite of the challenges such restrictions may pose within modern society. Careful attention to structures of ayahuasca use, including proper monitoring and opportunity for subsequent integration of the experience, should also be provided to increase the likelihood of optimal outcome.

We are faced with the challenge of how to incorporate these ancient technologies of consciousness exploration into our own modern healing paradigms. Although historically our culture was remarkably unaware of these plants and the profound effects they induce, this is no longer the case. The secret is out, and in this age of high-tech communication and ease of transport, the great mysteries of the remote forest are now being revealed. The implications for the modern age may indeed be profound. As we confront a world of widespread environmental destruction, and as we become increasingly aware of the growing menace of global climate change, it might be worthwhile to regard the traditional perspective of ayahuasca as communicator plants, representing a conduit between nature and humanity. Years ago, in the remote Amazon, I had an experience of hearing this call from Nature: that it was no accident that, after millennia of quiescence, these remarkable visionary plants are now revealing themselves. What I saw, or heard, or instinctively realized, was that it was no happenstance we were there; rather, we had been called to wake up, to pay attention, and to bring the message back to the modern world that our species is on the verge of destroying the earth, and with it the hopes and dreams of future generations.

The deep healing that the ayahuasca experience potentially offers, for both the individual and the collective, represents an extraordinary opportunity. Medical and psychiatric research into its myriad effects will provide an essential framework from which we may acquire a safe and practical structure to further explore these visionary plants and their potential to facilitate healing of our damaged planet as well as healing of the damaged people who inhabit the planet. There must be careful and scrupulous attention to safety parameters, with particular emphasis given to the knowledge and skills of those facilitating the experience. There is a great need to employ academic and ethical rigor in order to establish a strong and healthy foundation for the growing field of ayahuasca studies.

This volume of scientific explorations into the potential range of therapeutic effects of ayahuasca, ably edited by Beatriz Caiuby Labate and Clancy Cavnar, is a valuable contribution to this endeavor of establishing a rigorous field of ayahuasca studies. The range and mechanisms of ayahuasca and its putative capacity to facilitate states of both psychological and physical healing are explored. The potential of ayahuasca to be optimally employed as part of a treatment model for such difficult-to-treat clinical conditions as post-traumatic stress disorder, refractory mood, and anxiety disorders, and a variety of other psychiatric and even medical conditions, are methodically examined. The potential mechanisms of action, neurobiological as well as psychological, and their apparent facility to promote healing, are carefully scrutinized. Valuable input from a traditional indigenous healer, Taita Juan Bautista Agreda Chindoy from the Sibundoy Valley in Colombia, is included, providing lessons from an extant practitioner of the ancient art of ayahuasca healing. The area receiving the greatest attention is the treatment of drug and alcohol abuse, clinical conditions for which modern medicine and psychiatry lack effective treatment models, and which exert enormous costs to society: a natural area in which to apply the ayahuasca treatment model. Preliminary indications, from a variety of investigators in South America, North America, and Europe, are consistently positive. The implications of such findings, as they are replicated and expanded upon in the future, are enormous. Ultimately, ayahuasca may represent an entirely new medical paradigm; a model created for us by the ancients and the elders of the native peoples, who provide the link to the traditions and heritage of the earth.

Los Angeles
July 2013

Charles S. Grob

Preface

This book is inspired by the 2013 Psychedelic Science Conference, held in Oakland, California. The Multidisciplinary Association for Psychedelic Studies (MAPS) promoted the conference in cooperation with the Heffter Research Institute, the Beckley Foundation, and the Council on Spiritual Practices. The event convened over 1,900 people from all over the world, including anthropologists, medical doctors, lawyers, psychiatrists, and psychologists, and members of the general public. It was wide ranging, with a focus on the scientific research into the medical use of psychedelics. Research topics included MDMA-assisted therapy for post-traumatic stress disorder (PTSD), ibogaine for opiate addiction, and LSD and psilocybin for end-of life anxiety, among others. The conference was composed of three tracks: (1) the Clinical Research Track; (2) an Interdisciplinary Track, with a mix of topics, including psychedelic psychotherapy, non-clinical research, arts and culture, and medical marijuana; and (3) the Ayahuasca Track. Beatriz Caiuby Labate was the organizer of the Ayahuasca Track. This volume brings together a select collection of six presentations from this track, and is complemented by seven additional relevant contributions.

Ayahuasca (generally composed of *Banisteriopsis caapi* and *Psychotria viridis*) is a psychoactive brew of Amazonian origin that, over the last few decades, has caught the attention of many patients, healers, and researchers. The beverage's transformation into an internationally known "medicine" for physical, psychological, and spiritual ills has stirred up controversy over its use, and whether it ought to be banned or revered. The ritual and therapeutic uses of ayahuasca vary greatly by country; whereas different forms of the religious use of ayahuasca have been recognized as legitimate in some parts of the world, the therapeutic use of ayahuasca has not gained official acceptance beyond the limits of the Amazon rainforest.

This interdisciplinary collection presents a series of perspectives on the therapeutic potential of the ritual and clinical use of ayahuasca in the treatment and management of various diseases and ailments especially, its role in psychological well being and substance dependence. Anthropological and biomedical data on the use of ayahuasca for treating depression, PTSD, and substance dependence in different settings, such as indigenous contexts, neo-shamanic rituals, contemporary therapeutic circles, and in the ayahuasca religions of Santo Daime and União do Vegetal, in both South and North America, are presented and critiqued. The texts in this volume also discuss methodological, ethical, and political considerations for current and future research in this area.

With this work, we aim to bring the therapeutic use of ayahuasca to a new level of public examination and academic debate, as well as to fill in gaps in the current literature. Though multiple anecdotal reports on the therapeutic use of ayahuasca exist, there has been no systematic and dense reflection on the topic thus far. We hope this collection offers an important advancement in this discussion, and helps to inform international regulation on ayahuasca use based on the scientific study of this substance's relative benefits and harms. We also hope this book proves to be a source of inspiration for further research in this emergent field of studies.

We would like to thank the Center for Economic Research and Education—CIDE Región Centro in Aguascalientes, Mexico; MAPS in Santa Cruz, CA; and Anton Bilton, Tyringham, England, for their support. We would also like to express our gratitude to the contributors to the volume. Our colleagues Bob Jesse, Brian T. Anderson, Rafael Guimarães dos Santos, José Carlos Bouso, Michael Winkelman, and Mitchell B. Liester provided important help during the process of editing this collection. Finally, we are grateful to Springer for its openness to this frequently stigmatized topic.

Aguascalientes
San Francisco
October 2013

Beatriz Caiuby Labate
Clancy Cavnar

Contents

Contributors

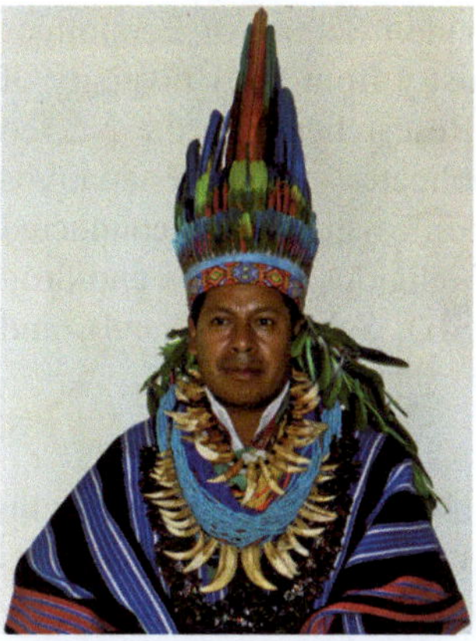

Taita Juan Bautista Agreda Chindoy is an indigenous Kametsa traditional healer from the Sibundoy Valley of the Alto Putumayo of Colombia. He is the son of Taita Martin, and comes from a recognized family of traditional yageceros. He is an established leader in his community and has over 25 years of experience working with Amazonian medicine, including yagé and other plants. He has been recognized by the Colombian Ministry of Health as a traditional healer and over the last few years has traveled abroad to share his knowledge and treat patients with various diseases.

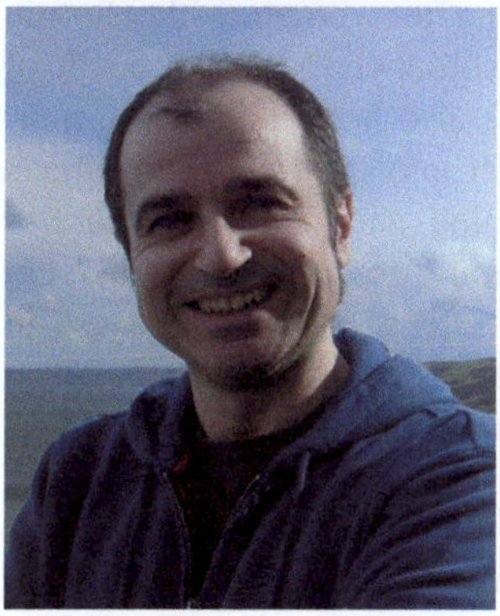

Miguel Ángel Alcázar is a Doctor of Psychology at the Ministry of Justice of Spain in the Juvenile Court in Toledo (Spain) and Associate Professor in the Department of Biological and Health Psychology of the Autonomous University of Madrid (Spain). He has a special interest in neuropsychology, psychopharmacology, personality, and forensic psychology. He has had many papers published on those subjects.

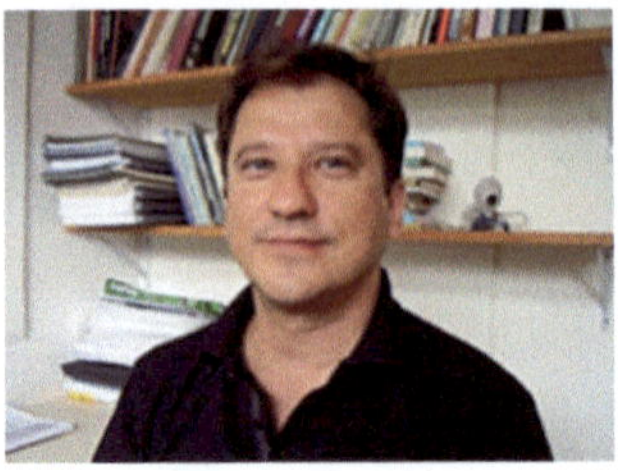

João Carlos Alchieri received his Ph.D. in Developmental Psychology from the University Federal do Rio Grande do Sul in 2004, with post-doctoral studies at the University of Brasilia. He is an Associate Professor at the Federal University of Rio Grande do Norte (UFRN), where he currently participates in post-graduate programs in health sciences and psychology. His activities focus on psychological assessment in health.

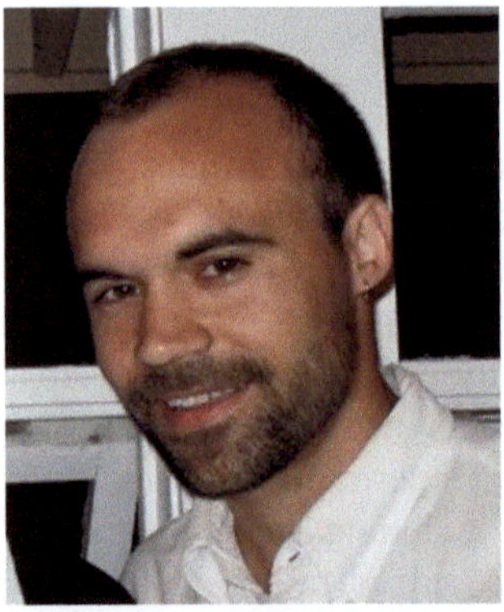

Brian T. Anderson is currently an M.D. candidate at the Stanford University School of Medicine. He holds an M.Sc. in Medical Sociology from the BIOS Centre at the London School of Economics and a B.A. in Biochemistry from the University of Pennsylvania. He is a Researcher with the Núcleo de Estudos Interdisciplinares sobre Psicoativos (NEIP, http://www.neip.info) and he has conducted ethnographic studies of religious practices and drug use in Philadelphia (USA), Salvador (Brazil), and Mexico City (Mexico).

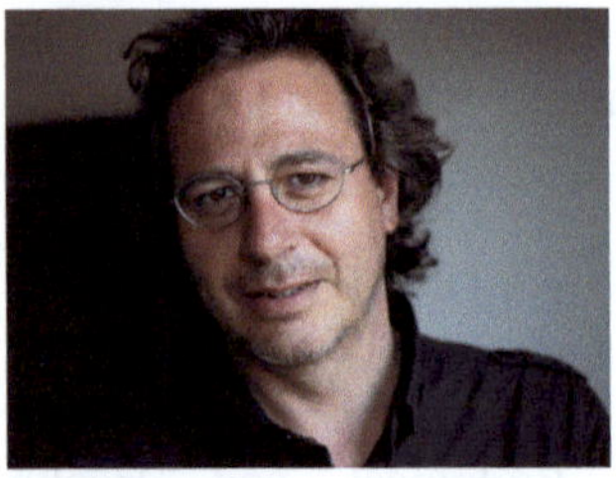

José Carlos Bouso is a Clinical Psychologist with a Ph.D. in Pharmacology. His current studies address preliminary data on the safety and efficacy of varying doses of MDMA administered in a psychotherapeutic setting to women with chronic post-traumatic stress disorder (PTSD) as a result of a sexual assault. He has also been conducting neuropsychological research into the long-term effects of drugs such as cocaine and cannabis. He has undertaken transcultural research, extensively studying the long-term effects of ayahuasca use in different cultures and ecosystems, both in Spanish and in Brazilian communities. José Carlos Bouso is co-author of several scientific papers and book chapters. He currently combines his activity as a Clinical Researcher at the Institut Hospital del Mar d'Investigacions Mèdiques (IMIM) with his work as scientific projects manager at International Center for Ethnobotanical Education, Research and Service (ICEERS—http://www.iceers.org).

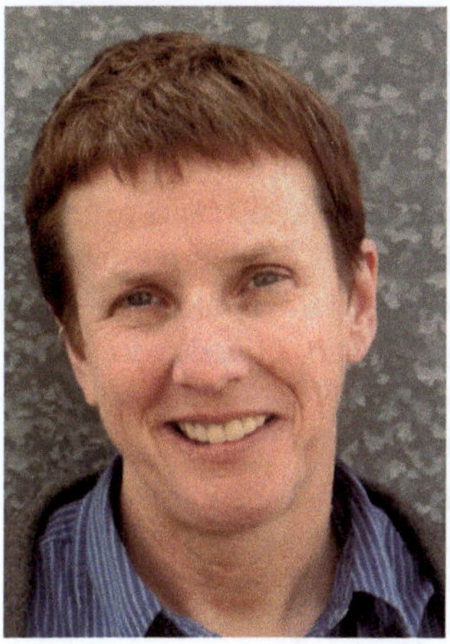

Clancy Cavnar is currently completing her post-doctoral hours in clinical psychology at the Marin Treatment Center, a methadone clinic in San Rafael, California. In 2011 she received a Doctorate in Clinical Psychology (PsyD) from John F. Kennedy University in Pleasant Hill, California, with a dissertation on gay and lesbian people's experiences with ayahuasca. She attended New College of the University of South Florida and completed an undergraduate degree in liberal arts in 1982. She attended the San Francisco Art Institute and graduated with a Master of Fine Art in painting in 1985. In 1993, she received a certificate in substance abuse counseling from the extension program of the University of California at Berkeley and, in 1997, she graduated with a Master's in Counseling from San Francisco State University. In that same year, she got in touch with the Santo Daime in the USA, and has traveled several times to Brazil since then. She is also co-editor, with Beatriz Caiuby Labate, of two books: *Ayahuasca Shamanism in the Amazon and Beyond* (Oxford University Press, in press), and *Prohibition, Religious Freedom, and Human Rights: Regulating Traditional Drug Use* (Springer, in press).

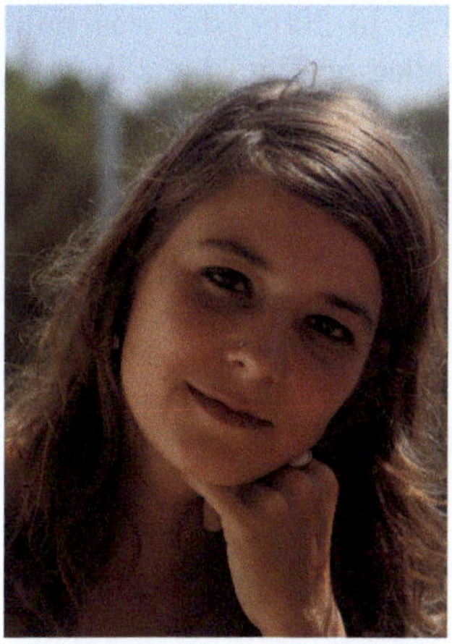

Marta Cutchet earned her Psychology degree in 2006 at Universidad Autónoma de Barcelona. In 2009, she earned a Clinical Psychopathology post-graduate degree at the same University. She collaborated in the project to assess addiction severity among ritual users of ayahuasca. Currently, she is working as a therapist in Centro de Investigación y Tratamiento de Adiciones (CITA).

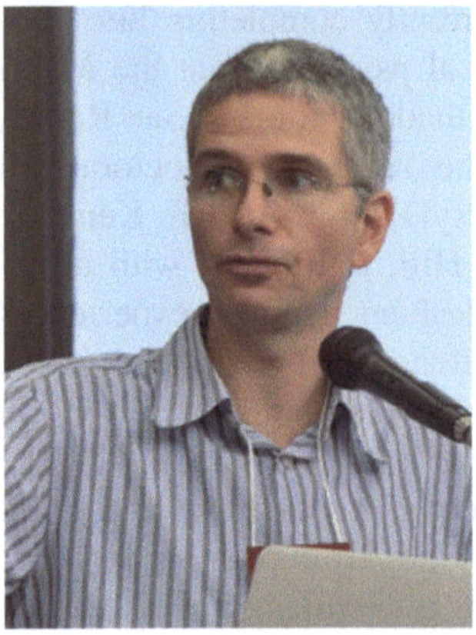

Dráulio Barros de Araujo received his Ph.D. in Physics Applied to Medicine and Biology from the University of São Paulo in Ribeirão Preto in 2002, where he engaged in postdoctoral studies on functional neuroimaging, became Assistant Professor, and then received the title of "livre-docente" (Associate). In 2009, he joined the Brain Institute at the Federal University of Rio Grande do Norte (UFRN), where he is currently Coordinator of the Graduate Program in Neuroscience, and Full Professor of Neuroimaging. His research deals with several aspects of neuroscience, using the methods of functional magnetic resonance imaging (fMRI), magnetoencephalography (MEG), and electroencephalography (EEG). In the last few years, Dr. Araujo has focused on the investigation of the cognitive and neural substrates of the ayahuasca experience.

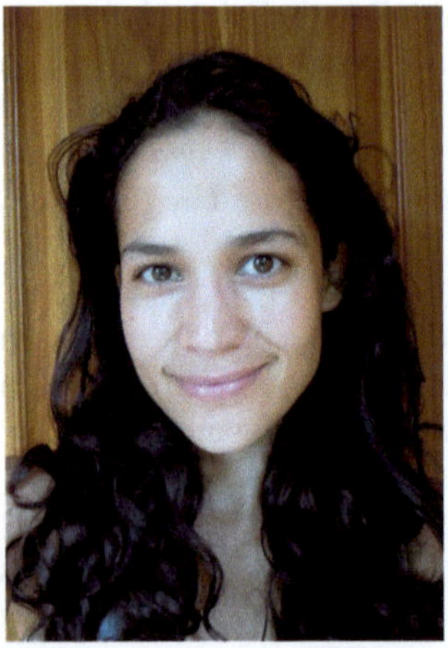

Celina M. De Leon is an independent researcher based in Oakland, California. She received a B.A. in Human Biology from Stanford University and was a US/India Fulbright Scholar in 2007. She is the co-founder of Posada Natura in Costa Rica, an interdisciplinary healing arts center dedicated to the practice and research of traditional medical systems (www.posadanatura.com). In 2009, she was initiated as a formal apprentice of Taita Juan Bautista Agreda Chindoy from the Cametsa indigenous lineage of the Sibundoy Valley, Alto Putumayo, Colombia.

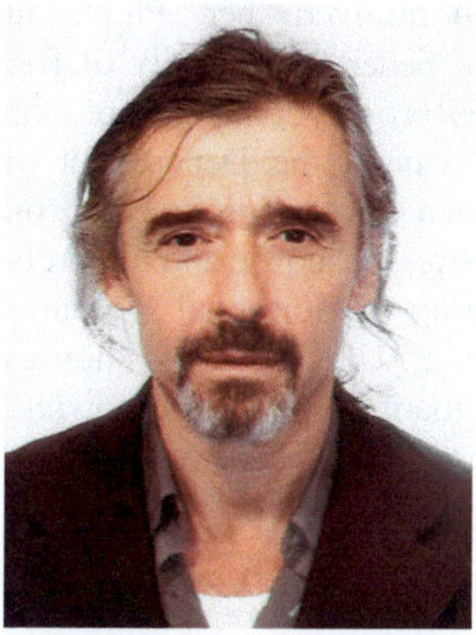

Josep María Fábregas graduated from the Central University of Barcelona with a degree in Medicine, specializing in psychiatry. He completed his studies at New York Staten Island Psychiatric Hospital. He was a Resident Physician at the Marmottan Hospital under Claude Olivenstain. He has been the Director of CITA (Addiction Research and Treatment Center) since 1981 and, in 2000, he founded IDEAA (Amazonian Ethnopsychology Applied Institute). He has lectured extensively on drug addiction and altered states of consciousness.

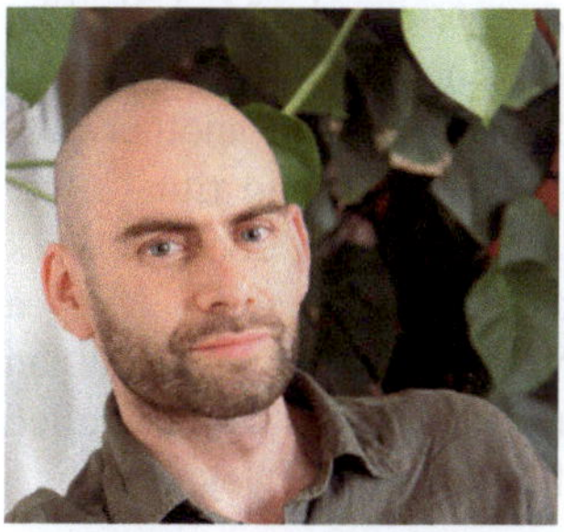

Xavier Fernández (Ashirvad) was a Psychologist and Ph.D. student at Universidad Santiago de Compostela. He had worked as a Psychotherapist and Researcher in Instituto de Etnopsicología Amazónica Aplicada (IDEAA). He was also an independent Researcher, transpersonal facilitator, and writer. Xavier passed away in 2011.

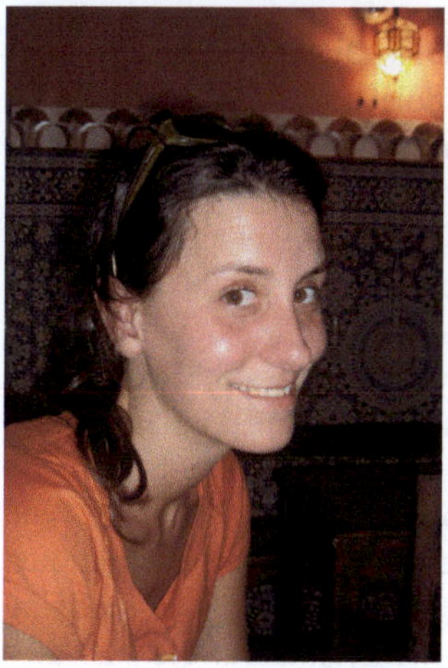

Sabela Fondevila graduated from the Department of Psychology at the Universidad Autónoma de Madrid in 2005. She completed a Master's degree in Psychodrama Therapy management between 2002 and 2004. She has been performing research in the Amazon Basin, studying the long-term neuropsychological and psychopathological conditions among ritual users of ayahuasca in the Mapiá and Rio Branco communities. Currently, she is doing her thesis on the cognitive science of religion under the direction of Prof. Manuel Martín-Loeches at the Center UCM-ISCIII for Human Evolution and Behavior.

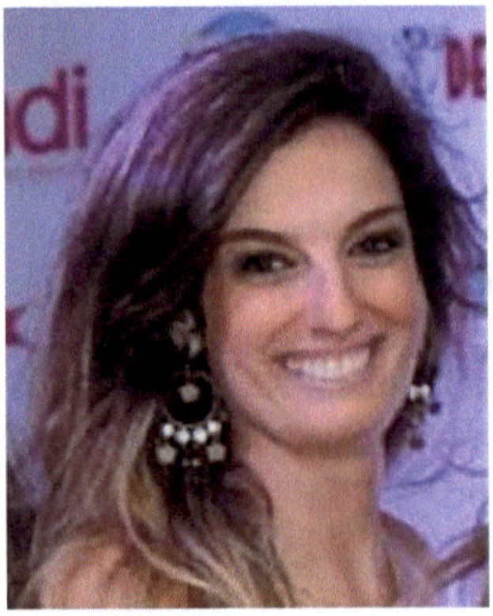

Nicole Galvao-Coelho received her Ph.D. in Psychobiology from the Federal University of Rio Grande do Norte (UFRN) in 2009, where she became Assistant Professor at the Department of Physiology. She has been developing research on neuroendocrinology of stress response and currently coordinates the Laboratory of Hormonal Measures and a Primate Center at UFRN, which houses around 200 common marmosets (*Callithrix jacchus*), a species that has been widely used as an animal model in neuroscience studies.

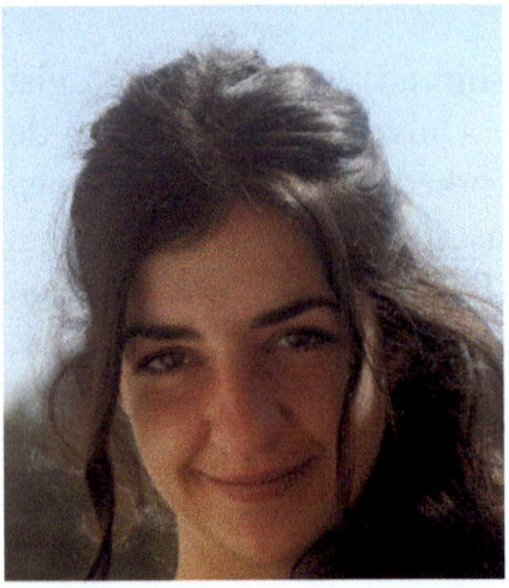

Débora González earned her Psychology degree in 2006 at Universidad Autónoma de Madrid. She published an article about the subjective effects of *Salvia divinorum* and collaborated on another project to assess addiction severity among ritual users of ayahuasca. Currently, she is doing doctoral work at Institut Municipal d`Investigació Médica (IMIM-Hospital del Mar), studying the human pharmacology and pattern of use of the so-called "research chemicals,"also known as "legal highs," in Spain.

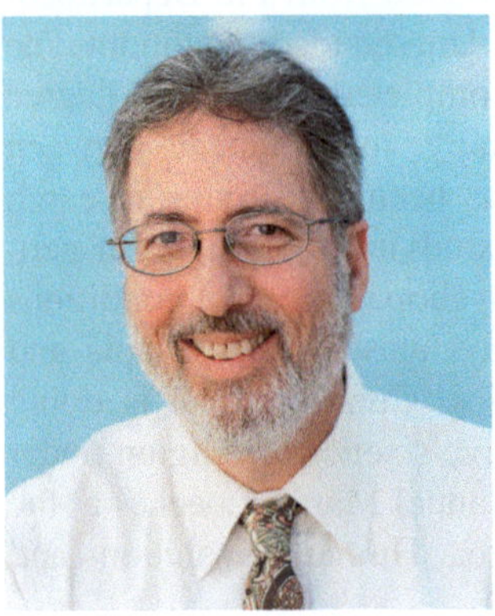

Charles S. Grob, M.D. is Director of the Division of Child and Adolescent Psychiatry at Harbor-UCLA Medical Center, and Professor of Psychiatry and Pediatrics at the UCLA School of Medicine. Prior to his appointment at UCLA, he held teaching and clinical positions at the University of California Irvine College of Medicine and the Johns Hopkins University School of Medicine, in the Departments of Psychiatry and Pediatrics. Dr. Grob conducted the first government-approved psychobiological research study of MDMA, and was the principal investigator of an international research project in the Brazilian Amazon studying the visionary plant brew, ayahuasca. He has also completed and published the first approved research investigation in several decades on the safety and efficacy of psilocybin treatment in terminal cancer patients with anxiety. Dr. Grob is the Editor of

Hallucinogens: A Reader (Tarcher/Putnam 2002) and co-editor of *Higher Wisdom: Eminent Elders Explore the Continuing Impact of Psychedelics* (SUNY Press 2005). He is also a founding board member of the Heffter Research Institute.

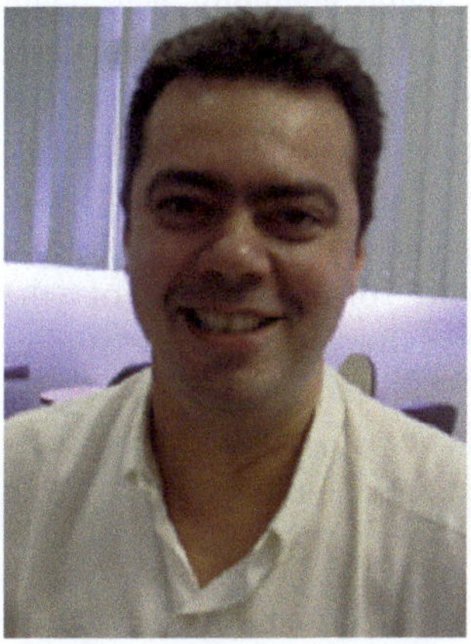

Jaime Hallak graduated with a degree in Medicine from the Federal University of Triangulo Mineiro in 1990, a Master of Medicine (mental health) from the University of São Paulo in 1998, a Ph.D. in Medicine (mental health) from the University of São Paulo in 2002, and then earned a postdoctoral degree from the University of Manchester in England in 2003. He is currently a Professor of Psychiatry, as a member of the Faculty of Medicine of Ribeirão Preto-University of São Paulo. His expertise is in psychiatry, with an emphasis on neuroimaging and psychopharmacology, particularly focusing on the following topics: schizophrenia, antipsychotics, temporal lobe epilepsy, and techniques of structural and functional neuroimaging.

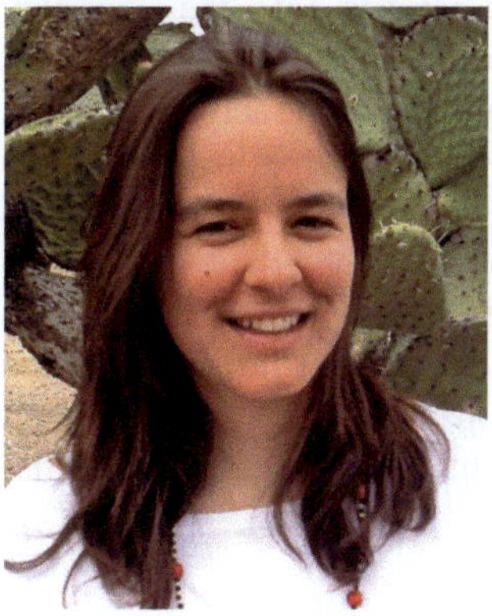

Beatriz Caiuby Labate has a Ph.D. in social anthropology from the State University of Campinas (Universidade Estadual de Campinas, UNICAMP), Brazil. Her main areas of interest are the study of psychoactive substances, drug policies, shamanism, ritual, and religion. She is visiting professor at the Drug Policy Program of the Center for Economic Research and Education (Centro de Investigación y Docencia Económicas, CIDE) in Aguascalientes, Mexico. She is also a research associate at the Institute of Medical Psychology, Heidelberg University, co-founder of the Nucleus for Interdisciplinary Studies of Psychoactives (NEIP), and editor of its site (http://www.neip.info). She is author, co-author, and co-editor of nine books, two with English translations, one journal special edition, and several peer-reviewed articles. For more information, see: http://bialabate.net.

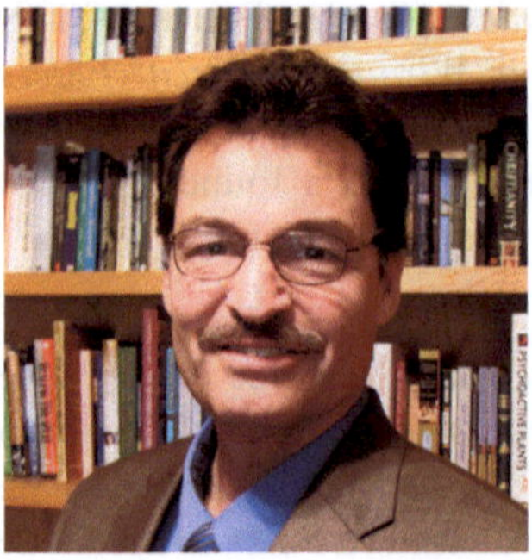

Mitchell B. Liester received his M.D. from the University of Colorado School of Medicine in 1985. He then completed a Psychiatric Residency at the University of California, Irvine where he co-authored a study investigating the phenomenology and sequelae of MDMA. He went on to publish in the fields of transpersonal psychology, near-death studies, and psychedelic medicines. He has lectured at universities, medical schools, and international conferences on shamanism, visionary experiences, near-death experiences, and the use of plant medicines in the treatment of addictions. He is a member of the Board of Directors of the International Association for Near-Death Studies (IANDS). For the last 24 years, Mitch has had a clinical psychiatric practice in Colorado. He currently resides in Monument, Colorado.

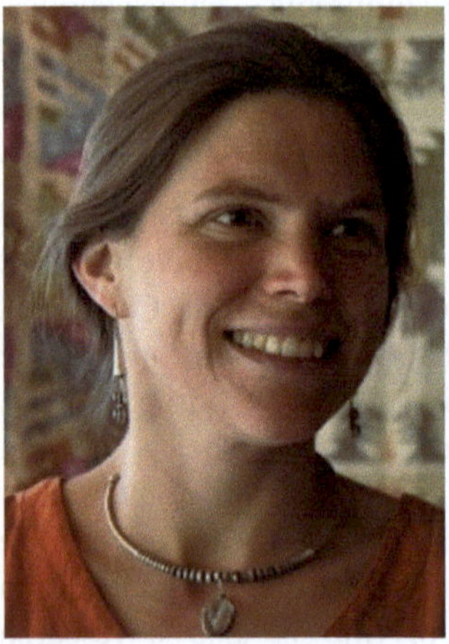

Anja Loizaga-Velder is a German–Mexican Clinical Psychologist who has been investigating the therapeutic potential of the ritual use of psychedelic plants for over 15 years. She is founding member and collaborating researcher of the Nierika, Multidisciplinary Association for the Preservation of the Indigenous Traditions of Sacred Plants in Mexico. She holds an M.A. degree in Psychology from the University of Koblenz/Landau in Germany and is currently a doctoral candidate in medical psychology at Heidelberg University. The study she discusses in her text is part of the work of the special research group "Ritual Dynamics and Salutogenesis" (RISA, http://www.risa.uni-hd.de).

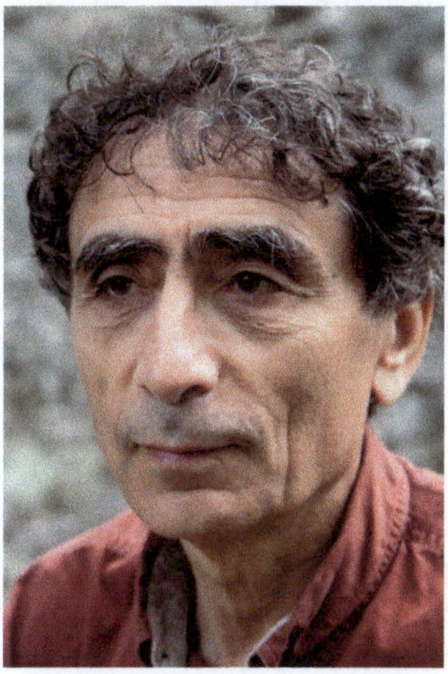

Gabor Maté M.D. is a Canadian physician, speaker, and the author of four bestselling books published in nearly 20 languages on five continents. His interests include the mind/body unity as manifested in health and illness, the effects of early childhood experiences in shaping brain and personality, the traumatic basis of addictions, and the attachment requirements for healthy child development. He has worked in family practice and palliative care, and for 12 years he worked in Vancouver's Downtown Eastside, notorious as North America's most concentrated area of drug use. Currently, he is Adjunct Professor in the Department of Criminology, Simon Fraser University, and teaches and leads seminars internationally. For more information, see: www.drgabormate.com.

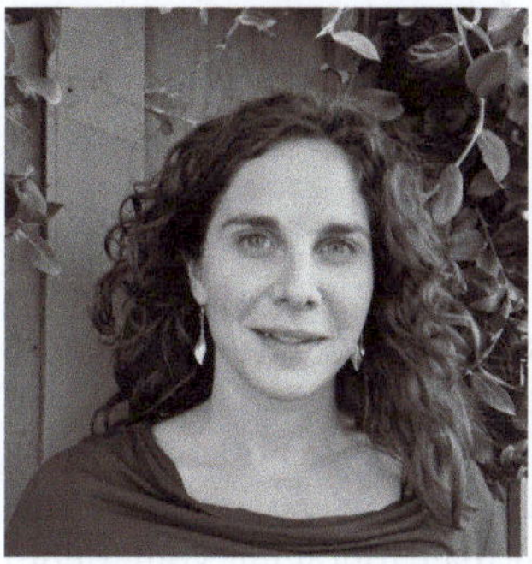

Julie D. Megler is a board-certified nurse practitioner in Psychiatry and Family Practice. She received her Master's of Science in Nursing from the University of Miami, Florida. After graduating, she worked at an emergency room (E.R.) in Detroit, Michigan. Her E.R. experience illustrated for her the gap between medical and psychiatric care, and how the mind/body connection is often ignored. These gaps in care inspired Julie to pursue a psychiatric-mental health nurse practitioner certificate at the University of California, San Francisco so that she could develop a practice that integrates medicine and mental health for the most effective treatment. Julie is now working with homeless veterans living in transitional housing. In addition to her work with veterans, Julie also has an integrative psychiatry practice in collaboration with therapists, an acupuncturist, a naturopath, a body worker, and a medical doctor.

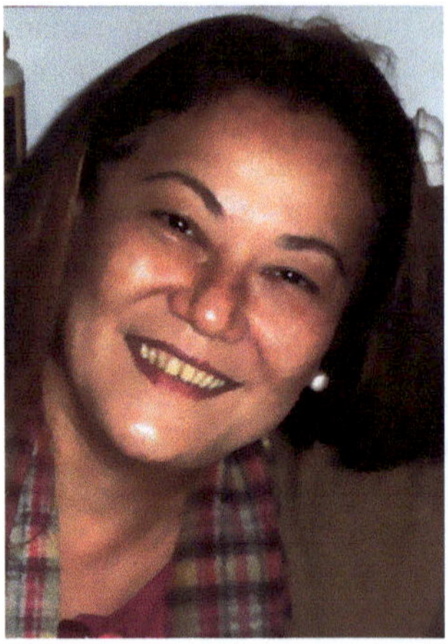

Suely Mizumoto is a Clinical Psychologist who has worked in the mental health field since 1978. She has had training in psychoanalysis, and has worked in hospitals as a clinician and as a Clinical Supervisor of a Therapeutic Community, and also at the Milênio Institute—Ipe Project of the Institute of Psychology of the University of São Paulo. She received her Master's of Science in Social Psychology from the University of São Paulo (IPUSP); her dissertation was "Dissociation, Religiosity, and Mental Health: A Study in Santo Daime and Umbanda." Since 1992, her clinical work has emphasized integration of spiritual and psychological issues, particularly relative to the use of psychoactive substances such as ayahuasca and marijuana. She is currently a member of the research team studying ayahuasca and psychoactive substances at the Psychiatry Department of the Federal University of São Paulo (UNIFESP) and of the Research Group on Mental Health, State University of Santa Cruz of Bahia (UESC-BA), also dedicated to studying ayahuasca.

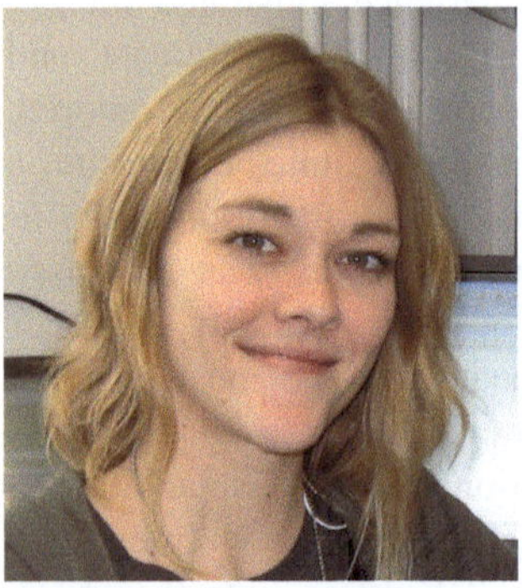

Jessica Nielson Ph.D. received her B.S. in Biology from Cal Poly Pomona in 2003, and her Ph.D. in Anatomy and Neurobiology from the University of California, Irvine, in 2010. During her doctoral work, she resolved a century-old controversy regarding the fate of the corticospinal tract following spinal cord injury, demonstrating definitively that this important motor pathway survives injury and is available in chronic cases for therapeutic interventions to promote regeneration and functional recovery. She joined the Brain and Spinal Injury Center at the University of California, San Francisco, in 2011 as a postdoctoral scholar, where she has been developing a novel bioinformatics approach to characterize syndromic features of spinal cord injury, with future plans to apply this approach to traumatic brain injury and post-traumatic stress disorder.

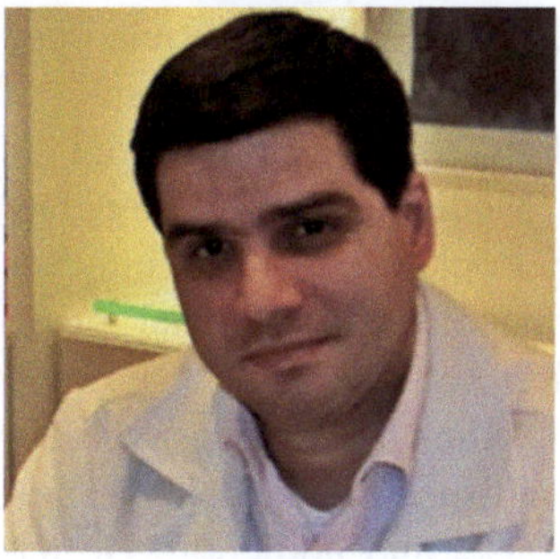

João Paulo Maia de Oliveira graduated in Medicine from the Federal University of Rio Grande do Norte (2003). He is a Psychiatrist, and received his Master's degree in Medicine, focusing on mental health, from the University of São Paulo. Now he is a Ph.D. student at the University of São Paulo and an Assistant Professor of Psychiatry at the Federal University of Rio Grande do Norte. His main research interests are schizophrenia, depression, and translational research.

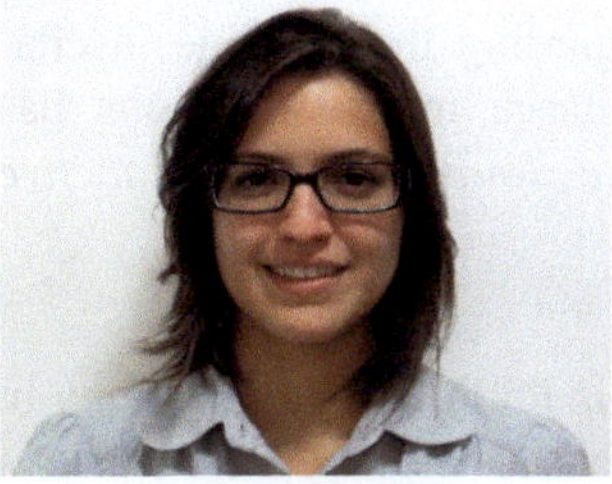

Fernanda Palhano-Fontes received her Master's degree in Neuroscience from the University of Rio Grande do Norte in 2012. She is currently a Ph.D. student at the Brain Institute at the Federal University of Rio Grande do Norte (UFRN), where she investigates, through functional magnetic resonance imaging (fMRI), cognitive, and therapeutic aspects of ayahuasca usage.

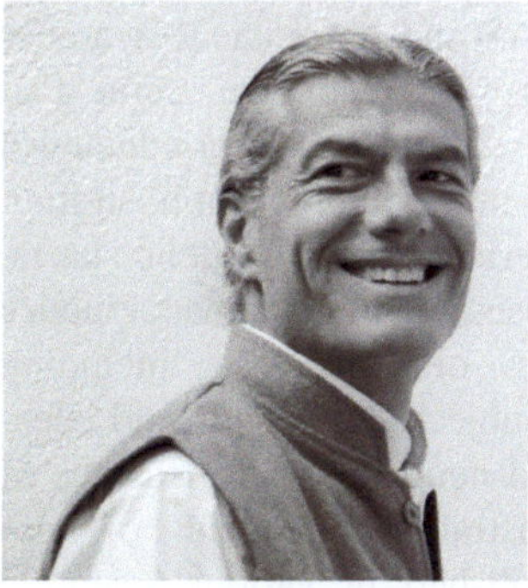

Armando Loizaga Pazzi is a Psychologist and certified chemical dependency counselor. He has worked in the substance abuse treatment and prevention field in Mexico since 1991. He has been Director and Coordinator of Diverse Clinical Addiction Treatment Programs and has also collaborated with traditional medicine associations in the study of transcultural treatments. He has been studying the therapeutic potential of ayahuasca-based treatment in this context since 1998. He is President of Nierika A.C., Multidisciplinary Association for Preservation of Sacred Plants. Currently, he is focusing his work on advancing multidisciplinary clinical research protocols in Mexico to evaluate the therapeutic potential of psychedelic plants used in ritual contexts.

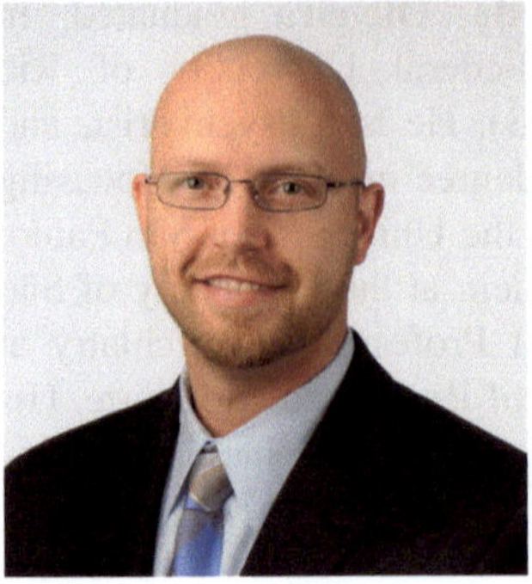

James Prickett, D.O, is a Resident Physician and a burgeoning Researcher at the University of Arizona Department of Psychiatry. He received his Doctor of Osteopathic Medicine degree from Des Moines University. Dr. Prickett's primary interests lie within psychopharmacology, traditional medicine, and the relationship between belief, spirituality, and mental health. He has been a guest speaker on topics including autism, psychedelic drugs, adolescent substance abuse, and addiction. He has traveled to Ecuador on several occasions to study traditional medicine in both the Andes and Amazon Basin. His research regarding the possible mechanisms by which ayahuasca treats addictions has been published in *The Journal of Psychoactive Drugs*.

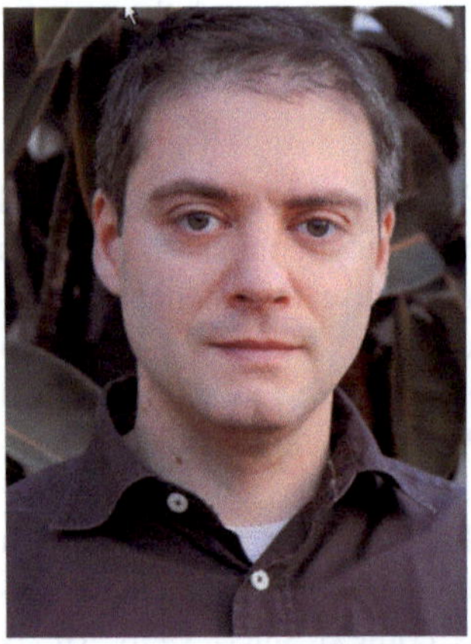

Jordi Riba received his Ph.D. in Pharmacology in 2003, at the Autonomous University of Barcelona (UAB), with a thesis on the human pharmacology of ayahuasca. He is currently an Associate Professor of Pharmacology at the UAB and Associate Researcher at the Drug Research Center of the Saint Pau Hospital in Barcelona, where he has conducted a series of clinical studies involving the administration of ayahuasca to experienced psychedelic users. These studies have assessed the phamacokinetics and pharmacodynamics of ayahuasca, including alkaloid disposition, subjective effects, and electroencephalography and neuroimaging measures of acute ayahuasca administration. The results of these studies have been published in various scientific journals such as *Psychopharmacology*, *The Journal of Pharmacology and Experimental Therapeutics*, *The British Journal of Clinical Pharmacology*, and *The Journal of Psychoactive Drugs*. He is currently the lead Researcher of a study assessing the effects of long-term ayahuasca use.

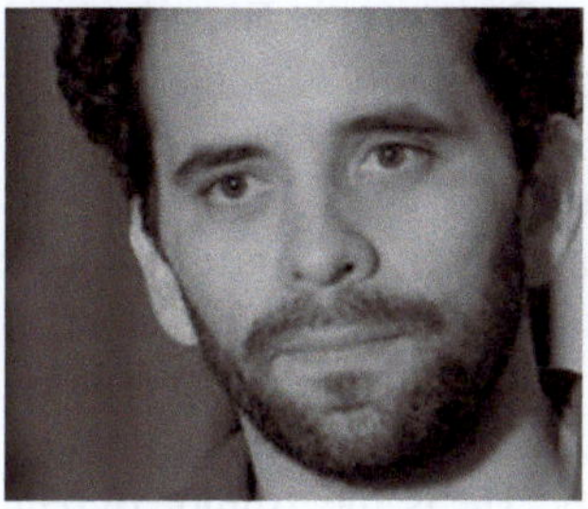

Rafael Guimarães dos Santos completed his undergraduate senior thesis in Biology at the Centro Universitário de Brasília—UniCEUB on the microbiology of ayahuasca and its effects on rat behavior and brain histomorphology. During his Master's in Psychology at the Universidade de Brasília (UnB), he investigated the acute effects of ayahuasca on regular ayahuasca users using psychometric measures of hopelessness, anxiety, and panic states. In his Ph.D. thesis in Pharmacology at Universidad Autónoma de Barcelona, he performed a comparison study of the acute subjective and physiological effects of ayahuasca and those produced by d-amphetamine, and also investigated the pharmacology of two consecutive doses of ayahuasca. Currently, he is member of the Advisory Board of the International Center for Ethnobotanical Education, Research and Service (ICEERS) in The Netherlands. For more information, see: http://banisteria.blogspot.com.

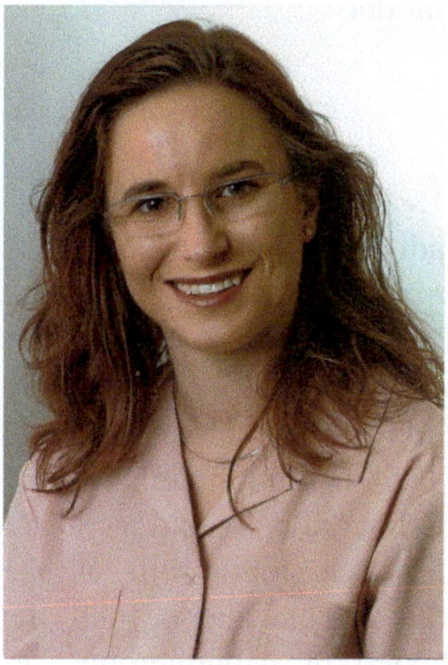

Janine Tatjana Schmid is a Psychologist currently working at a rehabilitation hospital supporting patients with chronic pain and cancer. She also gives lectures at the University of Heidelberg to medical students and training courses for patients, especially on rheumatic disorders and fibromyalgia. She earned a doctorate in Medical Psychology at the University of Heidelberg. Her doctoral thesis is entitled "Subjective Theories of Self Treatment with the Psychoactive Substance Ayahuasca." A summary of this research was published in the journal *Anthropology of Consciousness* in 2010. She has also written several articles for peer-reviewed journals and book chapters. Her special interests are in shamanism, psychotherapeutic methods, and the psychology of consciousness.

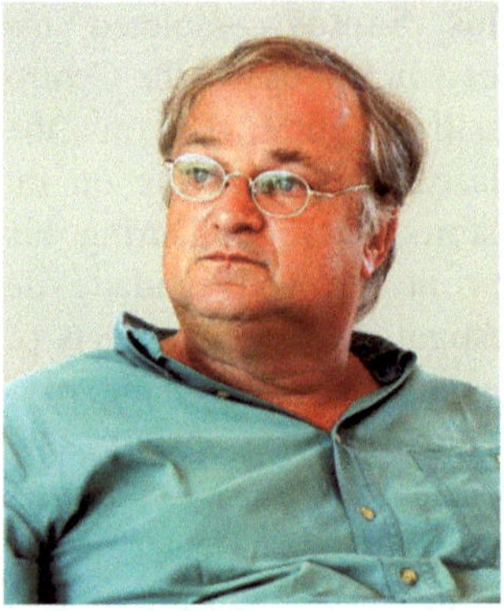

Benny Shanon earned a Doctorate in Experimental Psychology at Stanford University. He has been a Professor of Cognitive Psychology at the Hebrew University of Jerusalem since 1976. He has taught in various universities and research institutes in the United States and Europe. His areas of specialization are: the phenomenology of human consciousness and the pragmatics of language, thought processes, and creativity. He is the Author of *The Representational and the Presentational* (Haverster/Wheatsheaf/Prentice Hall 1993) and the *Antipodes of the Mind* (Oxford University Press 2002).

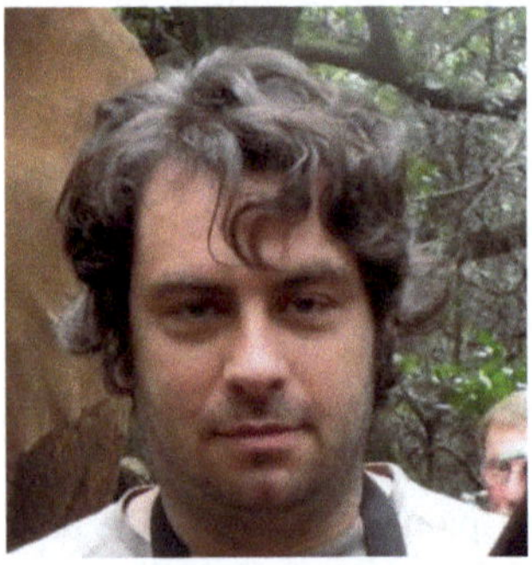

Bruno Lobão Soares is a Veterinary Doctor, and has received a Ph.D. in Neuroscience from the University of São Paulo. At the present, he is an Assistant Professor at Federal University of Rio Grande do Norte (UFRN). His current research is related to dopaminergic regulation of sleep and memory, and to new neuropharmacological tools in humans and in animal models.

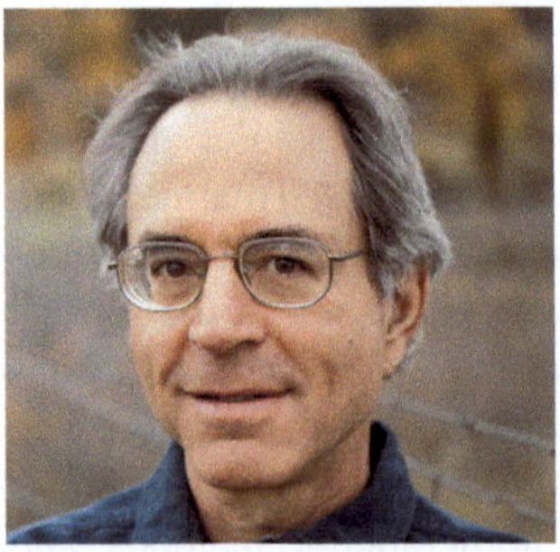

Rick Strassman graduated from Stanford University with a major in Biological Sciences, and received his Medical degree from the Albert Einstein College of Medicine of Yeshiva University in New York City. He did his internship and general psychiatry residency at the University of California, Davis, Medical Center in Sacramento, and a clinical psychopharmacology research fellowship at the University of California, San Diego. At the University of New Mexico in Albuquerque, Dr. Strassman's studies of the pineal melatonin documented the first known role of this hormone in humans. Later at UNM, he performed the first new US government-approved and funded clinical research with psychedelic drugs in over 20 years. Before leaving the university in 1995, he attained the rank of Tenured Associate Professor of Psychiatry, and received the UNM General Clinical

Research Center's Research Scientist Award. He is currently Clinical Associate Professor of Psychiatry at UNM and President and co-founder of the Cottonwood Research Foundation.

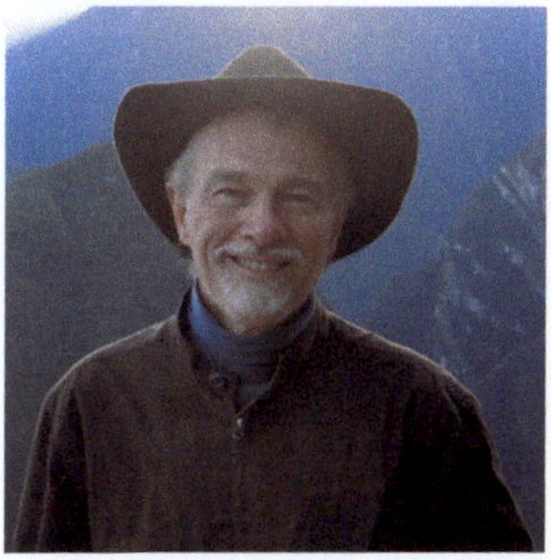

Michael Winkelman received his Ph.D. from the University of California-Irvine and a Master's in Public Health from the University of Arizona. He retired from the School of Human Evolution and Social Change at Arizona State University in 2009. He was President of the anthropology of consciousness and anthropology of religion sections of the American Anthropological Association. His cross-cultural and interdisciplinary research on shamanism and altered states of consciousness has focused on identifying the biological bases of religious experiences. His principal publications include *Shamans, Priests, and Witches* (1992), which provides a cross-cultural examination of shamanism; and *Shamanism: A Biopsychosocial Paradigm of Consciousness and Healing* (2nd edition 2010). This evolutionary approach to religion is expanded in his co-authored *Supernatural as Natural* (2008). Winkelman's work has shown that shamanism and psychedelics have a deep intersection in human evolution, and that these capacities for altering consciousness continue to be important today, as illustrated in his co-edited volumes *Psychedelic Medicine* (2007) and *Altering Consciousness* (2011). For more information, see: www.michaelwinkelman.com.

Chapter 1
Therapeutic Applications of Ayahuasca and Other Sacred Medicines

Michael J. Winkelman

Abstract Therapeutic applications of the psychedelics or hallucinogens found cross-culturally involve treatment of a variety of physical, psychological, and social maladies. Modern medicine has similarly found that a range of conditions may be successfully treated with these agents. The ability to treat a wide variety of conditions derives from variation in active ingredients, doses and modes of application, and factors of set and setting manipulated in ritual. Similarities in effects reported cross-culturally reflect biological mechanisms, while success in the treatment of a variety of specific psychological conditions points to the importance of ritual in eliciting their effects. Similar bases involve action on the serotonin and dopamine neurotransmitter systems that can be characterized as psychointegration: an elevation of ancient brain processes.

Therapeutic Application of Sacred Medicines in the Premodern and Modern World

Societies worldwide have discovered therapeutic applications of psychoactive plants, often referred to as sacred medicines, particularly those called psychedelics or hallucinogens. Hundreds of species of such plants and fungi were used for medicinal and religious purposes (see Schultes et al. 1992; Rätsch 2005), as well as for a variety of psychological and social conditions, culture-bound syndromes, and

Thanks to Ilsa Jerome for providing some updated references for this paper.

M. J. Winkelman (✉)
Retired from the School of Human Evolution and Social Change, Arizona State University
Tempe Arizona, Caixa Postal 62, Pirenópolis, GO 72980-000, Brazil
e-mail: michaeljwinkelman@gmail.com

B. C. Labate and C. Cavnar (eds.), *The Therapeutic Use of Ayahuasca*,
DOI: 10.1007/978-3-642-40426-9_1, © Springer-Verlag Berlin Heidelberg 2014

a range of physical diseases (see Schultes and Winkelman 1996). This review illustrates the range of uses and the diverse potential of these substances for addressing human maladies. The ethnographic data on indigenous uses of these substances, combined with a brief overview of some of the modern medical studies, illustrate that a wide range of effects are obtained with these plants. These cultural therapies involve both pharmacological and ritual manipulations. Highly developed healing traditions selectively utilized different species of the same genus, different preparation methods and doses, varying admixtures, and a variety of ritual and psychotherapeutic processes to obtain specific desired effects. The wide range of uses of these plants suggests that they can contribute new active ingredients for modern medicine, particularly in psychiatry.

As was illustrated by our illustrious contributors to *Psychedelic Medicine* (Winkelman and Roberts 2007a, b), there are a number of areas in which psychedelics have been established in treating what have been considered intractable health problems. While double-blind clinical trials have been sparse (but see Griffiths et al. 2006), this is not due to the lack of evidence for efficacy, but rather the administrative prohibitions that have drastically restricted clinical research. Nonetheless, using the criteria of phases of clinical evaluation, Winkelman and Roberts (2007c) concluded that there is at least Phase II[1] evidence for the effectiveness of most of these psychedelics, supporting the continuation of more advanced trials. Furthermore, their success with the often intractable maladies, ranging from depression and cluster headaches to posttraumatic stress disorder (PTSD), obsessive-compulsive disorders, wasting syndromes, and addictions justifies their immediate use with these desperate patient populations. In addition, the wide variety of therapeutic uses found for these substances in cultures around the world suggest the potential for far greater applications.

Therapeutic Uses of Psilocybin-containing "Magic Mushrooms"

The Aztecs called these fungi *teonanacatl*, meaning "food of the gods"; there is evidence of the use of psilocybin-containing mushrooms from many different genera in ritual healing practices in cultures around the world and deep in prehistory (see Rätsch 2005). One of the best documented therapeutic uses of psilocybin involves Maria Sabina, the Mazatec "Wise One" (Estrada 1981). Several different *Psilocybe* species are used by the Mazatec, as well as mushrooms of the *Conocybe* genera. In addition, other psychoactive plants are also employed, including *Salvia divinorum* Epl. and tobacco (*Nicotiana rustica* L., Solanaceae).

[1] Phase II studies or trials use small groups of selected patients to determine effectiveness and ideal doses for a specific illness after Phase I trials have established safety (lack of toxicity) and safe dose ranges.

Maria Sabina's life and practice illustrates typical shamanic features in the role of the mushrooms in selection and training. Mazatec shamans typically are self-initiated after being taught directly by the mushrooms. Maria Sabina discovered the "saintly children" alone in the forests as a starving child and ate them for sustenance; she encountered spirits in her experiences which taught her how to become a "wise one" (*sabia*) and heal. The wisdom and the ability to heal come from the "language of the mushrooms," which is central in the training and provides the means to diagnose and heal.

The mushrooms are ingested during an all-night vigil which is held in a house removed from other dwellings. The ingestion of the mushrooms by the healer and sometimes the patient permits diagnosis of the condition and guidance of the treatment. Patients seek remedies to illness, solutions to problems, to determine the possibility of recovery, to find lost animals or other objects of value, or to determine the condition of separated family members or loved ones. The healer's visions reveal the origin of the malady, wounds of the spirit, hexes, or how to recover the soul or spirit of the person that has been robbed or lost. The healer deals with illness caused by human enemies, as well as illness caused by malevolent spirits, driving them from the body. She calms the quarrels and disputes that disrupt the household, clears away bad air, purifies, undoes witchcraft, and restores peace. Cures are also directed to physical problems—to cure sick children, fever, chills, yellow skin, toothache, pimples, and physical pains—but with causes identified at the spiritual level.

Those participating in the ceremonies must maintain certain prohibitions, including fasting from breakfast on, no eggs or alcohol consumption for 4 days, and also no sexual acts for 4 days before and after the ceremony. Pregnant women are excluded from the ritual. Roman Catholic elements are incorporated into the indigenous Mazatec practices including, praying to Christ, Mary, and the saints while the mushrooms, the "saintly children," are cleansed in the smoke of copal incense. The mushrooms are generally eaten raw, accompanied with a cup of chocolate, and may be ground to release the juice, which is then drunk. Sometimes tobacco, mixed with lime and garlic, is rubbed on the arms of the sick person or placed in the mouth.

The healing ceremony involves chanting, whistling, humming, percussive artistry, ventriloquistic effects, and dancing by the healer; first in pitch darkness, and later by candlelight. The healer chants monophonically most of the night and sometimes hums. Saints are evoked, herbal remedies advised, pilgrimages directed, evil influences commanded to leave, and healing energies directed to the patient. The patients themselves experience visions, often of a terrifying and overpowering nature. Their vomiting, crying, and other emotional reactions reflect the cathartic nature of their experiences. Although the principal stated means of curing are the mushrooms and the chants, other therapeutic modalities are combined in the ceremony. Maria Sabina used the mushroom language in singing and chanting, percussive utterances, alliteration, and repetition of grammatical structures as part of the healing ritual. The chants' content suggests they also play a therapeutic role in establishing attitudinal postures and in encouraging positive motivation and expectation. The healer's performance indicates the enactment of roles that produce cathartic experiences in the patients.

Modern Medicinal Applications of Psilocybin

The use of psilocybin mushrooms in the successful treatment of the notorious cluster headaches has been documented by Sewell and Halpern (2007). The treatment of this condition was accidentally discovered by some of the victims of these headaches, who also noted the effectiveness of psilocybin and lysergic acid diethylamide (LSD) and shared their experiences online and eventually in conferences. In the case of cluster headaches, we see the clear ethical and moral necessity of supplying patients with these substances because of the virtually untreatable nature of this condition within biomedicine, and the desperate situation of the patients, illustrated by the other name of this ailment: suicide headaches. The research of Moreno and Delgado (2007) on "Psilocybin Treatment of Obsessive-Compulsive Disorder" illustrates another area where these ancient medicines offer promise for conditions that are often not effectively treated by conventional biomedical remedies. Grob (2007) and Grob et al. (2011, 2013) has researched psilocybin's applications in treating problems associated with terminal cancer, such as existential anxiety, despair, and fear often encountered by dying patients and their families. The spirituality-inducing effects of these substances go beyond conventional psychotherapies to facilitate core psychological processes involved in end-of-life issues. These studies demonstrate that psilocybin has the capacity to facilitate the emergence of experiences of spiritual transcendence that have powerful therapeutic impact and enhance emotional well being.

We should not, however, leave these profound psychological impacts for the end of life. Roland Griffiths and colleagues have provided an impressive series of publications (e.g., see Griffiths et al. 2006) on psilocybin that indicate that they not only induced mystical experiences but also long-term personality changes. Griffith's et al. (2006) carefully designed double-blind study showed that psilocybin has effects on participants' attitudes, moods, and experiences of spirituality that persist for months. In addition to significantly higher ratings on the scales used to assess mysticism, internal and external unity, sacredness, transcendence of time and space, ineffability, and experiences of oceanic boundlessness, the psilocybin sessions had significantly higher levels of positive mood, peace, harmony, joy, and intense happiness. There were lasting effects noted from the psilocybin experiences, including an enhanced positive attitude about life and themselves and positive altruistic social behaviors noted by third-party community observers. These effects point to the broader social implications of these substances as therapeutic agents.

The Mescaline-containing Cactaceae: Peyote (*Lophophora williamsii*) and San Pedro (*Trichocereus* spp.)

A number of different genera of the Cactaceae family are used in healing practices (see Schultes et al. 1992). The most important of these psychoactive Cactaceae are: peyote (*Lophophora williamsii*), the plant used in ancient Mexico and found today in the deserts of northern Mexico and across the Rio Grande in Texas; and the *Trichocereus* genus, particularly *Trichocereus pachanoi*, a cactus used for thousands of years in Peru and in mestizo traditions today (Sharon 1978; Joralemon and Sharon 1993). There are many alkaloids in these cacti, with the principal active ingredient being mescaline.

Peyote is the sacrament of the "Peyote Religion" or Native American Church (NAC), an organization founded more than 100 years ago in the wake of the complete domination of the indigenous peoples of North America. The peyote traditions were transferred from indigenous peoples of Mexico and given a new ritual format that blended the symbols of Christianity with indigenous beliefs. Aberle (1966) characterized the Peyote Religion as serving many different purposes, including religious, miraculous curing, transcendence, self-knowledge, incentive to work, release from guilt, and temperance from alcohol. In most cases, the initial recourse to peyote was for curing, and people stayed to maintain good health and mind, for:

> relief from feelings of aimlessness and helplessness, to overcome misfortunes, for future guidance and future good fortune, to access knowledge about causes of illness or misfortune, to foretell future occurrences, and to provide security against witches and ghosts. And so peyotism appeals to the person who seeks only a cure after crises, to the disorganized and unhappy, to the alienated and marginal, to the philosopher, to the mystic, and to the person who seeks guidance and a sense of purpose and sustaining motive (Aberle 1966, p. 194).

Modern Medicinal Perspectives on Peyote's Therapeutic Effectiveness

Therapeutic effects of peyote are widely attested to not only by Native American users, but also by anthropologists, social workers, addictions counselors, and physicians who have observed the effects of this sacred medicine. While further research is needed on specific physiological mechanisms of peyote, evidence exists regarding its relative safety and effectiveness (see Halpern et al. 2005; Halpern 1996). Evidence of acceptance equivalent to Phase III[2]—approved therapeutic

[2] Phase III studies use clinical trials, ideally with randomized controls, to confirm effectiveness, monitor adverse drug effects and interactions, and/or to compare to other commonly used treatments.

use—is found in the practice of the Indian Health Service, a branch of the U.S. Federal Government, of providing reimbursement for road men who use peyote for treatment of alcoholism among Native Americans (see Calabrese 2007).

The NAC has many effects on social, psychological, and emotional well being. Aberle points to the ability of peyote to induce a sense of connection with the spiritual world that was lost by many Native American individuals and groups in their forcible assimilation to European-American culture. The significance of spiritual experiences for rehabilitation of the addicted self has been noted in many therapeutic traditions, and may be particularly relevant for Native American groups deprived of their own spiritual traditions. The psychiatrist Jilek (1994) conveys the peyotists' perspective that the peyote ritual combats alcoholism by reducing physical and mental stress and enhancing mental and physical strength through contact with the supernatural. A widely noted effect involves management of cultural alienation experienced by young Native Americans, providing a context for a ritual death and rebirth and construction of a positive identification with one's culture. Peyotism provides internal peace and harmony instead of competition and conflict, and a reference group of close relations who meet needs for approval and esteem. Peyotism offers status, an assertion of self-worth, and a means of countering the effects of prejudice by providing validation of their separate identity. Peyotism is able to provide an alternative because it rejects dominant society values of acculturation and assimilation and the emphasis on materialism. The Peyote Church has been credited as an important factor towards the control of alcoholism amongst the participants.

Calabrese (1997, 2007, 2013) describes the Peyote Way as a cultural psychiatry involving "meaning-manipulative" therapies engaging social and intrapsychic processes. He characterizes peyote as a "desematicizing" agent that facilitates a reinterpretation of self. The cultural psychosocial therapies of the Native American Church treat alcoholism through a process of emplotment of their lives, a reintegration of the self into cultural patterns. These processes of meaning making take a significant role in the process of overcoming addictions; a recreation of the self in spiritual terms. Calabrese (1997, pp. 238–239) characterizes the effects in terms of a "social manipulation of consciousness states and symbols to support socially valued patterns of ritual experience, self-awareness, and emotional control… [rendering] adults more suggestible and thus more open to education and mental health interventions." In this sense, peyote rituals heal by shaping consciousness in ways that facilitate symbolic healing processes.

Ayahuasca: The Enigmatic Combination

The current international widespread use of ayahuasca reflects not only the wide range of its indigenous use across the Amazon Basin, but also the many modern adaptations in spiritual healing practices and organized churches. Medicinal and religious use of ayahuasca was widespread among hundreds of indigenous groups of South America, and provided the source for numerous urban adaptations in the mestizo populations, where the plant preparations are employed for sorcery, healing, and prophecy, as well as more mainstream religious purposes such as in the União do Vegetal and Santo Daime churches. Luna (1986) points to the widespread premodern use of ayahuasca for dealing with all aspects of life. The widespread use of ayahuasca may reflect some special properties derived from its enigmatic nature based in an unlikely combination of two plants: the *Banisteriopsis* vine, which provides a MAO inhibitor that allows the principal active ingredient, N,N-Dimethyltryptamine (DMT), from other plants (normally *Psychotria viridis* or *Diplopterys cabrerana*) to be active via oral administration. In addition, other plants were commonly added in prehistoric and premodern practices. McKenna et al. (1995) report more than 50 genera of plants that are added to the basic ayahuasca mixture as biodynamic constituents intended to have additional effects. Consequently a wide range of effects is reported, also varying as a function of mode of preparation, dosage, setting, and ceremonial processes.

Shamanic Training

Ayahuasca is used in the training of healers. Traditional training (see Luna 1986) requires extensive food restrictions and sexual abstinence and segregation from virtually all contact with women. Dietary prohibitions of alcohol, pork, chicken, fats, salt, sugar, condiments, fruit, vegetables, and cold beverages are widely reported. Plantains, smoked fish, and some jungle animals, occasionally augmented by rice and manioc, constitute the preferred diet. In traditional practice, the violations of these prohibitions are believed to cause illness or even death. Diet is viewed as a tool to help maintain the altered state of consciousness that permits the plant teachers to instruct, provide knowledge, and enable the initiate to acquire their power. The diet is viewed as a means of making the mind operate differently, providing access to wisdom and lucid dreams. The training period involves learning songs, chants, and medicinal recipes and enhancing the trainees' artistic and intellectual skills. The spirit-taught magical chants and songs which are central to the ayahuasquero's learning about the plant-teacher spirits and their powers. The chants learned serve many purposes: calling souls and spirits, affecting the actions of the ayahuasca or specific plant teachers, curing specific illnesses, and in love magic. In the practice of healing, ayahuasca is ingested along with tobacco juice in order to enable the healer to see into the patient's body and diagnose the cause of illness. In the visionary state, the healer can locate illness-causing darts within the patient's body and then suck them out. The visions also enable the healer to see the individual responsible for causing the patient's illness.

Premodern Amazonian Patterns of Ayahuasca Use

Andritzky (1989) notes two premodern Amazonian patterns of ayahuasca use, one involving the communal consumption by adult group members, and the other the ingestion by the healer in treatments of individual clients. When consumed in a group context, the consumption and intents are an individual issue, with no group leader or formal ceremony. Participants chant their own songs independently, without any coordination of the rhythm of the different chanters. The group context, including physical contact among the participants, is an important part of the modulation of the experiences. But each participant has their own focus of attention, a personal experience and search for knowledge or information of importance to the individual. Andritzky (1989) suggests that such ingestion by the adult members of the community strengthens social cohesion and identity. In individual healing sessions, the healers ingest ayahuasca, while the patients usually refrain. However, the interaction between healer and patient, as well as other ritual factors, serve to evoke visions and personal unconscious material in the patient. Andritzky suggests that the ayahuasqueros help people deal with the problems of acculturation. Their rituals mediate between the Euro-American and indigenous worlds, creating a synthesis of the traditional and the new through the use of emotionally relevant images of culture change from the indigenous point of view. The treatment and practices are a method of symbolic confrontation with psycho and sociotherapeutic effects. Ayahuasca apparently gives the user conscious access to the process of symbolization, with the effects shaped by songs, stories, and mythological worlds that structure visions. These prepare the patients for the experiences, and enable them to assimilate effects through collective motifs, rather than be flooded with unconscious personal material. The use of stories and their interpretations allow the healer to control the level of anxiety and the depth of regression of the individual. These and other factors contribute to the powerful set and setting effects that characterize experiences induced by ayahuasca.

Ayahuasca Among Contemporary Peruvian Vegetalistas

Dobkin de Rios (1992) summarizes uses of ayahuasca among Peruvian vegetalistas as including: acquiring protective spirits; determining the causes and cures of diseases; prophesizing the future; determining if wives were unfaithful; sending messages to other groups; discovering enemies and their plans; and in preparation for war or hunting expeditions. The illnesses treated are diverse, but those characterized as magical illnesses and culture-bound syndromes include: *susto* (fear), caused by an intense experience of fear interpreted as causing the loss of the person's soul; *dano* (harm), caused by sorcery of others who have feelings of envy or desire for vengeance; *mal de ojo* (evil eye), caused by envy, evil intentions or a glance; and *pulsario*, a painful abdominal ball believed to be caused by repressed emotions such as anger or sorrow. Dysfunctions in social or sexual relations, emotional problems, dependences and excesses, bad luck, as well as psychological, somatic and physical problems are also treated.

Dobkin de Rios also discusses urban adaptations of Peruvian vegetalistas to diagnose the cause of illness through analysis of the visionary experiences. The ayahuasquero channels the experiences through chants and whistling, which are followed by periods of silence alternated with chanting. These visions might reveal causes embodied in animal forms, the hate felt by others toward the patient, or a person carrying out harmful rituals against the patient. The determination of the cause then permits the ayahuasquero to effect a cure through neutralizing the influences which caused the illness. These treatments normally include many of the widely practiced healing techniques found throughout the Amazon Basin and many other parts of the world: singing, chanting, recitations, whistling, blowing smoke, and sucking on afflicted parts of the patient's body. The next morning as the effects fade, discussion and commentary about the experiences ensue. Sessions may be repeated several times over the next month or so, but there is very little or no follow-up by the ayahuasqueros.

My own recent unpublished research[3] reveals that the contemporary Peruvian neoayahuasquero practitioners conceptualize ayahuasca as a sacrament that has the ability to address physical, emotional, psychological, and spiritual conditions. Among the varied conceptions of the healing or "whole-ing" provided by ayahuasca is that it can heal the soul, the body, and past trauma. Ayahuasca is often seen as opening the heart, expanding love for others, and leading to healing of both self and relationships. Ingesting the brew is seen as expanding awareness, healing the personality, and providing the insight and energies to restore personal relations. The effects also enable people to better deal with anticipating their own death and dying, as well as that of their loved ones, and the grieving processes. Ayahuasca sometimes produces a radical rebirth that changes one's life for the better, helping people find their own true path with divine purpose. Using this sacrament is generally seen as opening one's mind to new possibilities, changing beliefs, particularly moving beyond the self-limiting beliefs regarding self and reality, and expanding one's understanding of life, God, and the universe. Some spoke of ayahuasca as putting one in touch with the god within and one's true self; opening the heart to spiritual healing. Others characterized ayahuasca as enabling the participants to control their own spiritual energies and integrate with the divine, mirroring God in their own lives; some specifically characterized the effects of ayahuasca as helping to establish a connection with Jesus. Ayahuasca is also seen as providing collective spiritual experiences and an experience of the divine. It may be used to create a communal connection while celebrating the cycles of the cosmos and nature, with special ceremonies to mark the cycles of the seasons, the

---

[3] This research was carried out in the Tarapoto and Iquitos areas of the Peruvian Amazon during May and June 2012 as part of services for a Peruvian neoayahuasquero evaluating contemporary practices and the nature of the clients in his retreats.

end of the year, and the full moons. The connection with a community of others is a significant feature of the ayahuasca experience, one that also elicits a sense of the need for service to others.

Western Ayahuasca Pilgrimages

The Western practice of pilgrimage to foreign sites for ayahuasca rituals is a relatively new phenomenon (see Foutiou 2010; Winkelman 2005), developing in the last few decades as knowledge about these ancient spiritual practices entered into the postmodern world. Foutiou's research on the globalization of ayahuasca practices in Peru involves what she calls "shamanic tourism," which is similar to other contemporary pilgrimages. This Western search for ayahuasca is not a pretext for drug abuse, but rather a spiritual quest that addresses an urgent need for self-transformation regarding fundamental religious and existential concerns. Foutiou characterizes this as an intercultural exchange that enables Westerners to adopt shamanic discourse, a view espoused by many contemporary sacred healers. These ayahuasca tourists seek self-exploration and spiritual growth, as well as physical and emotional healing. Ayahuasca is particularly attractive because it addresses both the spiritual component of healing as well as the physical diseases that result from a spiritual disconnect from nature, spirit, and other humans. Ayahuasca experiences are appealing to Westerners because they offer direct access to the spiritual and the "divine within," a more direct path to the divine than offered by their own religions, and a process of healing that is also part of a larger project for transforming humanity.

In one study (Winkelman 2005), participants in a retreat in Amazonia were queried in open-ended questions regarding their motivations for attending the retreat and their experience in the sessions. In contrast to the notion of ayahuasca use involving some form of drug use, only one respondent spoke of what might be considered hedonistic reasons for the retreat (to obtain artistic creativity, among other more spiritually oriented motivations). In direct contrast to the notion of drug-seeking behavior, a number of respondents saw this spiritual encounter as providing some assistance in addressing their personal substance abuse issues. Some saw ayahuasca as providing a tool for insight into personal abusive behaviors and motivation for ending alcohol abuse, a theme widely attested to in the varied literature on the use of these sacraments as tools for ending abusive drug behaviors.

While some spoke of seeking emotional healing, the vast majority of responses attested to a desire to establish greater spiritual awareness, direct spiritual relations, and enhanced spiritual development. Respondents spoke of imbibing ayahuasca to connect with some sacred dimension of nature, communing with God, engaging in a spiritual quest, and connecting with some spiritual dimension greater than them. Personal spiritual development was a main theme, with participants speaking of finding out about some true aspect of their selves, development of spirit mediumship abilities, obtaining spiritual healing, obtaining spiritual and philosophical insights, obtaining guidance and direction in life, and getting clarity about individual paths and purposes that could help with resolving personal problems.

The benefits that respondents obtained from the ayahuasca experiences echoed themes similar to their intents. They generally reported that the experiences increased their personal development, providing insights into their lives through access to deeper levels of the self, strengthening of the spiritual identity, and increasing self-awareness. Some spoke of personal enlightenment and enlightenment regarding the human condition, an increased capacity for meditation, calmness, and control of anxiety. In summary, the experiences speak to genuine spiritual and transpersonal concerns involving an increase in personal spiritual awareness and awareness of spiritual dimensions of the universe that contributed to enhanced personal spiritual development.

An assessment[4] of the motivation of Western ayahuasca pilgrims and the experiences they had found that the vast majority of the respondents ascribed spiritual, mystical, or metaphysical motivations as being moderately or very important reasons for their participation. All affirmed that their motivations included to "establish relations with the plants, their wisdom, God, spirits or a higher power" and to "enhance your relationship to the universe and acquire a better understanding of the unknown… [and to] establish a personal connection with the spiritual or sacred." Most also subscribed to the idea that ayahuasca enabled them to "learn about or experience the divine aspects of myself, some inner truth or divine immanence" and to "receive guidance or personal direction in life from the wisdom of the plant teachers, the spirits, the universe, God, etc." The respondents' experiences with ayahuasca also pointed to the central significance of spiritual themes in their responses, that ayahuasca gave "an increase in personal spiritual development." Their own personal spiritual development was attested to in an increased sense of awareness of the spiritual dimensions of the universe, an experience of the divine aspects of self, and an enhanced sense of personal connection with the spiritual or sacred.

Modern Medicinal Applications of Ayahuasca

Ayahuasca has also been examined in laboratory, clinical, and medicinal studies for its potentials to contribute to modern medicine. One of the primary areas of application is attested to in many of the papers of this volume: the field of addictions treatment (also see Mabit 2007). These applications constitute perhaps the most compelling reason for its' immediate medical use, given the general lack of long-term success of conventional addictions treatment programs. As is the case with peyote, ibogaine, and chemical substances such as LSD and ketamine, the

[4] See footnote 5.

psychedelics have been found to provide dramatic relief of symptoms of addiction and provide powerful forces for reorganizing the lives of addicts to help them achieve sobriety (see articles in Winkelman and Roberts 2007b; Winkelman 2009). The recognition of these potentials goes back to the 1960s, when the contributions of LSD to the treatment of alcoholism were first recognized. While the studies of the early period did not generally meet standards of research of today, they nonetheless established the dramatic initial increases in the sobriety of the LSD treatment groups as compared to controls, with effects tapering off over time. Recent retrospective studies and meta-analyses (e.g., Bogenschutz and Pommy 2012; Krebs and Johansen 2012; Ross 2012) continue to bear out the hypothesis that there are significant therapeutic mechanisms from these substances that can be applied to the treatment of addictions.

There is also a potential role for ayahuasca in the treatment of depression, as discussed in this volume in the paper by Palhano-Fontes et al. This possibility is supported by the research of Osório et al. (2011), who found that harmine, a β-carboline alkaloid that is found in the *Banisteriopsis* genus, has antidepressant effects in studies of both animals and humans. Harmine is a monoamine oxidase (MAO) inhibitor, an action that is one of the primary effects of the typical antidepressant drugs. Osório et al. research found evidence of antidepressant effects in the central nervous system of rodents, supporting further experimentation with harmine as a candidate for the pharmacological management of depression. Their exploratory study, using ayahuasca on nonpsychotic patients with clinical diagnoses of recurring depressive disorders, showed a decrease in depressive symptoms persisting for about 2 weeks.

Further applications of ayahuasca are suggested by several studies that have examined its usefulness in the treatment of Parkinson's disease, a currently incurable neurological disorder characterized by the loss of dopamine-producing neurons in the substantia nigra area of the brain. A study by Serrano-Dueñas (2001) using state-of-the art methodologies (double-blind, randomized, placebo-controlled trials) examined the effects of a single dose of *Banisteriopsis caapi* on the motor function of Parkinson's patients, using a standard assessment tool (Unified Parkinson's Disease Rating Scale). They found beneficial behavioral effects from the *Banisteriopsis* that they hypothesize were primarily due to the interaction of harmaline at glutamatergic receptors, specifically the glutamate receptor antagonist effects caused by the harmalines. They note evidence that harmaline binds to N-Methyl-D-aspartate (NMDA) receptors as an agonist which mimics the action of glutamate and postulate that it is this interaction of harmaline with the glutamatergic receptors that plays a central role in restoring the loss of motor function associated with Parkinson's disease. They postulate that these effects of harmaline may result from counter-acting the excitatory effects of glutamate and its roles in the neurodegeneration of dopaminergic neurons within the substantia nigra. They propose that this antiglutamate action of harmaline, which is responsible for the blockage of glutamatergic receptors, corrects imbalances caused by dopamine deficiency and consequently contributes to a restoration of normal motor function.

A more recent study conducted by Samoylenkoa et al. (2010) examined evidence of the effectiveness of compounds derived from aqueous extract of *Banisteriopsis caapi* stems in the treatment of Parkinson's disease by examining effects on MAO-A and MAO-B, with laboratory findings showing the presence of potent in vitro MAO-A inhibitory and antioxidant activities. Their tests for MAO inhibition found that an extract from *Banisteriopsis caapi*, as well as pure harmine, both exhibited an inhibitory effect on MAO-A, and increased release of dopamine. In addition, they concluded the evidence for inhibition by harmine and harmaline of MAO-B activity indicated that they provided protection against neurodegeneration, and consequently have potential for the treatment of Parkinson's diseases. Furthermore, they noted the potential therapeutic value of ayahuasca because of the presence of the potent antioxidants epicatechin and procyanidin B2. Since oxidative stress is associated with the pathogenesis found in neurodegenerative disorders such as Parkinson's and Alzheimer's diseases, they concluded that because of their selective MAO-B inhibitory activity, these antioxidants have significant potential in providing protection for neuronal cells that are damaged by oxidative free radicals.

Therapeutic Mechanisms of Psychoactive Sacramentals

How are such diverse effects obtained from relatively similar substances? The answer to this question involves a least three different mechanisms. First, in spite of similar chemical substances in diverse plants, there is also a broad range of different psychoactive substances in single plants and the combinations of plants characteristic of ayahuasca and the snuffs. There are dozens of different alkaloids in various psilocybin mushrooms, as well as the *Banisteriopsis*, *Psychotria*, and *Diplopterys* species and the additional plant teachers that may be included in ayahuasca combinations. Consequently, there are a variety of different pharmacological mechanisms that provide therapeutic effectiveness. Second, a range of effects is induced by factors that make set and setting influences very important. These plants have been known to produce a state of extreme susceptibility to ritual and other expectancy-based effects. This capacity of context and expectation to powerfully shape the effects of these substances has been widely recognized in the different psychiatric models described below (psychotic, psycholytic, and psychedelic) which were developed to explain the varied effects elicited by psychedelics.

Pharmacological Effects of the Sacred Medicines

A significant feature of the pharmacological effects of psychedelics in the treatment of addictions is manifested in an "after glow" effect of positive affect and increased openness to therapeutic intervention that lasts for several weeks following sessions. Furthermore, a crucial therapeutic role came to be attributed to the responses to large doses; the resultant "peak experience" that produced the personal transformation of the addict to attempt an engagement with sobriety. These transformative potentials were the basis for new views of the potentials of these substances embodied in the concept of the psychedelic paradigm of psychotherapy. The after-glow effects suggest the necessity of combining psycholytic and psychedelic mechanisms in addiction treatment.

These pharmacological effects are exemplified in the use of ibogaine and ketamine in the treatment of opioid, methamphetamine, and alcohol addictions. Iboga roots used in indigenous spiritual practices of the Bwiti of West Central Africa provided the original basis for the ibogaine extract. Both have a history of use in informal treatment of addiction in addict communities, functioning largely within the context of both addict and medical subcultures rather than in conventional medical settings. Ibogaine became an important element in heroin self-help groups and harm reduction movements among addicts in the Netherlands (Alper et al. 2008). Alper and Lotsof (2007) review the many forms of evidence regarding the efficacy of ibogaine in reducing withdrawal cravings, particularly the elimination of opioid and cocaine withdrawal symptoms and the lasting resolution of the acute withdrawal syndromes for several weeks to months. Alper and Lotsof indicate that the mechanisms of action of ibogaine are different from other addiction treatments: It is neither an opiate agonist nor an opiate antagonist, nor does it appear to operate on a serotonin model. They suggest that ibogaine causes a "resetting" or "normalization" of basic neuroadaptations that maintain dependence. Krupitsky and Kolp (2007) have documented the effectiveness of ketamine hydrochloride in psychedelic psychotherapy for the treatment of both alcoholics and heroin addicts. Ketamine represents an unusual case of a drug already approved by the FDA for use as an anesthetic now being applied off label for addictions. They review a history of studies showing ketamine's use for treating a range of conditions, as well as a powerful tool for catapulting psychedelic treatments beyond impasses experienced with LSD treatments. Krupitsky and Kolp review best uses and practices for applying ketamine's ability to induce ego-dissolving transpersonal peak experiences as a key part of treatment of addiction.

Psychointegration as a Pharmacological Mechanism

Therapeutic effects of sacred medicines are derived from the general principles underlying their effects of altering consciousness in general. In a series of publications (Winkelman 2001, 2007, 2010), I have provided a synthesis of laboratory, clinical, and ethnographic findings on the effects of sacred medicines that involve what I call "psychointegration." The central and common effects of these diverse substances involve the evocation of a similar response from the organism that elicits a serotonin-based triggering of slow and synchronized brainwaves, typically theta (3–6 cycles/s). This physiological elicitation of brain wave responses from the ancient levels of the brain evokes unconscious processes that are inherently therapeutic.

This concept of psychointegration reflects similar effects revealed by neurophysiologic, clinical, and cross-cultural studies, reflecting their action within the serotonin system, which has multiple roles, as reflected in its characterization as a neuromodulator that regulates the balance among many neurotransmitter systems. Psychointegrative effects are epitomized in the functions of serotonin in modulating the activities of dozens of bodily and brain processes and neurotransmitter systems; and by the psychointegrators' systemic effects on the serotonergic neurotransmitter system that enhances the integration of information across levels of the brain. This enhanced integrative function is manifested in the systemic effects at the level of the raphe and reticular formation, where there is an enhancement of excitatory effects, and the limbic brain, where emotions and memories are formed.

The effects of psychointegrators are reflected in synchronized alpha and theta brain wave hyperactivity across the neuraxis, the nerve bundle linking the structural levels of the brain from the brain stem to the frontal cortex. In the process of inducing synchronous discharges across this nerve bundle, psychointegrators elicit processes central to awareness and fundamental aspects of self, emotions, and attachments. These processes of psychointegration are revealed physiologically in the typical coherent theta wave discharges that produce a synchronization of brain waves across the neuraxis and lobes of the brain. Psychointegration is also manifested in psychological experiences, particularly those related to emotional healing and the sense of interconnectedness, such as in states of cosmic consciousness and other transpersonal experiences. Psychointegrators' effects on neural, sensory, emotional, and cognitive processes enhance consciousness by integrating normally unconscious emotional and self information into the frontal cortex and consciousness. This integration of the unconscious into consciousness underlies the general potentials of psychointegrators as therapeutic agents.

Set and Setting as Therapeutic Processes

The broad applications of psychointegrators are explained by studies that implicate individual and environmental factors in these substances' effects. The "set" (individual characteristics and expectations including attitude, motivation, mood, and personality) and "setting" (the physical and social context of use) produce quite varied experiences under psychedelics (see Passie et al. 2008). The primacy of set and setting effects is reflected in the different psychotherapeutic traditions in the clinical study of LSD, three different models of the nature of its effects. These three paradigms—called psychotomimetic, psycholytic, and psychedelic (see Grof 1975, 2001; Lukoff et al. 1990)—show that different effects may be derived from the same substance as a consequence of the state of extreme neurobiological flexibility produced. These different medical models help to establish that the rituals accompanying the sacred use of the substances are basic to their effects.

Roberts and Winkelman (2013) propose these primarily involve psycholytic, psychedelic, and entactogen effects.

The psycholytic model. The positive aspects of the LSD experience led to the psycholytic paradigm, based on recognition that LSD could aid psychotherapy. The psycholytic approach employs a series of low doses of LSD in conjunction with therapy sessions. The term "psycholytic" means "mind-dissolving," reflecting the hallucinogen-induced relaxation of the ordinary sense of self, altering the relationship between the conscious and unconscious, and allowing repressed material to become conscious (Passie 2007). This weakens psychological defenses and heightens emotional responsiveness, easing memory blocks and promoting catharsis. Doses are low enough for the patient and psychiatrist to discuss memories when they emerge. This discussion-type treatment may last several drug-free sessions, and new doses are used only if required to dislodge more memories. The ability to relive early life memories and to retain the memories for reflection in post-LSD sessions facilitates the progress of psychotherapy. Psycholytic therapy appears effective with psychosomatic problems and psychic rigidity; isolated individuals and those fixated at egocentric levels; concentration camp survivors with rigid defenses; patients with whom classic psychoanalysis has been unsuccessful; disorders rarely healed by psychotherapy, such as severe chronic compulsions and severe alcoholism; and severe character neuroses, depression, and compulsion (Passie 2007).

The psychedelic model. The subsequent LSD paradigm was referred to as psychedelic therapy, a term reflecting the "mind-manifesting" properties of the substances. The psychedelic model derived from the effects of large doses of LSD, particularly on alcoholics. These studies indicated that those who benefited most from LSD therapy had reported mystical experiences that produced profound personality changes, and suggested that the mystical insights were responsible for the therapeutic outcomes. The psychedelic approaches induce peak and mystical experiences that produce a profound sense of interconnectedness, unity, and meaningfulness that contribute to a feeling of rebirth. These experiences gave the patient a greater sense of self-control and the opportunity to make use of these insights for life changes.

Roberts and Winkelman (2013) propose that there are two main purposes of psychedelic, high dose therapy. The first is to produce a powerful, mystical experience in the client. Typically in mystical experiences, this includes a sense of ego-loss and self-transcendence. The mystical, peak experience is itself psychotherapeutic. Among the conditions that mystical experiences solve or ameliorate are: PTSD, alcoholism and addictions, obsessive–compulsive disorder, depression, death anxiety, and various neuroses and psychoses. Most contemporary research has used the psychedelic model, exemplified in the psilocybin research at Johns Hopkins that has found effects including mystical experiences, meaningfulness, spirituality, openness, and altruism (Griffiths et al. 2006, 2008).

The second type of psychedelic psychotherapeutic experience pushes the boundaries of transpersonal psychology even further, taking us into the realm of paranormal phenomena, past lives, and alternate realities. Material that emerges in these sessions goes beyond the normal ideas of objective reality, but may reflect an extraordinary "symptom" that can support the therapeutic responses when its significance is recognized. Grof (2009) proposes that these substances have the power to both identify a problem and its solution, guided by the power of the unconscious.

Entactogen or empathogen model. This model is derived from the effects of MDMA (3,4-methylenedioxy-N-amphetamine), a drug more commonly called "Ecstasy." MDMA has some properties typical of LSD-like psychedelics because it is a phenethylamine, but its effects are more related to the stimulants, as it also is an amphetamine. The use of MDMA in psychotherapy facilitates connections with the traumatic memories necessary for engaging in therapeutic resolution of the trauma. MDMA allows the client to reduce or even wholly disconnect from the fear associated with memories of a traumatic event or other stressors. Mithoefer (2007), Mithoefer et al. (2013) has used MDMA in the treatment of PTSD. MDMA's ability to facilitate PTSD therapy involves its ability to reduce acute stress reactions and anxiety, curtailing the cycle of the body's stress response. By reducing anxiety-provoking feelings, conditioned fear responses, and avoidance of feelings, MDMA makes it easier for patients to trust the validity of their own feelings and release the associated emotional blockages. As illustrated in the chapter in this volume by Nielson and Megler, ayahuasca is also a promising candidate for treatment of PTSD.

Future Directions and Conclusions

Perhaps one of the most significant, yet heretofore unexplored, areas of medicinal application of the psychointegrators involves the snuffs. There are a variety of indigenous South American traditions involving the use of *Virola* and *Anadenanthera* species, combined with other plants (see Altschul 1972; De Smet 1985; Schultes et al. 1992). The principal active ingredients of both genera involve a number of different forms of DMT and other tryptamines, with the *Anadenanthera* species characterized by the presence of 5-methoxy-N,N-dimethyltryptamine, as well as bufotenine (Torres and Repke 2006). The snuffs are normally snorted, although some are also smoked, and some preparations may be made for oral ingestion. The nasal application may make it particularly useful for experimentation with cocaine and methamphetamine users accustomed to this route of drug administration.

In some of the indigenous groups, the snuffs have been employed primarily by shamans, who use it ritualistically for a variety of purposes. In addition, the *Virola* snuffs are used in a variety of communal functions in the Amazon region. Typically, groups of men from different villages take snuffs together as a part of building and solidifying alliances. These experiences are seen as occasions for men to relieve frustrations without personal responsibility for their behaviors. Under the influence of the snuff, many of the usual avoidance taboos are overlooked, permitting a release of the emotions and strains of everyday life. Chagnon (1983) suggests that one of the primary functions of the snuff-induced experiences is to allow snuffers to work off pent up antagonisms and frustrations by being fierce and expressing passions they are not ordinarily able to exhibit. It may, however, also release antisocial behavior, including violence and homicide. However, the use in intercommunity ceremonies clearly serves to reduce inter-group tensions. Those who have grievances against others may seek them out for vengeance through a chest-pounding exchange. The snuff is believed to enable them to withstand the pain. This chest-pounding exchange is followed by squatting together with arms around each other's neck in an extended period of shouting as they gradually reduce their excitement.

As illustrated in Schultes et al. (1992) *Plants of the Gods*, humanity still has an immense unexplored pharmacological bounty. The generations of shamans who tested these plants have provided guidelines for humanity in this exploration. The evidence available indicates that these sacred medicines have efficacy in treating a wide range of conditions, physical as well as psychological and social. While a variety of factors have impeded effective research, the many forms of evidence available, including the contributions to this volume, illustrate the therapeutic efficacy and potentials of these plants. Physicians and governments have a moral obligation to make the psychointegrators available for clinical use. Activists may find useful guidelines for promoting these changes in a variety of political, bureaucratic, and policy-making endeavors outlined in *Psychedelic Medicine*, particularly Winkelman and Roberts (2007c).

References

Aberle, D. (1966). *The peyote religion among the Navaho*. Chicago, IL: Aldine.

Alper, K. R., & Lotsof, H. S. (2007). The use of ibogaine in the treatment of addictions. In M. Winkelman & T. Robert (Eds.), *Psychedelic medicine: New evidence for hallucinogenic substances as treatments* (Vol. 2, pp. 43–66). Westport, CT: Praeger Perspectives.

Alper, K. R., Lotsof, H. S., & Kaplan, C. D. (2008). The ibogaine medical subculture. *Journal of Ethnopharmacology, 115*, 9–24.

Altschul, S. (1972). *The genus anadenanthera in Amerindian cultures*. Cambridge, MA: Botanical Museum Harvard University.

Andritzky, W. (1989). Sociopsychotherapeutic functions of ayahuasca healing in Amazonia. *Journal of Psychoactive Drugs, 21*(1), 77–89.

Bogenschutz, M. P., & Pommy, J. M. (2012). Therapeutic mechanisms of classic hallucinogens in the treatment of addictions: From indirect evidence to testable hypotheses. *Drug Testing and Analysis, 4*(7–8), 543–555.

Calabrese, J. (1997). Spiritual healing and human development in the Native American Church: Toward a cultural psychiatry of peyote. *Psychoanalytic Review, 84*(2), 237–255.

Calabrese, J. (2007). The therapeutic use of peyote in the Native American Church. In M. Winkelman & T. Roberts (Eds.), *Psychedelic medicine: New evidence for hallucinogenic substances as treatments* (Vol. 2, pp. 29–42). Westport, CT: Praeger Perspectives.

Calabrese, J. (2013). *A different medicine: Postcolonial healing in the Native American Church*. New York, NY: Oxford University Press.

Chagnon, N. (1983). *Yanomamo: The fierce people*. New York, NY: Holt, Rinehart and Winston.

De Smet, P. A. G. M. (1985). *Ritual enemas and snuffs in the Americas*. Amsterdam: CEDLA.

Dobkin de Rios, M. (1992). *Amazon healer: The life and times of an urban healer*. Bridport, Dorset, UK: Prism Press.

Estrada, A. (1981). *Maria Sabina: Her life and chants*. (H. Munn, Trans.). Santa Barbara, CA: Ross-Erickson.

Fotiou, E. (2010). *From medicine men to day-trippers: Shamanic tourism in Iquitos, Peru*. (Unpublished doctoral dissertation). Department of Anthropology, University of Wisconsin-Madison.

Griffiths, R. R., Richards, W. A., McCann, U., & Jesse, R. (2006). Psilocybin can occasion mystical-type experiences having substantial, sustained personal meaning and spiritual significance. *Psychopharmacology, 187*(3), 268–283.

Grob, C. (2007). The use of psilocybin in patients with advanced cancer and existential anxiety. In M. Winkelman & T. Roberts (Eds.), *Psychedelic medicine: New evidence for hallucinogenic substances as treatments* (Vol. 1, pp. 205–216). Westport, CT: Praeger Perspectives.

Grob, C., Danforth, A. L., Chopra, G. S., Hagerty, M., McKay, C. R., Halberstadt, A. L., et al. (2011). Pilot study of psilocybin treatment for anxiety in patients with advanced-stage cancer. *Archives of General Psychiatry, 68*, 71–78.

Grob, C., Bossos, A., & Griffiths, R. (2013). Use of the classic hallucinogen psilocybin for treatment of existential distress associated with cancer. In B. Carr & J. Steel (Eds.), *Psychological aspects of cancer: A guide to emotional and psychological consequences of cancer, their causes, and their management* (pp. 291–308). New York, NY: Springer.

Grof, S. (1975). *Realms of the human unconscious: Observations from LSD research*. New York, NY: Viking Press. Republished in 2009 as *LSD: Doorway to the numinous*. Rochester, VT: Park Street Press.

Grof, S. (2001). *LSD psychotherapy*. Sarasota, FL: Multidisciplinary Association for Psychedelic Studies.

Grof, S. (2009). *LSD: Doorway to the numinous*. Rochester, VT: Inner Traditions.

Halpern, J. (1996). The use of hallucinogens in the treatment of addiction. *Addiction Research, 4*(2), 177–189.

Halpern, J. H., Sherwood, A. R., Hudson, J. I., Yurgelun-Todd, D., & Pope, H. G., Jr. (2005). Psychological and cognitive effects of long-term peyote use among Native Americans. *Biological Psychiatry, 58*(8), 624–631.

Jilek, W. G. (1994). Traditional healing in the prevention and treatment of alcohol and drug abuse. *Transcultural Psychiatric Research Review, 31*, 219–258.

Joralemon, D., & Sharon, D. (1993). *Sorcery and shamanism curanderos and clients in northern Peru*. Salt Lake City, UT: University of Utah Press.

Krebs, T. S., & Johansen, P. Ø. (2012). Lysergic acid diethylamide (LSD) for alcoholism: Meta-analysis of randomized controlled trials. *Journal of Psychopharmacology, 26*(7), 994–1002.

Krupitsky, E., & Kolp, E. (2007). Ketamine psychedelic psychotherapy. In M. Winkelman & T. Robert (Eds.), *Psychedelic medicine: New evidence for hallucinogenic substances as treatments* (Vol. 2, pp. 67–86). Westport, CT: Praeger Perspectives.

Lukoff, D., Zanger, R., & Lu, F. (1990). Transpersonal psychology research review: Psychoactive substances and transpersonal states. *Journal of Transpersonal Psychology, 22*, 107–147.

Luna, L. E. (1986). *Vegetalismo: Shamanism among the Mestizo populations of the Peruvian Amazon*. University of Stockholm Studies in Comparative Religion 27. Stockholm, Sweden: Almqvist and Wiksell International.

Mabit, J. (2007). Ayahuasca in the treatment of addictions. In M. Winkelman & T. Robert (Eds.), *Psychedelic medicine: New evidence for hallucinogenic substances as treatments* (Vol. 2, pp. 87–105). Westport, CT: Praeger Perspectives.

McKenna, D. J., Luna, L. E., & Towers, G. N. (1995). Biodynamic constituents in ayahuasca admixture plants: An uninvestigated folk pharmacopeia. In R. E. Schultes & S. von Ries (Eds.), *Ethnobotany: Evolution of a discipline* (pp. 349–361). Portland: Dioscorides Press.

Mithoefer, M. C. et al. (2013). Durability of improvement in post-traumatic stress disorder symptoms and absence of harmful effects or drug dependency after 3,4-methylenedioxymethamphetamine-assisted psychotherapy: A prospective long-term follow-up study. *Journal of Psychopharmacology, 27*(1), 28–39.

Mithoefer, M. (2007). MDMA-assisted psychotherapy for the treatment of post-traumatic stress disorder. In M. Winkelman & T. Roberts (Eds.), *Psychedelic medicine: New evidence for hallucinogenic substances as treatments* (Vol. 1, pp. 155–176). Westport, CT: Praeger Perspectives.

Moreno, F. A., & Delgado, P. L. (2007). Psilocybin treatment of obsessive-compulsive disorder. In M. Winkelman & T. Roberts (Eds.), *Psychedelic medicine: New evidence for hallucinogenic substances as treatments* (Vol. 1, pp. 125–140). Westport, CT: Praeger Perspectives.

Nielson, J. L., & Megler, J. D. Ayahuasca as a candidate therapy for PTSD. In this volume.

Osório, F. L. et al. (2011). The therapeutic potential of harmine and ayahuasca in depression: Evidence from exploratory animal and human studies. In R.G. dos Santos (Ed.), *The ethnopharmacology of ayahuasca* (pp. 75–85). Kerala, India: Transworld Research Network.

Palhano-Fontes, F. P., Alchieri, J. C., Oliveira, J. P. M., Lobao Soares, B., Hallak, J. E. C., Galvao-Coelho, N., & de Araujo, D. B. The therapeutic potentials of ayahuasca in the treatment of depression. In this volume.

Passie, T. (2007). Contemporary psychedelic therapy: An overview. In M. Winkelman & T. Roberts (Eds.), *Psychedelic medicine: New evidence for hallucinogenic substances as treatments* (Vol. 1, pp. 45–68). Westport, CT: Praeger Perspectives.

Passie, T., Halpern, J., Stichtenoth, D., Emrish, H., & Hintzen, A. (2008). The pharmacology of Lysergic acid diethylamide: A review. *CNS Neuroscience & Therapeutics, 14*, 295–314.

Rätsch, C. (2005). *The encyclopedia of psychoactive plants: Ethnopharmacology and its applications* (J. Baker, Trans.). Rochester, VT: Park Street Press. (Originally published Enzyklopädie der psychoaktiven Pflanzen. Aarau, Switzerland: AT Verlag, 1998).

Roberts, T., & Winkelman, M. (2013). Psychedelic induced transpersonal experiences, therapies, and their implications for transpersonal psychology. In H. Freedman & G. Hartelius (Eds.), *The Wiley-Blackwell handbook of transpersonal psychology* (pp. 459–479). West Sussex, UK: John Wiley and Sons.

Ross, S. (2012). Serotonergic hallucinogens and emerging targets for addiction pharmacotherapies. *Psychiatric Clinics of North America, 35*(2), 357–374.

Samoylenkoa, V. et al. (2010). Banisteriopsis caapi, a unique combination of MAO inhibitory and antioxidative constituents for the activities relevant to neurodegenerative disorders and Parkinson's disease. *Journal of Ethnopharmacology 127,*(2), 357–367.

Schultes, R., Hofmann, A., & Rätsch, C. (1992). *Plants of the gods: Their sacred, healing and hallucinogenic powers*. Rochester, VT: Healing Arts Press.

Schultes, E., & Winkelman, M. (1996). The principal American hallucinogenic plants and their bioactive and therapeutic properties. In M. Winkelman & W. Andritzky (Eds.), *Yearbook of cross-cultural medicine and psychotherapy* (pp. 205–240). Berlin: Verland und Vertrieb.

Serrano-Dueñas, M., Cardozo-Pelaez, F., & Sánchez-Ramos, J. R. (2001). Effects of Banisteriopsis caapi extract on Parkinson's disease. *The Scientific Review of Alternative Medicine, 5*, 127–132.

Sewell, A., & Halpern, J.H. (2007). Response of cluster headaches to psilocybin and LSD. In M. Winkelman & T. Roberts (Eds.), *Psychedelic medicine: New evidence for hallucinogenic substances as treatments* (Vol. 1, pp. 97–124). Westport, CT: Praeger Perspectives.

Sharon, D. (1978). *Wizard of the four winds*. New York, NY: Macmillan Press.

Torres, C.M., & Repke, D. (2006). *Anadenanthera: Visionary plant of ancient South America*. New York, NY: Haworth Herbal Press.

Winkelman, M. (2001). Psychointegrators: Multidisciplinary perspectives on the therapeutic effects of hallucinogens. *Complementary Health Practice Review, 6*(3), 219–237.

Winkelman, M. (2005). Drug tourism of spiritual healing? Ayahuasca seekers in Amazonia. *Journal of Psychoactive Drugs, 37*(2), 209–218.

Winkelman, M. (2007). Therapeutic bases of psychedelic medicines: Psychointegrative effects. In M. Winkelman and T. Roberts (Eds.), *Psychedelic medicine: New evidence for hallucinogenic substances as treatments* (Vol. 1, pp. 1-20), Westport, CT: Praeger Perspectives.

Winkelman, M. (2009). Sacred medicines for harm reduction and substance abuse rehabilitation. In A. Browne-Miller (Ed.), *The Praeger international collection on addictions* (Vol. 3, pp. 377–401). Westport, CT: Praeger Perspectives.

Winkelman, M. (2010). *Shamanism: A biopsychosocial paradigm of consciousness and healing* (2nd ed.). Santa Barbara, CA.: ABC-Clio.

Winkelman, M., & Roberts, T. (Eds.). (2007a). *Psychedelic medicine: New evidence for hallucinogenic substances as treatments* (Vols. 1–2). Westport, CT: Praeger Perspectives.

Winkelman, M., & Roberts, T. (Eds.). (2007b). *Psychedelic medicine: New evidence for hallucinogenic substances as treatments* (Vols. 1–2). Westport, CT: Praeger Perspectives.

Winkelman, M., & Roberts, T. (2007c). Conclusions: Guidelines for implementing the use of psychedelic medicines. In M. Winkelman and T. Roberts (Eds.), *Psychedelic medicine: New evidence for hallucinogenic substances as treatments* (Vol. 1, pp. 271–298). Westport, CT: Praeger Perspectives.

Chapter 2
The Therapeutic Potentials of Ayahuasca in the Treatment of Depression

Fernanda Palhano-Fontes, Joao C. Alchieri, Joao Paulo M. Oliveira, Bruno Lobao Soares, Jaime E. C. Hallak, Nicole Galvao-Coelho and Draulio B. de Araujo

Abstract Major depressive disorder (MDD) is generally classified as a mood disorder with a profound effect on the individual's behavior and quality of life. According to the World Health Organization, in about 20 years, depression will be the disorder with the most significant repercussions, both socially and economically. Despite the substantial progress in the development of new antidepressants, their effectiveness remains low, with remission of about 50 % after a single regime of treatment. The most common form of pharmacological treatment of MDD is based

---

F. Palhano-Fontes · D. B. de Araujo (✉)
Brain Institute/Onofre Lopes University Hospital, Federal University of Rio Grande do Norte (UFRN), Av. Nascimento Castro, Natal, RN 2155, Brazil
e-mail: draulio@neuro.ufrn.br

F. Palhano-Fontes
e-mail: fernandapalhano@neuro.ufrn.br

J. C. Alchieri
Department of Psychology, Federal University of Rio Grande do Norte (UFRN), Natal, Brazil
e-mail: jcalchieri@gmail.com

J. P. M. Oliveira
Department of Internal Medicine, Federal University of Rio Grande do Norte (UFRN), Natal, Brazil
e-mail: j.p@usp.br

B. L. Soares
Department of Biophysics, Federal University of Rio Grande do Norte (UFRN), Natal, Brazil
e-mail: brunolobaosoares@gmail.com

J. E. C. Hallak
Department of Neuroscience and Behavior, University of Sao Paulo, Ribeirao Preto, Brazil
e-mail: jhallak@fmrp.usp.br

N. Galvao-Coelho
Department of Physiology, Federal University of Rio Grande do Norte (UFRN), Natal, Brazil
e-mail: galvaonic@hotmail.com

B. C. Labate and C. Cavnar (eds.), *The Therapeutic Use of Ayahuasca*,
DOI: 10.1007/978-3-642-40426-9_2,

on selective serotonin reuptake inhibitors (SSRIs), designed to increase extracellular levels of the neurotransmitter serotonin. Unfortunately, antidepressants currently available based on SSRIs may take several weeks to achieve the desired therapeutic effects. Therefore, massive effort has been devoted to find alternative treatments for MDD. For example, the use of ketamine, of ($\pm$)-1-(2,5-Dimethoxy-4-iodophenyl)-2-aminopropane (DOI), and β-carbolines is under current investigation. Based on evidence from the literature and a pilot study conducted by our group, we speculate about the possible therapeutic potential of ayahuasca for MDD. In part, such conjecture is based on the fact that ayahuasca combines N,N-dimethyltryptamine (DMT), acting particularly on serotonin neurotransmission through 5-HT_{2A} receptors and monoamine oxidase inhibitors (MAOI), both involved, at least indirectly, with pharmacological formulations intended for MDD treatment. In this chapter, we will review the major aspects of MDD such as diagnosis, current pharmacological treatments, and the motivations to use ayahuasca as a novel alternative.

Major Depressive Disorder: Causes and Diagnosis

Major depressive disorder (MDD) is generally classified as a mood disorder with a profound effect on the individual's behavior and quality of life. It has a prevalence of 17 % throughout life, being twice as common in women as it is in men and usually begins in the third decade of life. For most people, MDD presents itself in recurrent episodes. However, about 20–25 % of patients are chronically ill. According to the World Health Organization (WHO), MDD is the fourth leading cause of morbidity, and they predict that by 2020, it will be ranked second disease burden worldwide (Fava and Kendler 2000).

MDD is associated with intense personal suffering, high morbidity, and increased mortality (Ebmeier et al. 2006). The Diagnostic and Statistical Manual of Mental Disorders of the American Psychiatric Association (DSM-IV-TR) defines this condition based on the presence of depressed mood (irritable mood in children and adolescents) and/or loss of interest or pleasure (anhedonia) for at least 2 weeks, accompanied by at least four of the following symptoms: (a) considerable change in weight (5 % of body weight), (b) frequent insomnia or hypersomnia, (c) psychomotor agitation or retardation, (d) fatigue or loss of energy, (e) low self-esteem or inappropriate guilt, (f) diminished capacity to think, concentrate, or make decisions, (g) recurrent thoughts of death, suicidal ideation, or suicide attempts. In addition, the diagnosis requires that the symptoms cause significant distress and/or impairment in social, occupational, or other areas of life, and should not be directly caused by another general medical condition or psychoactive substance use and must not meet the criteria for mixed episode (in which the diagnostic criteria of depression and mania occur concurrently) (American Psychiatric Association [APA] 2000b).

Multiple theories attempt to explain the etiology of depression, but the most widely accepted one is the monoamine hypothesis. This theory suggests that MDD is a result of decreased brain levels of monoamines, such as dopamine, norepinephrine, and serotonin (Wong and Licinio 2001). Among these, serotonin has received the most attention. Besides the reduction of serotonin levels found in depression, studies also point to an altered expression of $5HT_{1A}$ autoreceptors and heteroreceptors. The most consistent finding is an increase in pre-synaptic $5HT_{1A}$ autoreceptors, which inhibit the release of serotonin, and consequently reduce serotonin levels in the synaptic cleft. A reduced number of postsynaptic $5HT_{1A}$ heteroreceptors in the hippocampus and prefrontal cortex, presumably induced by high cortisol levels also found in these patients, is also associated with MDD.

On the other hand, the monoamine hypothesis does not explain important matters such as the causes of the monoaminergic disturbance and the elevated refractoriness to the treatment of MDD with antidepressant drugs that target the increase of the monoamine levels in the synaptic cleft. In this scenario, several alternative hypotheses were brought to focus such as hypothalamic–pituitary–adrenal (HPA) axis dysfunctions and the inflammatory and neurodegenerative hypotheses.

One of the most common HPA abnormalities observed in depressed patients is an increase in reactivity of this axis. Scientific evidence indicates that MDD patients have impaired glucocorticoid receptor (GR) function, which results in reduced negative feedback in the HPA system, leading to chronically high levels of adrenocorticotrophic hormone-releasing factor (CRF), and increased cortisol in the plasma, urine, and cerebrospinal fluid (Zunszain et al. 2011).

Complementarily, the inflammatory theory is based on the strong mutual regulation and communication between the immune and HPA systems (Leuchter et al. 2010). Chronic activation of the HPA axis also provokes GR resistance in immune cells (Leonard 2007). Normally, basal cortisol induces the production of lymphocytes T CD4 Th2, but chronicle GR resistance leads to an imbalance in the immune system, displacing the production of these lymphocytes to a Th1 subtype, thus reducing the concentration of anti-inflammatory cytokines (IL-4, IL-10), and increasing the pro-inflammatory cytokines (IL-1, IL-6, TNF-a) (Leuchter et al. 2010; Li et al. 2011). In turn, the massive liberation of pro-inflammatory cytokines induces a decrease in GR function (Pace et al. 2007).

Taken together, a link between these three theories has been observed: The excess of circulating corticosteroids and pro-inflammatory cytokines increases activity of indoleamine 2,3-dioxygenase (IDO), an enzyme which induces formation of kynurenine in the tryptophan-kynurenine pathway, resulting in the deficiency of serotonin commonly observed in depression (Miura et al. 2008).

The neurodegenerative hypothesis is based on the fact that many depressed patients have reduced hippocampal volume (Bremner et al. 2000). Studies suggest that such reduction does not come only as a consequence of neuronal death (Sapolsky 2004). Instead, it can be a result of a reduction in neurogenesis induced by high glucocorticoid, pro-inflammatory cytokine levels and reduced serotonin availability, which in turn can inhibit the production of cell growth factors such as brain derived neurotropic factor (BDNF) (Shimizu et al. 2003). Animals models of depression (Berry et al. 2012) have shown that social deprivation in mice leads to increased depressive-like behaviors, elevated corticosterone levels, and reduced BDNF levels (Zhou et al. 2008).

Despite the dysregulation of the inflammatory proteins, stress hormones, and brain factors associated with depression, one of the main challenges regarding MDD diagnosis is the absence of a specific biomarker related to this disease. The use of biomarkers has an important role in understanding and monitoring conventional and alternative treatments (Leuchter et al. 2010). The current consensus is that no biomarker alone is sufficient to predict and identify individuals at risk, make the diagnosis, or direct clinical treatment decisions concerning depression. Accordingly, the construction of a multimodal panel of biomarkers is recommended to obtain the accuracy required in clinical practice or research protocols (Lakhan et al. 2010). For MDD, there are several candidates for identifying biomarkers, including neuropsychological assessment, electroencephalography (EEG), polysomnography (PSG), biochemical markers, medical imaging, genomics, proteomics, and metabolomics, among others.

Biochemical Markers

Information on biochemical markers is accessed indirectly by measurements of the cerebrospinal fluid (CSF), saliva, or blood. In this scenario, CSF may be considered the source that best reflects brain activity. However, it is not easily accessible on a risk-free basis. On the other hand, although urine and feces are easily collected, it is difficult to associate levels of metabolites present in these two vehicles with the ones found in the brain. Saliva has also been used with success for the measurement of steroid hormones, such as cortisol (Dziurkowska et al. 2013). However, this is generally not considered a reliable strategy for use with depressed patients (Knorr et al. 2010). Therefore, biochemical markers have been sought in the blood, both for its easy accessibility and for the fact that many molecules found in the brain are excreted via the route of blood circulation.

Curiously, plasmatic factors which target the serotoninergic system are not considered good biomarkers for chronic depression (Pivac et al. 2002). On the other hand, high concentration of cortisol in the plasma has frequently been read as a biomarker indicative of depression, in agreement with the hypercortisolemia theory (Leonard 2007; Tadić et al. 2011). Moreover, plasmatic pro-inflammatory cytokine levels, which are reported to be increased in MDD, are also considered reliable biomarkers, in accordance with inflammatory theory (Li et al. 2011).

Polysomnographic Markers

Sleep abnormalities are consistently revealed in EEG findings in patients suffering from MDD. Although there is no single marker of sleep specifically associated with depression, many studies have found differences in sleep between MDD patients and healthy control subjects. The use of polysomnography (PSG) in these patients has revealed impaired sleep continuity, reduced latency to REM sleep (interval between sleep onset and the occurrence of the first REM period), increased amount of REM sleep, longer first REM period, increased REM density (number of eye movements during REM), and reduced slow-wave sleep (Benca et al. 1992; Riemann et al. 2001; Tsuno et al. 2005).

The reduction in the latency to REM sleep associated with depression has been observed since the 1970s. Several studies have reported that this change is related to the secretion of cortisol at night, suggesting that dysregulation of mood, sleep, and HPA may be interconnected (Poland et al. 1992). An inverse relationship is observed between cortisol level and the latency shortening: Subjects showing the shortest REM latency also have the greatest degree of HPA activity (Asnis et al. 1983). Asnis and colleagues speculate that the association between REM latency and the HPA axis is caused by a dysregulation of the muscarinic cholinergic system, which exerts a role in both physiologic systems (Asnis et al. 1983).

In addition, it has been proposed that the decreased latency to REM sleep associated with depression may be a familiar trait (Giles et al. 1987). Giles and her co-researchers investigated risk factors in patients with a lifetime history of depression. They reported that the relative risk for MDD in relatives with reduced REM latency was almost three times greater than for relatives with non-reduced REM latency (Giles et al. 1988). They also found shortened REM latency, even in psychiatrically asymptomatic first-degree relatives of depressed probands (Giles et al. 1989). Other investigators reported sleep disorders (Lauer et al. 1995) and dysregulation of the HPA axis (Mannie et al. 2007) in otherwise healthy adults, but whose first-degree relatives had a history of depressive disorder.

Furthermore, the connection between REM sleep and depression has been demonstrated by the fact that acute sleep deprivation (total, partial, or specifically REM sleep) alleviates depressive symptoms (Benca et al. 1992; Riemann et al. 2001). Pharmacological treatment also influences REM sleep. It has been shown that antidepressants decrease the amount of REM sleep. In addition, such changes in the initial stages of antidepressant treatment are a predictor of treatment outcome (Riemann et al. 2001).

Magnetic Resonance Imaging Markers

The use of magnetic resonance imaging has helped to identify the psychopathological mechanisms underlying MDD. Recent studies show that depressed patients present neuroanatomical and functional alterations when compared to healthy controls. One of the most consistent results is the reduction of hippocampal volume in MDD (Bremner et al. 2000; Lorenzetti et al. 2009; MacQueen 2009). Another common finding is the volume reduction in some of the basal ganglia structures, such as the caudate and putamen (Lorenzetti et al. 2009). Although the results are not always convergent, such morphological changes are an indication that structural images can provide information relevant to the characterization of depression.

In addition to brain anatomy changes, some studies used functional neuroimaging techniques to evaluate the brain function of MDD patients. The amygdala, a medial temporal lobe structure that is highly sensitive to emotional stimuli, has been repeatedly implicated in depression symptoms. Studies using functional magnetic resonance imaging (fMRI) showed hyperactivity of the amygdala of depressed patients (Davey et al. 2011; Sheline et al. 2001).

Moreover, the ventromedial prefrontal cortex, the anterior cingulate cortex, and the inferior parietal cortex have been the subject of many studies on depression. These regions constitute a network known as the Default Mode Network (DMN), which is characterized by greater activity during rest than during the execution of a goal-specific task (Raichle et al. 2001). The DMN has been implicated in processes involving self-judgments, recall of autobiographical memories, mental simulations, mind-wandering, and daydreaming (Buckner et al. 2008; Northoff et al. 2006). Using an emotional regulation task, Sheline and colleagues examined the functionality of the DMN in patients with MDD, investigating whether the ability to regulate its activity, and therefore the self-referential processing, was impaired. The results showed that the individuals with depression failed to modulate different regions of the DMN, including the anterior cingulate cortex, lateral parietal cortex, the medial prefrontal cortex, and the lateral temporal cortex. Furthermore, some studies showed alterations in the functional connectivity patterns of the DMN. For instance, Greicius et al. (2007) reported a significant increase in functional connectivity in the subgenual cingulate cortex and precuneus in depressed patients when compared with healthy controls. These results are consistent with clinical symptoms, such as rumination, in which MDD patients are impulsively focused on the past and/or future negative consequences, rather than reflecting on the present moment (Devilbiss et al. 2012).

Abnormalities in functional connectivity of other networks were also found in depressive patients (Anand et al. 2005; Sheline et al. 2010; Veer et al. 2010). For example, Veer and colleagues showed that there is: (1) a decrease in connectivity between the amygdala and the left anterior insula, structures related to affection; (2) reduction in the connectivity of the left frontal pole, a network associated with attention and working memory; and (3) a decrease in bilateral connectivity of lingual gyrus and ventromedial visual areas (Veer et al. 2010). The connectivity has also been related to the response to antidepressant treatment. A study by Anand et al. (2005), evaluated the effect of sertraline, a commonly used antidepressant, in cortico-limbic connectivity. After treatment, patients showed increased connectivity between the anterior cingulate cortex and the limbic regions, a circuit that has been linked to emotional regulation.

Pharmacological Treatments

Several alternatives are available for treatment of MDD. The most common ones are the use of antidepressant medications (Uppal et al. 2010), psychotherapy (Cuijpers et al. 2011), electroconvulsive therapy (Andrade et al. 2010), and other somatic therapies (Segal et al. 2010). The goal of treatment is the remission of the depressive episodes, defined by the DSM-IV as the absence of MDD symptoms for at least 2 months (Kennedy et al. 2001). A treatment response is considered when depressive symptoms are reduced by 50 % or more, usually evaluated by the Hamilton Scale (HAM-D), and not necessarily mean remission (Ebmeier et al. 2006).

In general, pharmacological treatment has a number of phases. The first, known as acute, lasts about 8 weeks, and is essential to evaluate the patient's response to the treatment (Bolland and Keller 2004). If this first step is successful, there is another period that lasts 16–20 weeks and aims to prevent possible recurrence of depressive episodes (Kennedy et al. 2001). Some cases go through the maintenance phase indefinitely, for example, individuals at high risk of recurrence, such as those who have had multiple episodes or partial response to treatment, and patients who have episodes of high severity with psychotic symptoms and suicidal risk (APA 2000a).

The discovery of antidepressants in the 1950s drastically transformed the treatment of depression, and they remain the leading strategy (Ebmeier et al. 2006). Several classes of antidepressants are available, classified according to their chemical structure, effect on the synapses, and action on reuptake and metabolism of neurotransmitters.

The first generation of antidepressants can be divided into tricyclics (TCA) and monoamine oxidase inhibitors (MAOI). Both act by increasing extracellular levels of monoamines; TCA by inhibiting the reuptake of dopamine, noradrenaline, and serotonin, and MAOI by preventing the action of MAO, thereby avoiding the degradation of monoamine neurotransmitters (Bolland and Keller 2004).

In addition to the therapeutic action, TCA acts on several other receptors, leading to antimuscarinic, antihistaminic, and anti-$\alpha 2$ adrenergic effects that lead to undesirable outcomes such as urinary retention, constipation, orthostatic hypotension, weight gain, and somnolence. Furthermore, TCA block sodium channels interfering with nerve conduction, becoming potentially arrhythmogenic. Although recently questioned, it is classically believed that the main side effect of MAOI is the high risk of hypertensive crisis triggered by its combined ingestion with foods containing tyramine, a sympathomimetic amine, which is metabolized by MAO (Grady and Stahl 2012).

Given the low selectivity of classic antidepressants, newer antidepressants were developed. Among these are the selective serotonin reuptake inhibitors: SSRIs (fluoxetine, paroxetine, etc.), selective noradrenaline reuptake inhibitors (reboxetine), and serotonin and norepinephrine reuptake inhibitors (venlafaxine, duloxetine, and desvenlafaxine). Moreover, there are antidepressants with multiple action mechanisms, such as mirtazapine, which acts as a noradrenergic pre-synaptic $\alpha 2$-receptor antagonist and serotonin ($5HT_2$ and $5HT_3$) antagonist, and nefazodone which act by inhibiting the reuptake of serotonin and norepinephrine, and as a 5HT and $\alpha 2$ antagonist (Cipriani et al. 2009).

The newer antidepressants, such as SSRIs, have essentially the same mechanism of action as the first generation, i.e., they increase the level of monoamines in the brain (Zarate 2011; Zarate et al. 2006). However, this new generation offers more safety. Side effects, although milder, are still present, and are specific to different classes of medications. For example, sexual dysfunction and gastrointestinal disorders are common with the use of SSRIs, and sleepiness and weight gain are associated with the use of mirtazapine (Cipriani et al. 2009). Given that the effectiveness of the various antidepressants is similar, the choice of medication is made based on side effects, safety, tolerability, patient's individual preferences, quantity and quality of clinical trial data, and cost (APA 2000a).

With respect to the modulation on the HPA axis made by different antidepressants, evidence indicates that it depends on the type of antidepressant and length of treatment. Increased adrenocorticotropic hormone (ACTH) and cortisol levels have been reported 5 hours after a single oral administration of reboxetine, and a decrease of these hormones after a single oral administration of mirtazapine in both healthy individuals and in subjects with depression (Schüle 2006). Moreover, a gradual and significant reduction of HPA activity has been found after 5 weeks of treatment with reboxetine in depressed patients (Schüle et al. 2006). On the other hand, treatment with mirtazapine only reduces HPA activity during the first week; after that, HPA activity increases again (Pariante et al. 2004).

Despite substantial progress in the development of new drugs, less than 50 % of patients achieve remission as a result of antidepressant use, even after four different pharmacological treatment regimes (Warden et al. 2007). Besides low effectiveness, the pharmacological treatments that are currently available carry another limitation associated with the chronology of the drug action: It takes several weeks to reach the desired therapeutic effects (Zarate 2011; Zarate et al. 2006). Thus, enormous effort has been devoted to the search for alternative pharmacological treatments that could improve treatment efficiency and accelerate the onset of therapeutic effects (Uppal et al. 2010). For instance, studies conducted with ketamine, an NMDA antagonist, showed antidepressant effects after a single intravenous injection, which persisted significantly after 1 week (Liebrenz et al. 2007). Furthermore, the use of (±)-1-(2,5-Dimethoxy-4-iodophenyl)-2-aminopropane (DOI), a powerful $5HT_{2A/2C}$ agonist, resulted in positive responses in two models of anxiety in mice (Dhonnchadha et al. 2003). In another study, mice subjected to the forced swimming test, a common paradigm used to study depression in rodents, exhibited decreased immobility time 6 h after receiving DOI, an effect that is considered predictive of antidepressant response (Masuda and Sugiyama 2000).

Another serotonergic agonist, N,N-dimethyltryptamine (DMT), has also been considered a potential antidepressant. Some hypotheses have emerged that, at low doses, the anxiolytic mechanism associated with DMT would be mediated by a trace amine receptor, which could be one of the sites of action of endogenous DMT (Jacob and Presti 2005).

Anxiolytic and antidepressant effects are also related to β-carbolines. In a recent study, the use of harmane, norharmane, and harmine in an animal model was capable of reducing the time of immobility in the forced swimming test (Farzin and Mansouri 2005). Similar effects were observed in animal models using the elevated plus maze test, a common paradigm for the study of anxiety in rodents (Aricioglu and Altunbas 2003). It has recently been found that the use of harmine alone in rodent models leads to the reduction of various signs and symptoms associated with depression, such as anhedonia, and regulation to normal levels of ACTH and hippocampal BDNF (Fortunato et al. 2010).

Based on the evidence presented here, and in a pilot study conducted by our group, described below, the question arose regarding the use of substances that combine DMT and MAOI, as is the case of ayahuasca, in MDD treatment. There are several anecdotal reports that the ritual use of ayahuasca is associated with the relief of depression symptoms.

Ayahuasca tea is traditionally prepared by decoction of the bark and stem of the *Banisteriopsis caapi* vine with leaves of the *Psychotria viridis* bush. The *B. caapi* contains the alkaloids harmine, tetrahydroharmine (THH), and harmaline; the three belonging to the β-carbolines group, and corresponding to 0.05–1.95 % of the dry weight of the plant. In addition, *P. viridis* provides the hallucinogenic tryptamine DMT, which corresponds to 0.1–0.66 % of the dry weight of the plant (McKenna et al. 1984; Riba et al. 2003).

Ayahuasca's activity is dependent on the synergistic interaction between these components. β-carbolines are potent reversible and competitive MAOI (Mckenna et al. 1984) and can increase serotonin levels, blocking its deamination. Their main action in ayahuasca is apparently to protect DMT from peripheral degradation, preventing oxidative deamination of the orally ingested DMT and enabling it to reach the central nervous system (McKenna 2004). The pharmacological effects of DMT also depend on its interaction with the serotoninergic system. DMT is the substrate for both cell-surface serotonin uptake transporters (SERTs) and neuronal vesicle monoamine transporters (VMAT2). Unlike drugs that are uptake inhibitors, DMT is transported into the cytosol or vesicle by SERT or VMAT2, respectively (Cozzi et al. 2009). Therefore, high intracellular and vesicular concentrations of DMT may be achieved inside of neurons, and can interact with intracellular sigma-1 receptors located in the mitochondria-associated endoplasmic reticulum membrane (Su et al. 2009). Hence, the DMT can be released into the synaptic cleft upon vesicular fusion to interact with cell-surface sigma-1 receptors or serotonin post-synaptic receptors (Cozzi et al. 2009).

The effects of ayahuasca are heterogeneous (Riba et al. 2001), and encompass sensory, cognitive, and affective changes (Prado et al. 2009), rich visual experiences (de Araujo et al. 2011), and entheogenic experiences (Shanon 2003). These effects begin between 35 and 40 min after tea ingestion, reaching their height between 90 and 120 min, and lasting for 4 h (Riba et al. 2003). Thus far, all studies to date have demonstrated the safety of ayahuasca, with reports of individuals who have used it for more than 30 years without evidence of harm to health (Callaway et al. 1999; Grob et al. 1996; Riba et al. 2001; Riba et al. 2003). Changes in both blood pressure—systolic, diastolic, and mean—and heart rate are not significant (Riba et al. 2003). Furthermore, a recent study showed that the ritual use of the tea is not associated with the psychosocial problems that are usually found with other drugs (Fábregas et al. 2010).

Preliminary evidence of its potential use as an antidepressant is encouraging. A double blind, placebo controlled experiment indicated that the use of ayahuasca significantly reduces the scores of behavioral scales of panic and hopelessness in participants who were under the influence of the tea compared to a control group (Santos et al. 2007).

Ayahuasca and MDD Biomarkers

In addition to the pharmacological evidence described previously, other evidence might also support the use of ayahuasca as an antidepressant. Recent studies have indicated that regular ayahuasca use is involved in long-term modulation of the serotonin systems in the brain, specifically in SERTs levels. Such modulation can increase the serotoninergic system's function, which might be a mechanism for its possible positive effect in depressed patients. Ayahuasca also has significant effects on the endocrine system, mainly in the HPA axis, and the immune system. Studies have found increases in prolactin and cortisol levels approximately 2 hours after a single ayahuasca dose. This increase of cortisol has an impact on cell immunity and reduces CD3 and CD4 lymphocytes after ayahuasca use (Dos Santos et al. 2011). Another study used two sequential doses of ayahuasca with an interval of 4 hours and found endocrine and immunomodulatory effects analogous to those previously reported (Dos Santos et al. 2012). In line with this evidence, rapid increase in cortisol levels was observed in a single acute treatment with antidepressants like reboxetine that act on the serotoninergic system (Schüle 2006).

Barbanoj and colleagues investigated the effect of ayahuasca on sleep. They evaluated sleep quality, polysomnography, and spectral analysis in 22 healthy volunteers following a unique ayahuasca dose administration during the day. Results indicated that ayahuasca had no significant effects on sleep initiation or continuity as assessed by subjective and objective measures. Furthermore, it was found that the tea inhibits REM sleep, decreasing its duration in absolute values and in percentage of REM sleep. A trend increase in REM latency was also reported (Barbanoj et al. 2008). Based on these results, one can further speculate that ayahuasca might have therapeutic potential, as evidence from the literature points out that PSG changes in depression (increased amount of REM sleep and reduction in REM latency) go in the opposite direction from the changes induced by ayahuasca (Benca et al. 1992; Riemann et al. 2001; Tsuno et al. 2005).

There is also fMRI evidence of the potential antidepressant effects of ayahuasca. In a study conducted by our group, which aimed at evaluating the changes induced by ayahuasca in the DMN, 10 healthy subjects submitted to two fMRI sessions: one before and one right after tea intake. It was observed that ayahuasca caused a reduction in the fMRI signal of central nodes of the DMN, such as the anterior cingulate cortex, the medial prefrontal cortex, the posterior cingulate cortex, the precuneus, and the inferior parietal lobe. Moreover, changes in connectivity patterns of the DMN were observed (Fig. 2.1), especially a decrease in

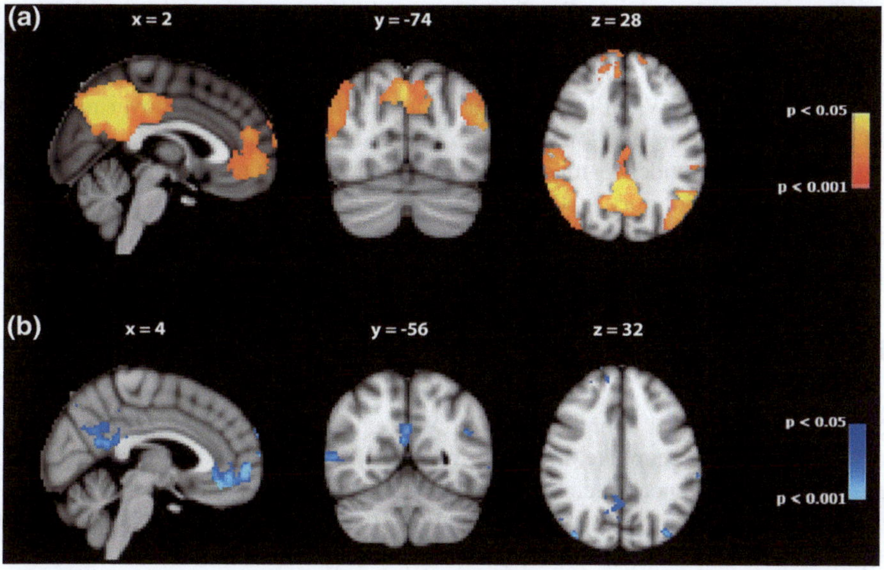

Fig. 2.1 Ayahuasca effects on the DMN. **a** An fMRI image showing the set of regions that comprise the DMN. **b** Regions where ayahuasca caused a BOLD signal reduction. Statistical maps were obtained comparing the groups before and after ayahuasca intake ($p < 0.05$ uncorrected)

the functional connectivity of the precuneus (Fontes et al. 2012). However, some studies show an opposite modulation in patients with depression, i.e., increased DMN activity and functional connectivity (Greicius et al. 2007; Sheline et al. 2009).

Our group has been conducting an exploratory study of the feasibility of the use of ayahuasca as an antidepressant. The ethics committee of the Clinical Hospital of Ribeirao Preto approved this study (No. 2484/2008). Preliminary evaluations were conducted in three female subjects with a clinical diagnosis of recurrent depressive disorder and current mild to severe depressive episodes without psychotic symptoms. The subjects were in the washout period between medication changes, and had been without antidepressant medication for 2 weeks.

Patients received a single oral dose of 2 ml/Kg of ayahuasca tea and were assessed using psychiatric scales, including the HAM-D, 10 min before administration of tea, and 40, 80, 140, and 180 min after ingestion, and on days 1, 2, 7, 14, and 28 after the experimental session. Results showed a significant decrease of HAM-D scores over time, beginning at 40 min after intake and lasting for 14 days (de Lima Osório et al. 2011).

It is interesting to notice that the improvement observed in HAM-D scale can also be further corroborated by the patient's testimonials. One patient stated: "I stayed huddled and crying softly, I was completely huddled and I could not answer because I felt as if the devil and Our Lady were battling for my soul and I could not interfere. After a long battle Our Lady won and pulled me to her side and I felt an intense joy." Another said: "I felt as if I was trying to hold a ball of blue energy. I did not succeed because it was like my hands were different poles of a magnet, moving them apart. When I finally got to hold it, the energy came over me and it all made sense. From then on, I was no longer feeling depressed."

Although this evidence must be considered with caution due to the inherent limitations of exploratory studies, the results suggest that ayahuasca has antidepressant properties presenting an interesting acute effect.

Final Remarks

New pharmacological approaches to MDD treatment have expanded beyond the model of serotonin reuptake, including the use of ketamine as well as the potential use of novel substances such as ayahuasca. Different aspects related to the identification of biomarkers and theories about the psychophysiological action of ayahuasca were characterized and presented as part of the *zeitgeist* of depression. Although the evidence presented herein was supported by international studies, more research is necessary to support the pharmacological use of ayahuasca and of similar DMT/MAOI combinations in the treatment of MDD. Based on that evidence, and on studies conducted by our group, it is possible to glimpse promising pharmacological implications for the use of ayahuasca in treating depression.

There is an interesting aspect to consider about the use of ayahuasca in depression: A closer look at our preliminary results reveals that the depressive signs and symptoms are reduced after a single ayahuasca intake, and that the effects last for about 14 days. Curiously, in the context of the Brazilian ayahuasca religions, the interval between sessions is exactly 2 weeks. One must also consider the number of anecdotal reports from experienced ayahuasca drinkers, and also from naïve ayahuasca drinkers, supporting the notion that ayahuasca has antidepressant potentials. From a broader reflection on how knowledge is transformed, the discovery of ayahuasca's antidepressant effects might be considered a thought-provoking example of a successful dialog between science and cultural tradition.

References

American Psychiatric Association. (2000a). *American Psychiatric Association practice guidelines for the treatment of psychiatric disorders: Compendium 2000*. Washington, DC: Author.

American Psychiatric Association. (2000b). *Diagnostic criteria from DSM-IV-TR*. Arlington, VA: Author.

Anand, A., Li, Y., Wang, Y., Wu, J., Gao, S., Bukhari, L., Mathews, V. P., et al. (2005). Antidepressant effect on connectivity of the mood-regulating circuit: An FMRI study. *Neuropsychopharmacology, 30*(7), 1334–1344. doi:1300725 [pii] 10.1038/sj.npp.1300725.

Andrade, P., Noblesse, L. H., Temel, Y., Ackermans, L., Lim, L. W., Steinbusch, H. W., et al. (2010). Neurostimulatory and ablative treatment options in major depressive disorder: A systematic review. *Acta Neurochir (Wien), 152*(4), 565–577. doi:10.1007/s00701-009-0589-6.

Aricioglu, F., & Altunbas, H. (2003). Harmane induces anxiolysis and antidepressant-like effects in rats. *Annals of the New York Academy of Sciences, 1009*, 196–201.

Asnis, G. M., Halbreich, U., Sachar, E. J., Nathan, R. S., Ostrow, L. C., Novacenko, H., et al. (1983). Plasma cortisol secretion and REM period latency in adult endogenous depression. *American Journal of Psychiatry, 140*(6), 750–753.

Barbanoj, M. J., Riba, J., Clos, S., Gimenez, S., Grasa, E., & Romero, S. (2008). Daytime ayahuasca administration modulates REM and slow-wave sleep in healthy volunteers. *Psychopharmacology, 196*(2), 315–326. doi:10.1007/S00213-007-0963-0.

Benca, R. M., Obermeyer, W. H., Thisted, R. A., & Gillin, J. C. (1992). Sleep and psychiatric disorders: A meta-analysis. *Archives of General Psychiatry, 49*(8), 651–668 (discussion 669–670).

Berry, A., Bellisario, V., Capoccia, S., Tirassa, P., Calza, A., Alleva, E., et al. (2012). Social deprivation stress is a triggering factor for the emergence of anxiety-and depression-like behaviours and leads to reduced brain BDNF levels in C57BL/6 J mice. *Psychoneuroendocrinology, 37*(6), 762–772.

Boland, R. J., & Keller, M. B. (2004). Antidepressants. In A. F. Schatzberg & C. B. Nemeroff (Eds.), *Textbook of Psychopharmacology* (3rd ed., pp. 847–864). Washington, DC: American Psychiatric Press.

Bremner, J. D., Narayan, M., Anderson, E. R., Staib, L. H., Miller, H. L., & Charney, D. S. (2000). Hippocampal volume reduction in major depression. *American Journal of Psychiatry, 157*(1), 115–117.

Buckner, R. L., Andrews-Hanna, J. R., & Schacter, D. L. (2008). The brain's default network: Anatomy, function, and relevance to disease. *Annals of the New York Academy of Sciences, 1124*, 1–38. doi:1124/1/1 [pii] 10.1196/annals.1440.011.

Callaway, J. C., McKenna, D. J., Grob, C. S., Brito, G. S., Raymon, L. P., Poland, R. E., et al. (1999). Pharmacokinetics of Hoasca alkaloids in healthy humans. *Journal of Ethnopharmacology, 65*(3), 243–256.

Cipriani, A., Furukawa, T. A., Salanti, G., Geddes, J. R., Higgins, J. P. T., Churchill, R., et al. (2009). Comparative efficacy and acceptability of 12 new-generation antidepressants: A multiple-treatments meta-analysis. *Lancet, 373*(9665), 746–758. doi:10.1016/s0140-6736(09)60046-5.

Cozzi, N. V., Gopalakrishnan, A., Anderson, L. L., Feih, J. T., Shulgin, A. T., Daley, P. F., et al. (2009). Dimethyltryptamine and other hallucinogenic tryptamines exhibit substrate behavior at the serotonin uptake transporter and the vesicle monoamine transporter. *Journal of Neural Transmission, 116*(12), 1591–1599.

Cuijpers, P., Geraedts, A. S., van Oppen, P., Andersson, G., Markowitz, J. C., & van Straten, A. (2011). Interpersonal psychotherapy for depression: A meta-analysis. *American Journal of Psychiatry, 168*(6), 581–592. doi:appi.ajp.2010.10101411 [pii] 10.1176/appi.ajp.2010.10101411.

Davey, C. G., Allen, N. B., Harrison, B. J., & Yucel, M. (2011). Increased amygdala response to positive social feedback in young people with major depressive disorder. *Biological Psychiatry, 69*(8), 734–741. doi:S0006–3223(10)01275–8 [pii] 10.1016/j.biopsych.2010.12.004.

de Araujo, D. B., Ribeiro, S., Cecchi, G. A., Carvalho, F. M., Sanchez, T. A., Pinto, J. P., et al. (2011). Seeing with the eyes shut: Neural basis of enhanced imagery following ayahuasca ingestion. *Human Brain Mapping, 33*(11), 2550–2560. doi:10.1002/hbm.21381.

de Lima Osório, F., de Macedo, L. R. H., de Sousa, J. P. M., Pinto, J. P., Quevedo, J., de Souza Crippa, J. A., et al. (2011). The therapeutic potential of harmine and ayahuasca in depression: Evidence from exploratory animal and human studies. In R. E. Dos Santos (Ed.), *The ethnopharmacology of ayahuasca* (pp. 75–85). Trivandrum, India: Transworld Research Network.

Devilbiss, D. M., Jenison, R. L., & Berridge, C. W. (2012). Stress-induced impairment of a working memory task: Role of spiking rate and spiking history predicted discharge. *PLoS Computational Biology, 8*(9), e1002681.

Dhonnchadha, B., Bourin, M., & Hascoet, M. (2003). Anxiolytic-like effects of 5-HT2 ligands on three mouse models of anxiety. *Behavioural Brain Research, 140*(1–2), 203–214. doi:PII S0166–4328(02)00311-X.

Dos Santos, R. G., Grasa, E., Valle, M., Ballester, M. R., Bouso, J. C., Nomdedéu, J. F., et al. (2012). Pharmacology of ayahuasca administered in two repeated doses. *Psychopharmacology (Berl), 219*(4), 1039–1053. doi: 10.1007/s00213-011-2434-x.

Dos Santos, R. G., Valle, M., Bouso, J. C., Nomdedéu, J. F., Rodríguez-Espinosa, J., McIlhenny, E. H., et al. (2011). Autonomic, neuroendocrine, and immunological effects of ayahuasca: A comparative study with d-amphetamine. *Journal of Clinical Psychopharmacology, 31*(6), 717–726. doi:10.1097/JCP.0b013e31823607f6.

Dziurkowska, E., Wesolowski, M., & Dziurkowski, M. (2013). Salivary cortisol in women with major depressive disorder under selective serotonin reuptake inhibitors therapy. *Archives of Women's Mental Health, 16*(2), 139–147. doi:10.1007/s00737-013-0329-z.

Ebmeier, K., Donaghey, C., & Steele, J. (2006). Recent developments and current controversies in depression. *Lancet, 367*(9505), 153–167.

Farzin, D., & Mansouri, M. (2005). Anti-immobility effects of beta-carbolines in the mouse forced-swim test. *Behavioural Pharmacology, 16*, S41–S42.

Fava, M., & Kendler, K. (2000). Major depressive disorder. *Neuron, 28*(2), 335–341.

Fontes, F. P., Ribeiro, S. T. G., Pinto, J. P., Hallak, J. E. C., Crippa, J. A. S., & De Araujo, D. B. (2012). *Default Mode Network changes induced by ayahuasca*. New Orleans, LA: Paper presented at the Society for Neuroscience Annual Meeting.

Fortunato, J. J., Réus, G. Z., Kirsch, T. R., Stringari, R. B., Fries, G. R., Kapczinski, F., et al. (2010). Effects of beta-carboline harmine on behavioral and physiological parameters observed in the chronic mild stress model: Further evidence of antidepressant properties. *Brain Research Bulletin, 81*(4–5), 491–496. doi:S0361–9230(09)00304–9 [pii] 10.1016/j.brainresbull.2009.09.008.

Fábregas, J. M., González, D., Fondevila, S., Cutchet, M., Fernández, X., Barbosa, P. C. R., et al. (2010). Assessment of addiction severity among ritual users of ayahuasca. *Drug and Alcohol Dependence, 111*(3), 257–261.

Giles, D. E., Biggs, M. M., Rush, A. J., & Roffwarg, H. P. (1988). Risk factors in families of unipolar depression. I. Psychiatric illness and reduced REM latency. *Journal of Affective Disorders, 14*(1), 51–59.

Giles, D. E., Kupfer, D. J., Roffwarg, H. P., Rush, A. J., Biggs, M. M., & Etzel, B. A. (1989). Polysomnographic parameters in first-degree relatives of unipolar probands. *Psychiatry Research, 27*(2), 127–136.

Giles, D. E., Roffwarg, H. P., & Rush, A. J. (1987). REM latency concordance in depressed family members. *Biological Psychiatry, 22*(7), 910–914. doi:0006–3223(87)90090–4 [pii].

Grady, M. M., & Stahl, S. M. (2012). Practical guide for prescribing MAOIs: Debunking myths and removing barriers. *CNS Spectrums, 17*(1), 2–10. doi:10.1017/S109285291200003X.

Greicius, M. D., Flores, B. H., Menon, V., Glover, G. H., Solvason, H. B., Kenna, H., et al. (2007). Resting-state functional connectivity in major depression: Abnormally increased contributions from subgenual cingulate cortex and thalamus. *Biological Psychiatry, 62*(5), 429–437. doi:10.1016/j.biopsych.2006.09.020.

Grob, C., McKenna, D., Callaway, J., Brito, G., Neves, E., Oberlaender, G., et al. (1996). Human psychopharmacology of hoasca, a plant hallucinogen used in ritual context in Brazil. *Journal of Nervous and Mental Disease, 184*(2), 86–94.

Jacob, M., & Presti, D. (2005). Endogenous psychoactive tryptamines reconsidered: An anxiolytic role for dimethyltryptamine. *Medical Hypotheses, 64*(5), 930–937. doi:10.1016/j.mehy.2004.11.005.

Kennedy, S., Lam, R., Cohen, N., Ravindran, A., & CANMAT Depression Workgroup (2001). Clinical guidelines for the treatment of depressive disorders IV. Medications and other biological treatments. *Canadian Journal of Psychiatry, 46,*(Suppl. 1), 38S–58S.

Knorr, U., Vinberg, M., Kessing, L. V., & Wetterslev, J. (2010). Salivary cortisol in depressed patients versus control persons: A systematic review and meta-analysis. *Psychoneuroendocrinology, 35*(9), 1275–1286. doi:10.1016/j.psyneuen.2010.04.001.

Lakhan, S. E., Vieira, K., & Hamlat, E. (2010). Biomarkers in psychiatry: Drawbacks and potential for misuse. *International Archives of Medicine, 3*(1). doi:10.1186/1755-7682-3-1.

Lauer, C. J., Schreiber, W., Holsboer, F., & Krieg, J. C. (1995). In quest of identifying vulnerability markers for psychiatric disorders by all-night polysomnography. *Archives of General Psychiatry, 52*(2), 145–153.

Leonard, B. E. (2007). Inflammation, depression, and dementia: Are they connected? *Neurochemical Research, 32*(10), 1749–1756. doi:10.1007/s11064-007-9385-y.

Leuchter, A. F., Cook, I. A., Hamilton, S. P., Narr, K. L., Toga, A., Hunter, A. M., et al. (2010). Biomarkers to predict antidepressant response. *Current Psychiatry Reports, 12*(6), 553–562. doi:10.1007/s11920-010-0160-4.

Li, M., Soczynska, J. K., & Kennedy, S. H. (2011). Inflammatory biomarkers in depression: An opportunity for novel therapeutic interventions. *Curr Psychiatry Rep, 13*(5), 316–320. doi:10.1007/s11920-011-0210-6.

Liebrenz, M., Borgeat, A., Leisinger, R., & Stohler, R. (2007). Intravenous ketamine therapy in a patient with a treatment-resistant major depression. *Swiss Medical Weekly, 137*(15–16), 234–236.

Lorenzetti, V., Allen, N. B., Fornito, A., & Yucel, M. (2009). Structural brain abnormalities in major depressive disorder: A selective review of recent MRI studies. *Journal of Affective Disorders, 117*(1–2), 1–17. doi:S0165-0327(08)00476-X [pii] 10.1016/j.jad.2008.11.021.

MacQueen, G. M. (2009). Magnetic resonance imaging and prediction of outcome in patients with major depressive disorder. *Journal of Psychiatry and Neuroscience, 34*(5), 343–349.

Mannie, Z. N., Harmer, C. J., & Cowen, P. J. (2007). Increased waking salivary cortisol levels in young people at familial risk of depression. *American Journal of Psychiatry, 164*(4), 617–621. doi:164/4/617 [pii] 10.1176/appi.ajp.164.4.617.

Masuda, Y., & Sugiyama, T. (2000). The effect of globopentaosylceramide on a depression model, mouse forced swimming. *Tohoku Journal of Experimental Medicine, 191*(1), 47–54.

McKenna, D. J. (2004). Clinical investigations of the therapeutic potential of ayahuasca: Rationale and regulatory challenges. *Pharmacology & Therapeutics, 102*(2), 111–129.doi:2004/03/002 [pii] 10.1016/J.Pharmathera.2004.03.002.

McKenna, D. J., Towers, G. H., & Abbott, F. S. (1984). Monoamine oxidase inhibitors in South American hallucinogenic plants part 2: Constituents of orally-active myristicaceous hallucinogens. *Journal of Ethnopharmacology, 12*(2), 179–211. doi:0378-8741(84)90048-5

Miura, H., Ozaki, N., Sawada, M., Isobe, K., Ohta, T., & Nagatsu, T. (2008). A link between stress and depression: Shifts in the balance between the kynurenine and serotonin pathways of tryptophan metabolism and the etiology and pathophysiology of depression. *Stress: The International Journal on the Biology of Stress, 11*(3), 198–209.

Northoff, G., Heinzel, A., Greck, M., Bennpohl, F., Dobrowolny, H., & Panksepp, J. (2006). Self-referential processing in our brain: A meta-analysis of imaging studies on the self. *Neuroimage, 31*(1), 440–457. doi:10.1016/J.Neuroimage.2005.12.002.

Pace, T. W., Hu, F., & Miller, A. H. (2007). Cytokine-effects on glucocorticoid receptor function: Relevance to glucocorticoid resistance and the pathophysiology and treatment of major depression. *Brain, Behavior, and Immunity, 21*(1), 9–19. doi:10.1016/j.bbi.2006.08.009.

Pariante, C. M., Thomas, S. A., Lovestone, S., Makoff, A., & Kerwin, R. W. (2004). Do antidepressants regulate how cortisol affects the brain? *Psychoneuroendocrinology, 29*(4), 423–447.

Pivac, N., Mück-Seler, D., Sagud, M., & Jakovljević, M. (2002). Platelet serotonergic markers in posttraumatic stress disorder. *Progress in Neuro-Psychopharmacology & Biological Psychiatry, 26*(6), 1193–1198. doi:S0278-5846(02)00261-0 [pii].

Poland, R. E., McCracken, J. T., Lutchmansingh, P., & Tondo, L. (1992). Relationship between REM sleep latency and nocturnal cortisol concentrations in depressed patients. *Journal of Sleep Research, 1*(1), 54–57.

Prado, D. A., Pinto, J., Crippa, J., Santos, A., Ribeiro, S., Araujo, D., et al. (2009). Effects of the Amazonian psychoactive plant beverage ayahuasca on prefrontal and limbic regions during a language task: An fMRI study. *European Neuropsychopharmacology, 19,* S314–S315.

Raichle, M. E., MacLeod, A. M., Snyder, A. Z., Powers, W. J., Gusnard, D. A., & Shulman, G. L. (2001). A default mode of brain function. *Proceedings of the National Academy of Sciences of the United States of America, 98*(2), 676–682.

Riba, J., Rodriguez-Fornells, A., Urbano, G., Morte, A., Antonijoan, R., Montero, M., et al. (2001). Subjective effects and tolerability of the South American psychoactive beverage ayahuasca in healthy volunteers. *Psychopharmacology, 154*(1), 85–95.

Riba, J., Valle, M., Urbano, G., Yritia, M., Morte, A., & Barbanoj, M. J. (2003). Human pharmacology of ayahuasca: Subjective and cardiovascular effects, monoamine metabolite excretion, and pharmacokinetics. *Journal of Pharmacology and Experimental Therapeutics, 306*(1), 73–83. doi:10.1124/Jpet.103.049882.

Riemann, D., Berger, M., & Voderholzer, U. (2001). Sleep and depression—results from psychobiological studies: An overview. *Biological Psychology, 57*(1–3), 67–103.

Santos, R. G., Landeira-Fernandez, J., Strassman, R. J., Motta, V., & Cruz, A. P. M. (2007). Effects of ayahuasca on psychometric measures of anxiety, panic-like and hopelessness in Santo Daime members. *Journal of Ethnopharmacology, 112*(3), 507–513. doi:10.1016/J.Jep.2007.04.012.

Sapolsky, R. M. (2004). Is impaired neurogenesis relevant to the affective symptoms of depression? *Biological Psychiatry, 56*(3), 137–139.

Schüle, C. (2006). Neuroendocrinological mechanisms of actions of antidepressant drugs. *Journal of Neuroendocrinology, 19*(3), 213–226.

Schüle, C., Baghai, T. C., Eser, D., Zwanzger, P., Jordan, M., Buechs, R., et al. (2006). Time course of hypothalamic-pituitary-adrenocortical axis activity during treatment with reboxetine and mirtazapine in depressed patients. *Psychopharmacology (Berl), 186*(4), 601–611.

Segal, Z. V., Bieling, P., Young, T., MacQueen, G., Cooke, R., Martin, L., et al. (2010). Antidepressant monotherapy vs sequential pharmacotherapy and mindfulness-based cognitive therapy, or placebo, for relapse prophylaxis in recurrent depression. *Archives of General Psychiatry, 67*(12), 1256–1264. doi:67/12/1256 [pii] 10.1001/archgenpsychiatry.2010.168.

Shanon, B. (2003). Altered states and the study of consciousness: The case of ayahuasca. *Journal of Mind and Behavior, 24*(2), 125–153.

Sheline, Y. I., Barch, D. M., Donnelly, J. M., Ollinger, J. M., Snyder, A. Z., & Mintun, M. A. (2001). Increased amygdala response to masked emotional faces in depressed subjects resolves with antidepressant treatment: An fMRI study. *Biological Psychiatry, 50*(9), 651–658. doi:S000632230101263X [pii].

Sheline, Y. I., Barch, D. M., Price, J. L., Rundle, M. M., Vaishnavi, S. N., Snyder, A. Z., et al. (2009). The Default Mode Network and self-referential processes in depression. *Proceedings of the National Academy of Sciences USA, 106*(6), 1942–1947. doi:0812686106 [pii] 10.1073/pnas.0812686106.

Sheline, Y. I., Price, J. L., Yan, Z. Z., & Mintun, M. A. (2010). Resting-state functional MRI in depression unmasks increased connectivity between networks via the dorsal nexus. *Proceedings of the National Academy of Sciences of the United States of America, 107*(24), 11020–11025. doi:10.1073/Pnas.1000446107.

Shimizu, E., Hashimoto, K., Okamura, N., Koike, K., Komatsu, N., Kumakiri, C., et al. (2003). Alterations of serum levels of brain-derived neurotrophic factor (BDNF) in depressed patients with or without antidepressants. *Biological Psychiatry, 54*(1), 70–75.

Su, T. P., Hayashi, T., & Vaupel, D. B. (2009). When the endogenous hallucinogenic trace amine N,N-dimethyltryptamine meets the sigma-1 receptor. *Science Signaling, 2*(61), pe12.

Tadić, A., Wagner, S., Gorbulev, S., Dahmen, N., Hiemke, C., Braus, D. F., & Lieb, K. (2011). Peripheral blood and neuropsychological markers for the onset of action of antidepressant drugs in patients with Major Depressive Disorder. *BMC Psychiatry, 11,* 16. doi:1471-244X-11-16 [pii] 10.1186/1471-244X-11-16.

Tsuno, N., Besset, A., & Ritchie, K. (2005). Sleep and depression. *Journal of Clinical Psychiatry, 66*(10), 1254–1269.

Uppal, A., Singh, A., Gahtori, P., Ghosh, S. K., & Ahmad, M. Z. (2010). Antidepressants: Current strategies and future opportunities. *Current Pharmaceutical Design, 16*(38), 4243–4253. doi:BSP/CPD/E-Pub/000292 [pii].

Veer, I. M., Beckmann, C. F., van Tol, M. J., Ferrarini, L., Milles, J., Veltman, D. J., et al. (2010). Whole brain resting-state analysis reveals decreased functional connectivity in major depression. *Frontiers in Systems Neuroscience, 4.* doi:10.3389/fnsys.2010.00041.

Warden, D., Rush, A. J., Trivedi, M. H., Fava, M., & Wisniewski, S. R. (2007). The STAR*D Project results: A comprehensive review of findings. *Current Psychiatry Reports, 9*(6), 449–459.

Wong, M., & Licinio, J. (2001). Research and treatment approaches to depression. *Nature Reviews Neuroscience, 2*(5), 343–351.

Zarate, C. (2011). A randomized trial of an N-methyl-D-aspartate antagonist and neural correlates of rapid antidepressant response in treatment-resistant bipolar depression. *Biological Psychiatry, 69*(9), 115S–115S.

Zarate, C., Singh, J., Carlson, P., Brutsche, N., Ameli, R., Luckenbaugh, D., et al. (2006). A randomized trial of an N-methyl-D-aspartate antagonist in treatment-resistant major depression. *Archives of General Psychiatry, 63*(8), 856–864.

Zhou, J., Li, L., Tang, S., Cao, X., Li, Z., Li, W., et al. (2008). Effects of serotonin depletion on the hippocampal GR/MR and BDNF expression during the stress adaptation. *Behavioural Brain Research, 195*(1), 129–138.

Zunszain, P. A., Anacker, C., Cattaneo, A., Carvalho, L. A., & Pariante, C. M. (2011). Glucocorticoids, cytokines, and brain abnormalities in depression. *Progress in Neuro-Psychopharmacology and Biological Psychiatry, 35*(3), 722–729. doi:10.1016/j.pnpbp.2010.04.011.

Chapter 3
Ayahuasca as a Candidate Therapy for PTSD

Jessica L. Nielson and Julie D. Megler

Abstract Posttraumatic stress disorder (PTSD) is a syndrome that affects a substantial portion of both the civilian and military populations, and is often underdiagnosed due to complications with delayed onset and co-occurring psychiatric disorders. The prevalence of this devastating disorder is growing as more people come forward with traumatic events in their past. It is crucial that we develop a more comprehensive diagnostic and therapeutic framework for PTSD in order to reduce harm and aid in long-term functional recovery. Currently accepted therapeutic options for PTSD are proving to be insufficient as increasing numbers of people present with treatment-resistant PTSD, and alternative avenues for diagnosis and treatment are currently being investigated to improve standards of patient care. This chapter focuses on the rationale for why ayahuasca may be successful in treating certain kinds of PTSD, and reviews the previously reported pathophysiology of PTSD and its current treatments, and the new, experimental therapies being explored. This chapter also proposes a novel method known as "syndromics," which aims to characterize the full syndrome of PTSD using bioinformatics and multivariate pattern detection, in the hopes that by understanding the full complexity of this syndrome, we will be able to identify more efficient therapeutic targets, such as ayahuasca, to cure it.

The original version of this chapter was revised: The citation of "John Pasquina" name has been removed. The correction to this chapter is available at https://doi.org/10.1007/978-3-642-40426-9_14

J. L. Nielson (✉)
Department of Neurological Surgery, University of California, San Francisco,
1001 Potrero Avenue, Building 1, Room 101, San Francisco, CA 94110, USA
e-mail: nielsonj@neurosurg.ucsf.edu
URL: http://www.brainandspinalinjury.org/member.php?id=148

J. D. Megler
The Well Clinic, San Francisco, CA, USA
e-mail: juliemeglernp@gmail.com
URL: http://www.wellsanfrancisco.com/staff/julie-megler

B. Caiuby Labate and C. Cavnar (eds.), *The Therapeutic Use of Ayahuasca*,
https://doi.org/10.1007/978-3-642-40426-9_3,

Relevance

> It is to our detriment that we live in a culture that does not honor the internal world. In many cultures, the internal world of dreams, feelings, images, and sensations is sacred. Yet, most of us are only peripherally aware of its existence. We have little or no experience of finding our way around in this internal landscape. Consequently, when our experience demands it, we are unprepared (Levine and Frederick 1997).

Posttraumatic stress disorder (PTSD) is a debilitating syndrome that causes extreme states of fear as the result of a deeply distressing experience (American Psychological Association 1994; Yehuda 2002). It is estimated that approximately 40–60 % of adults have been exposed to a traumatic experience, and approximately 7–12 % of them will develop PTSD (Stein et al. 2000). However, among combat veterans, this statistic increases to 22–31 % (Prigerson et al. 2002), and may be an under-representation of the actual prevalence of PTSD, as symptoms often go unrecognized for years as clinicians and patients struggle to conceptualize the intrinsic experience of the patient. Diagnosis is further complicated because PTSD symptoms often remain undetected under co-morbid conditions such as substance abuse, major depressive disorder, somatization disorder, and other anxiety spectrum disorders (Johnson 2009). PTSD is underdiagnosed in both medical and psychiatric clinical practice (Zimmerman and Mattia 1999). This is confounded by the harsh reality of the rapidly increasing suicide rate among members of the military (Dao and Lehren 2013). This is a wake-up call to us all to develop a better framework for diagnosing and treating these patients to maximize long-term recovery and quality of life, and reduce the risk of abuse, relapse, and suicide.

Within both the military and civilian populations, the stigma of PTSD is a serious issue preventing help-seeking and reducing quality of life (Gould et al. 2007). Often the most stigmatized and difficult to treat mental illnesses are also the ones best managed by controlled substances. When prescribing controlled substances, clinicians are faced with an ethical battle. Because of the potential for misuse of these medications, leading to substance abuse, clinicians often under-treat patients well managed by controlled substances (Longo and Johnson 2000; Longo et al. 2000). This results in misdiagnosis and neglectful treatment of those with complicated mental health disorders like PTSD. Additionally, federal regulation of controlled substances makes using them for research purposes difficult (Dolan 2011), and slows progress toward exploring the therapeutic potential that some of these substances may have for complicated disorders of the mind and body. Although this does not suggest that every substance should be used in medicine, it does suggest that exploration of these substances may hold the key to unleashing what current medicine has failed to provide a solution.

There are a number of controlled substances being tested by a growing number of researchers for the treatment of PTSD, including 3,4-methylenedioxymethamphetamine (MDMA)-assisted psychotherapy (Mithoefer et al. 2011, 2013; Oehen et al. 2013) and agonists of the endocannabinoid system (Neumeister et al. 2013).

However, this chapter focuses on the potential of ayahuasca as a candidate for treatment of PTSD. Ayahuasca is an Amazonian tea that contains dimethyltryptamine (DMT), among other constituents. Ironically, DMT is a controlled substance in the Western world, and its potential production in the human body has been thoroughly reviewed (Barker et al. 2012), though its source and function are still poorly understood.

We hypothesize that the mechanism of ayahuasca's therapeutic benefits mimic currently available psychotherapies. Different than therapy that requires communication with a clinician, an added value of the ayahuasca journey is that it takes individuals into a realm where they can be without pressure to explain what is beyond their intellectual capacity. In this realm, victims can be fully present to experience all emotional and sensational elements of their traumatic patterns, allowing them to finally find resolution with their past without the distraction of having to articulate details they struggle to comprehend on a conscious level. Here, we review the pathophysiology that has previously been reported about PTSD and the rationale for the potential therapeutic benefits ayahuasca may provide for PTSD, based on the psychopharmacologic and psychotherapeutic aspects of ayahuasca.

What is PTSD?

A review of the involvement in memory formation and the development of PTSD and the pathology of trauma is required to understand the pharmacologic and therapeutic potential of ayahuasca for PTSD.

The memory system. Human memory, formed by the limbic system, can most simply be divided into implicit and explicit memories. Once the memories are formed, they are stored in the prefrontal cortex for future retrieval. Implicit memories are processed by the amygdala. These are somatic memories that do not require conscious awareness, such as remembering how to ride a bike or tie one's shoelaces. Explicit memory is our conscious memory; it is where we make cognitive sense of our memories and are able to recall previous experiences and information. The hippocampus is where explicit memories are processed so that they can later be retrieved from storage in the prefrontal cortex (Stickgold 2002). Traumatic experiences create an implicit memory without an explicit memory to consciously make sense of it. The body remembers what the conscious mind cannot. Therefore, when a victim experiences stimuli reminiscent of the traumatic event, she or he has sensations similar to those associated with the original experience. This can be re-traumatizing for the subject when overwhelming fear and anxiety return as if they were in the initial moment of victimization all over again. However, this type of response can also lead to catharsis in the form of extinction, which is the purpose of exposure therapies. By experiencing the memory of the trauma in a safe and therapeutic environment, subjects can tune themselves to respond differently to the triggers and move past their debilitating side effects

(Ursano et al. 2004). The primary goal of treatment for PTSD is to free subconscious memories to be meaningfully processed and integrated into the victim's life without replicating the disorienting emotional intensity.

The development of PTSD. The hypothalamus-pituitary-adrenal (HPA) axis is the body's stress response system. Its primary functions, in relation to trauma, are to guide emotions that stimulate instinctual behavior for survival (the "fight or flight" response), and to process memories. Stressful stimuli are first sensed by a part of the limbic system called the amygdala, which goes on to activate the HPA axis. In a normal response to stress, there is a negative feedback mechanism to turn the HPA axis off when there is no longer a threat. Trauma, however, disrupts the negative feedback mechanisms of the HPA axis, so that the body is in a chronic state of arousal. This chronic arousal state suppresses the hippocampus, preventing the formation of explicit memory, thus trapping traumatic memories in the implicit system. This is what underlies PTSD. The images, emotions, and somatic sensations can all be provoked, but without explicit memory, they cannot be articulated or understood. The persistent arousal of the stress response system leaves the body and brain unable to differentiate past from present (Johnson 2009).

Symptoms of PTSD are a manifestation of a victim's attempt to interpret internal states that are often difficult for the patient to describe, and even more difficult for the clinician to interpret and treat, resulting in a barrier against translating the internal state of these patients for those trying to treat them. PTSD poses another challenge to psychiatry, with its high rates of treatment resistance, both in the form of ineffective therapies and due to subjects' hesitation to accept treatment for a highly stigmatized disorder (Gould et al. 2007). This resistance to treatment often leads trauma survivors to develop their own maladaptive coping mechanisms, such as substance abuse and antisocial behaviors, to suppress debilitating symptoms. In turn, these coping mechanisms often lead to an exacerbation of their symptoms, creating a negative feedback loop that can be like a runaway train of fear and anxiety, leading those who suffer from PTSD toward extreme ends, including suicide. This is known as "maladaptive plasticity," and functions as a strong opposition to the positive feedback loop needed to promote functional recovery.

Maladaptive patterns of PTSD cease when subjects slow down and experience all of the elements of sensation and the feelings that accompany them. If victims allow themselves to acknowledge the thoughts and sensations associated with their traumas, the perceptions will have their natural flow, peak, and then begin to diminish and resolve, allowing the nervous system to regain its capacity for self-regulation (Levine and Frederick 1997). Maladaptive plasticity has been extensively modeled at the preclinical level in trauma paradigms, both in learned helplessness (LH) animal models of PTSD (Grau et al. 1981; Petty et al. 1992; van der Kolk et al. 1985) and following attempts to understand spinal learning following spinal cord injury (SCI) (Ferguson et al. 2012a, b; Grau et al. 2012). Maladaptive spinal learning following SCI shows the same physiological responses as the maladaptive coping mechanisms seen after a psychological trauma, leading to the development of PTSD. Adaptive plasticity occurs as the nervous system attempts to adapt after a severe trauma has occurred. The goal is to learn from the limitations, re-tune the neural connections, and identify behavioral modifications that will strengthen and reinforce these connections to maximize recovery and reduce additional harm. Due to the fact that the serotonergic system is affected by trauma, we believe that targeting this system therapeutically may be the key for modulating the downstream effects of trauma, as reviewed below. We hypothesize that this puts the nervous system into a "tuning" state where physiological patterns can be modified. The process of modulating the nervous system is known as "plasticity" and has been extensively studied within the contexts of learning and memory (Shepherd and Bear 2011), and response to trauma (Wang and Sun 2011). In understanding how the nervous system adapts, we can unlock the mechanisms that are necessary to steer those adaptations toward the direction of healing, recovery, and growth.

This tuning occurs both after trauma, when maladaptive plasticity takes control after serotonergic activity is reduced, and following treatment with serotonergic agonists, which may promote "metaplasticity" (the plasticity of plasticity). This is what we are referring to as "tuning': The ability to change the way the system changes in response to a stimulus. If this is done during a time of plasticity (i.e., tuning), there is an opportunity to modify the connections of the system (e.g., learn a new task), and establish a new pattern of activation that will reinforce the new behavior (integration). For PTSD, the addictive and antisocial behaviors can be seen as the maladaptive component of this plasticity. If gone improperly treated and unchecked, it can spin out of control and away from healing. However, this tuning period can also be directed toward positive reinforcement. In the tuning phase, the subject has the opportunity to choose a path to integrate what is being set forth during this stage. They can choose to walk down the path of coping mechanisms, including drug addiction and antisocial behaviors, solidifying their debilitating symptoms. Or they can choose the more difficult, yet more rewarding path of establishing new patterns reinforced with integrative exercises, such as psychotherapy, to implement the changes in their life needed to move through the downstream effects of their trauma.

This translation of maladaptive plasticity in both SCI and PTSD taps into the core nature of trauma itself, whether physical or psychological, and involves the serotonergic system as a key modulator of this plasticity.

Serotonin and PTSD. Following PTSD (Murrough et al. 2011) and SCI (Hains 2002), there is decreased serotonergic activity that reduces the effects of naturally occurring serotonin (5HT) signaling. Decreased serotonin affects the body's ability to modulate arousal, resulting in an exaggerated startle response to stimuli. In addition, it leads to further dysfunction in regulation of the amygdala, hippocampus, and prefrontal cortex. The goal of most therapies targeting this effect is to flood the system with serotonin using selective serotonin reuptake inhibitors (SSRIs), boosting the function of this system, which is involved in the activation of stress (Jones and Moller 2011) and modulation of pain (Hains et al. 2002), both of which greatly contribute to the debilitating consequences of physical and psychological trauma. Drugs that target the serotonergic system are already being tested to treat depression, PTSD (Murphy 2010), and pain (Dharmshaktu 2012). Serotonergic agonists like MDMA, DMT-containing ayahuasca, and 2,5-dimethoxy-4-iodoamphetamine (DOI) have shown promising results to treat a wide range of complications from trauma, including PTSD (Bouso et al. 2008; Mithoefer et al. 2011, 2013; Oehen et al. 2013), drug addiction (Thomas et al. 2013), and spinal cord injury (Lyalka et al. 2011), respectively. Therefore, psychedelic substances like DMT-containing ayahuasca should be explored as candidates to test serotonergic-mediated adaptive plasticity on recovery from trauma.

Treatment of PTSD

Current treatments for PTSD. Antidepressants are the first line psychopharmacologic treatment for PTSD (Johnson 2009). Specifically, selective serotonin reuptake inhibitors (SSRIs) and serotonin-norepinephrine reuptake inhibitors (SNRIs) manage symptoms that result from alteration in serotonin pathways. Modulation of the serotonergic system has been shown to be effective in both psychological and physical models of trauma. Somatic-based therapies also play a prominent role in healing trauma. A blockage of undischarged arousal in the body's somatic nervous system is a result of the memory disruption in PTSD. Symptoms of anxiety arise to contain and discharge the blocked arousal. However, anxiety does not resolve the underlying somatic freeze. In order to achieve resolution of traumatic events, arousal symptoms must be discharged on the somatic sensory level where the information was first stored (Johnson 2009). Levine suggests that the first step toward resolving trauma is to work with unresolved impacts through the felt sense (Levine and Frederick 1997). The felt sense is perceived by bringing awareness inside the body to the sensory and emotional landscape. It moves focus to the present internal experience. The awareness of the felt sense provides victims with a gentle energetic discharge just as effective as that which is accessed through action in non-pathological reactions to threat (Levine and Frederick 1997).

Exposure therapy is the fastest acting psychotherapy, and one of the most effective, targeting traumatic memories of PTSD (Johnson 2009). During exposure therapy, patients are exposed to a feared object, or context, without the danger. The exposure allows them to re-experience the traumatic event in a safe and controlled environment, creating an opportunity to integrate information and resolve the pathological memory. The intensity of distress associated with disturbing implicit memories is decreased through the confrontation of situations, people, and emotions associated with traumatic triggers. The confrontation allows victims to identify, reorganize, and neutralize environmental cues (Johnson 2009). Eye Movement Desensitization and Reprocessing (EMDR) is a Food and Drug Administration approved evidence-based therapy for PTSD with an exposure component (Ursano et al. 2004). In EMDR, the patient is asked to focus on eye movements, hand taps, and sounds while the disturbing images, negative cognitions, and bodily sensation associated with the traumatic memory are brought to mind. EMDR helps change the reaction to memories by reducing the disturbing thoughts that have not been discharged or released.

We believe that current therapeutic options for those who suffer from PTSD are insufficient, due to the high incidence of treatment resistance and suicide already discussed, suggesting that new treatment options need to be explored. Conventional medicine has shifted its focus to rely on the intellect as the agency of care (Lewis et al. 2000). Because humans are most aware of their intellect, it is falsely assumed that the problem lies within the intellect, and this is where it can be solved (Levine and Frederick 1997). Emotions are rarely considered in pathophysiology; however, the very core of the traumatic reaction is emotional. Progress cannot be made with the PTSD patient until he or she is able to discuss the traumatic event without replaying the memory accompanied by its sensory and affective intensity.

Embarking on the journey to transformation requires courage, as it is not possible to escape reliving the emotional experiences victims most wish to rid themselves of. Due to the emotional volatility that accompanies resolving trauma symptoms, PTSD interventions must prioritize a safe and secure environment. The type of integrative therapy that is used must also be determined prior to treatment, since certain triggers may prevent recovery. Although it may seem intuitive for people who have been paralyzed by SCI to maintain an active stretching routine in physical therapy to reduce muscle pathology, this method has not proven to be beneficial, and animal models suggest it may even prevent recovery (Caudle et al. 2011), perhaps due to activation of maladaptive patterns that cause more harm than good. This suggests that the kind of therapy that triggers this kind of stimulation in PTSD (i.e., re-experiencing, exposure therapy) may prevent victims from recovering. This reaction is so strong that it could explain why some people are treatment resistant.

Ayahuasca for PTSD Treatment

Experimental therapies currently under investigation for PTSD include MDMA-assisted psychotherapy (Bouso et al. 2008; Mithoefer et al. 2011, 2013; Oehen et al. 2013), modulation of the endocannabinoid system (Neumeister et al. 2013), and anecdotal (Fig. 3.1a) and complementary (Thomas et al. 2013) evidence for ayahuasca for PTSD. The treatment of addiction with ayahuasca is considered complementary to treatment of PTSD in consideration of the fact that many PTSD patients have substance abuse disorders (SUDs) (Saladin et al. 1995). Brain imaging studies in humans suggest that ayahuasca significantly activates frontal and paralimbic brain regions, specifically the left amygdala and parahippocampal gyrus (Riba et al. 2006). These regions play a prominent role in emotional processing and memory formation. As reviewed earlier, the amygdala processes implicit memories and the hippocampus explicit memories. Ayahuasca's activation of the hippocampus can allow for implicit memory formation previously disrupted by a traumatic event. During an ayahuasca journey, victims have the opportunity to

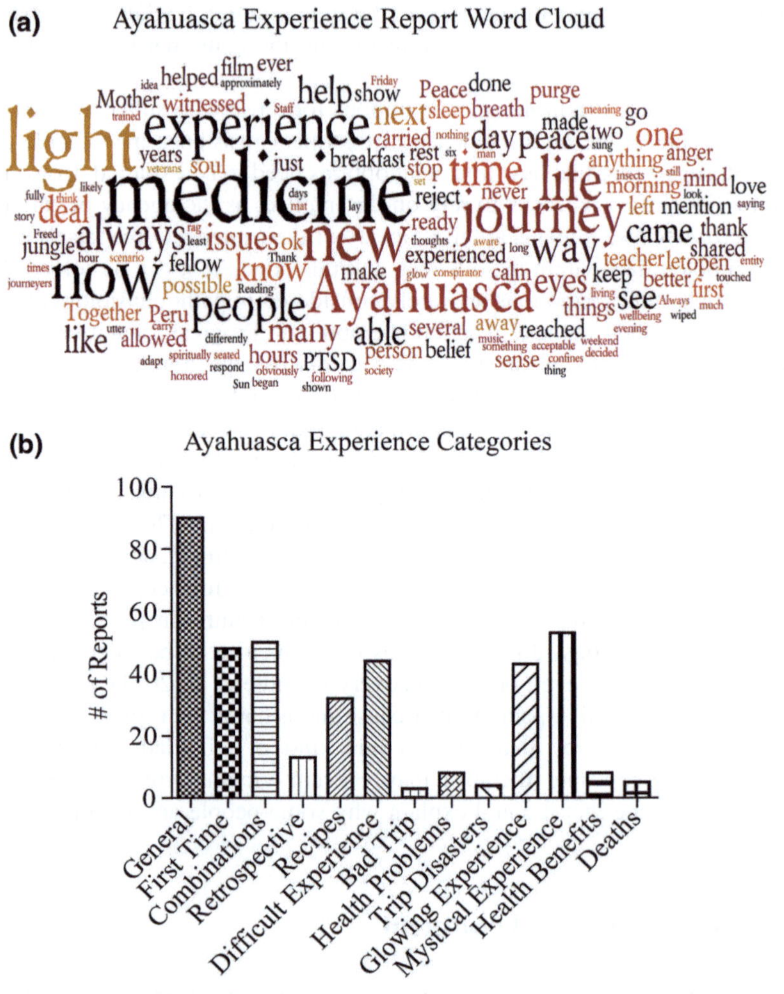

Fig. 3.1 Quantification of ayahuasca experience reports. Word frequency clouds (**a**) generated from Wordle™ from reports posted on Facebook by war veterans using ayahuasca to treat their PTSD ($n = 3$). Subjects taking ayahuasca for PTSD generally had a positive description of their experience and specifically referred to ayahuasca as "medicine." To get a better sense of anecdotal experiences of ayahuasca, regardless of the intentions of the experience, additional ayahuasca experience reports were mined from Erowid (2012) and plotted as a number of reports per experience category (**b**). Classification of experiences showed a trend towards positive experiences (e.g., glowing, mystical), with a comparable number of difficult experiences. However, there were far less "bad trips" reported, as opposed to difficult experiences, and the number of deaths affiliated with ayahuasca use were also minimal (Erowid 2013)

change how they react to memories in ways similar to exposure therapy and EMDR. The following is an account of a trauma victim's ayahuasca experience, reproduced with permission:

> A major aspect of working with aya [ayahuasca], is reliving trauma. The beauty of the experience of the medicine is that while the environment is contained and quite safe, especially while under the guidance of a healer, it is still psychologically compelling and transformative. For example, the idea that you are about to die or are dying is quite common while using aya. The individual has a choice to accept and make peace with this. Now, despite the fact the individual was not actually dying, the psychological result is the same: He faced death and made peace with it and can now incorporate this into life. I had a very powerful experience where I was forced to relive a traumatic memory repeatedly until I no longer held any negative energy toward it. It resulted in my ability to view the memory without the negative reaction I previously held (2013, Personal Communication).

Although it may seem counterintuitive to reactivate the HPA axis to aid in healing, as described in exposure therapies, if done in a safe, controlled environment, it creates the opportunity to identify, reorganize, and neutralize triggers and symptoms. Preliminary evidence from several war veterans with PTSD who participated in ayahuasca ceremonies at a healing center in Peru ($n = 3$) suggests that ritualized ayahuasca therapy can be a beneficial treatment for PTSD symptoms. Experience reports posted on Facebook by these subjects were mined and assessed in a word frequency cloud developed in Wordle™ (Feinberg 2013) to determine whether a healing theme could be derived from their experience of their treatment (Fig. 3.1a). This word cloud suggests that they viewed ayahuasca as a form of medicine to treat their PTSD, and the general theme trended toward positive experiences. Additional experience reports mined from Erowid and plotted as number of reports per category (Fig. 3.1b) reveal a comparable number of difficult experiences compared to both glowing and mystical experiences, as well as equal numbers of health problems and benefits, though these trended on the lower scale of total reports (Erowid 2012). Prior studies have shown ayahuasca to be safe under the appropriate conditions (McKenna 2004), however a handful of deaths have been associated with the use of ayahuasca (Fig. 3.1b) (Erowid 2013), and therefore appropriate measures, such as screening for contraindicated drugs and preparedness for this kind of therapy, should be utilized prior to consideration of this as a therapy.

Previous research indicates that ayahuasca administration causes robust activation of the HPA axis (Dos Santos et al. 2011), and thus may further aid in healing trauma. Studies have shown that ayahuasca is a serotonergic agonist (Riba et al. 2002), similar to SSRIs and SNRIs. Additional research has also found that regular ayahuasca use results in long-term modulation of serotonin systems in the brain (Callaway et al. 1994). Since the serotonin transporter is involved in multiple mental health disorders, it is hypothesized that there is a link between the elevation of serotonin transporters seen with long-term ayahuasca use and positive behavior changes.

Sensation is the language of the reptilian brain (Levine and Frederick 1997), and emotion the language of the mammalian brain. Through the activation of the limbic system and the HPA axis, ayahuasca communicates fluently with areas of the human brain that need nurturing to heal. During the ayahuasca journey, individuals can explore sensations, emotions, and thoughts associated with trauma, so that symptoms are discharged and resolved. Ayahuasca also guides victims to resolve events that predispose them to PTSD. "Complex trauma" is chronic interpersonal trauma in childhood that occurs within the caregiving system, such as with sexual and domestic violence. It is a significant risk factor for the sequela of PTSD with exposure to future traumatic events (Blaustein et al. 2003). The impact of prior traumas on resilience indicates that psychotherapeutic interventions aimed at integrating and diminishing the effects of traumatic experience must target not only the precipitating trauma, but remote trauma as well (Ursano et al. 2004). Complex trauma is an important target for intervention, as proper neurodevelopment is achieved through synchronizing the nervous system with attachment figures. After birth, the mother and child communicate and exchange with each other via the regulation of each other's limbic minds (Lewis et al. 2000). Emotional learning happens implicitly. Without synchronization with primary attachment figures, children lose their capacity to adequately regulate physical and emotional states (Blaustein et al. 2003). Similar to the limbic regulation that may occur between mother and child, successful therapeutic interventions are achieved when patient and therapist interact on an emotional level to develop and strengthen pathways that were dysregulated or insufficiently developed. Psychotherapy changes people because one person can help restructure the limbic brain of another, leading to greater emotional health (Lewis et al. 2000). Ayahuasca opens the limbic pathways of the brain to affect the emotional core of the trauma in a way similar to affective psychotherapy for trauma, and also impacts higher cortical areas (de Araujo et al. 2012; Riba et al. 2006) to allow the patient to assign a new context to their trauma to help them understand and move through it. Physiologically, we see activation of the same emotional brain centers with ayahuasca administration as we do in attachment relationships. Ayahuasca has the capacity to go a step beyond the event that precipitated PTSD. It can resolve remote childhood traumas that predispose survivors to the disorder. Assisted by the guidance of a trained healer, the ingestion of ayahuasca provides individuals with the opportunity to reestablish limbic connections and revise pathological ones.

Ayahuasca facilitates healing by emphasizing emotions and sensations, thus it requires consideration of the mental state, and the physical and social environment. To prevent exacerbation of pathological symptoms, ayahuasca should be avoided in individuals with severe mental illness (in particular mania and psychosis), self-injurious behavior, or high suicidality. It is also imperative that therapeutic use of ayahuasca be in a well-supported and contained environment. As with exposure therapies, ayahuasca runs the risk of re-traumatization by introducing traumatic memories or triggers. An appropriate mind state and setting maximizes the individual's ability to look at each aspect of the self to resolve traumatic symptoms during their journeys. Individuals can then work toward a harmonious whole by integrating their ayahuasca experience into daily life.

A Paradigm Shift

What needs to be improved? Modern psychiatry is in a medical renaissance. Central to the current approach to psychiatry is Engel's biopsychosocial model, which suggests that illness and health are the result of an interaction between biological, psychological, and social dimensions (Engel 1977). The highly popularized field of integrative medicine is an expansion of Engel's model. Integrative medicine is a multidisciplinary approach that combines conventional treatments with alternative therapies. It uses the biopsychosocial model to look at each aspect of the self and move toward a harmonious whole. However, it also includes a critical piece missing in Engel's model: spirituality. Religion and spirituality have a significant impact on health behaviors, coping, physical and emotional symptoms, and quality of life. Ayahuasca has a tremendous therapeutic potential in this context, as its implementation weaves together all dimensions at the core of mental health: psychopharmacology, psychotherapy, psycho-education, psychosocial rehabilitation, and spirituality.

There are several barriers PTSD patients must grapple with on the road toward receiving the best treatment possible. One of these barriers is the stigma associated with having a mental disorder such as PTSD. Another barrier is that imposed upon the research community that is beginning to identify currently scheduled substances that are potentially beneficial for treating PTSD (Mithoefer et al. 2011, 2013; Oehen et al. 2013), yet are experiencing difficulty navigating research into scheduled substances (Dolan 2011). Researchers and clinicians should be allowed access, under the appropriate peer-reviewed protocols, to investigate the therapeutic potential of certain socially stigmatized substances like psychedelics. Substantial progress is being made regarding researchers' ability to explore these substances for their therapeutic potential, thanks to the hard work of the Multidisciplinary Association for Psychedelic Studies (MAPS) (Multidisciplinary Association for Psychedelic Studies 2013).

Yet another barrier touches at the very core of trying to diagnose PTSD using the current standardized diagnostic tool known as the DSM. The director of the National Institute of Mental Health (NIMH) recently stated that research into mental health should not be confined to the DSM categories, and that research should be steered toward finding better ways to diagnose mental health disorders from experimental research information (Ledford 2013). As a result, an NIMH strategy called the Research Domain Criteria Project (RDoC) was founded in 2009, aimed at promoting studies that will design novel methods for classification of mental disorders using metrics related to behavioral, genetic, neurobiological, and other potential mental health predictors (National Institute of Mental Health 2011). In line with this, a set of common data elements (CDEs) was defined in an attempt to standardize data collected in PTSD research (Kaloupek et al. 2010), which may prove useful in attempting to accurately diagnose and treat PTSD. Once we can properly diagnose PTSD, we can understand better how existing and experimental therapies will treat, and hopefully cure, PTSD.

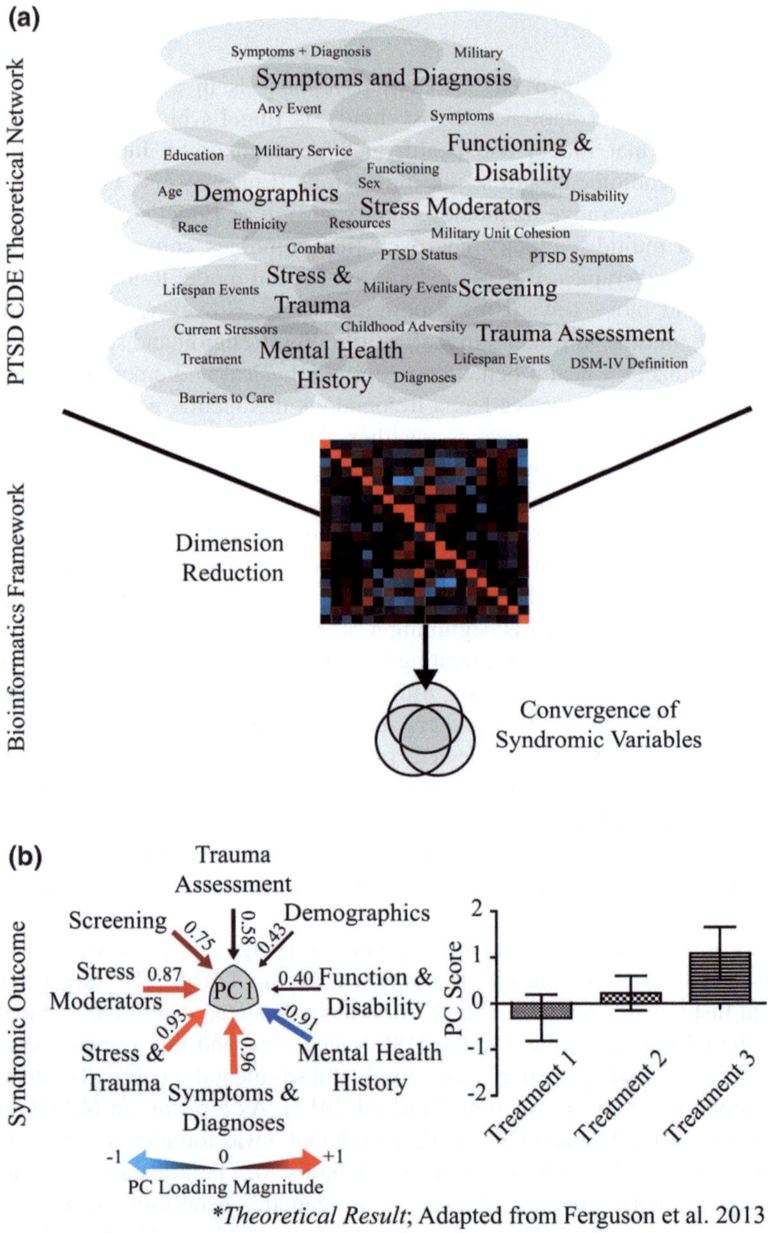
(a)
PTSD CDE Theoretical Network
Symptoms + Diagnosis
Military
Symptoms and Diagnosis
Any Event
Symptoms
Education
Military Service
Functioning &
Disability
Functioning
Sex
Age
Demographics
Stress Moderators
Disability
Race
Ethnicity
Resources
Military Unit Cohesion
Combat
PTSD Status
PTSD Symptoms
Stress &
Trauma
Lifespan Events
Military Events
Screening
Current Stressors
Childhood Adversity
Trauma Assessment
Treatment
Mental Health
History
Lifespan Events
DSM-IV Definition
Diagnoses
Barriers to Care
Bioinformatics Framework
Dimension
Reduction
Convergence of
Syndromic Variables
(b)
Syndromic Outcome
Trauma
Assessment
Screening
0.75
0.58
0.43
Demographics
Stress
Moderators
0.87
PC1
0.40
Function &
Disability
-0.91
0.93
Stress &
Trauma
0.96
Mental Health
History
Symptoms &
Diagnoses
-1
0
+1
PC Loading Magnitude
PC Score
2
1
0
-1
-2
Treatment 1
Treatment 2
Treatment 3
*Theoretical Result; Adapted from Ferguson et al. 2013

◀**Fig. 3.2** Theoretical syndromic framework to define the syndrome of PTSD, and how to test candidate treatments on this syndrome. Common data elements (CDE) have been developed to standardize data collection and interpretation for PTSD studies (Kaloupek et al. 2010). However, this large array of variables produces a complex matrix of correlations that may be difficult to analyze and interpret using conventional methods of analysis (**a**). By applying this type of data to our bioinformatics framework (Ferguson et al. 2013, 2011), we can leverage the correlation matrix for all variables in a PTSD drug trial, and apply pattern detection algorithms to reduce the dimensionality of this dataset to reveal new syndrome variables that describe the intersection between multiple variables simultaneously. Syndrome variables (**b**, PC1) can be defined as the collective contribution of multiple variables that contribute to a given amount of variance in the dataset. Each sub-variable loads onto their respective syndrome variable with the magnitude dictated by the correlation between that sub-variable and the entire syndrome variable. Posthoc testing of various predictor variables, including treatment categories, can then be tested on the syndrome variable to understand how these syndromic patterns move together as a response to treatments

Syndromic approach to PTSD. Although our current research at University of California San Francisco (UCSF) is not focused on psychiatric disorders per se, we are developing a novel approach known as syndromics (Ferguson et al. 2011) to better characterize and diagnose complex neurotrauma disorders like brain and spinal cord injury (Ferguson et al. 2013). This involves taking a data-driven, rather than hypothesis-driven, approach in order to more accurately assess existing and candidate therapeutic effects on complex syndromes of the nervous system, including PTSD. We hypothesize that by collecting and analyzing data using these criteria, and incorporating it into the bioinformatics framework we are developing (Ferguson et al. 2011, 2013), we will be able to identify the appropriate risk factors for PTSD, characterize the entire syndrome of PTSD, and more accurately test therapeutic efficacy in ongoing and future clinical trials (Fig. 3.2).

We propose that the notion of "set and setting," first coined by Leary in the 1960s, and specifically tested on the DMT experience (Leary 1966), applies to assessing the complex task of understanding and treating PTSD. While there may not be a universal treatment protocol for PTSD, there is a diverse framework of therapeutic avenues that can be tailored based on the multivariate nature of PTSD. This could include specific components in medical and personal history (set), as well as intentions for recovery and type of therapist and therapy that is administered (setting). The current diagnostic criteria for PTSD do not account for this complex constellation of symptoms, and the validity and usefulness of the current tools are being called into question (Ledford 2013). However, recent efforts have been made to harmonize and coordinate the information collected for patients with PTSD in an attempt to better characterize and treat it. These are known as common data elements (CDE), and are created by a consensus of clinicians and researchers in an attempt to standardize data collection for PTSD studies (Kaloupek et al. 2010). We aim to incorporate these standardized protocols of data collection specific for PTSD, and assess their role in the PTSD syndrome, and how they move together with respect to treatment (Fig. 3.2b).

Set and setting could be tested as predictor variables for therapeutic efficacy of existing and candidate therapies. This can take into account the mind state, intentions, and medical history of the patient, and variables involved in the administration of the therapy, such as location, ceremonial context, medicine, healer components, and integration methods can also be considered. The relevance of this has been shown in psychiatric research where questions were raised regarding the relative influence of the psychiatrist being a driving force in their patient's recovery, as opposed to the treatment alone. In fact, there was a substantial influence on recovery due to the method of administering the therapy (McKay et al. 2006).

Once the syndrome of PTSD is defined and subjects are reclassified based on their syndromic scores, simple univariate tests of predictor variables can be assessed. This can be used to screen risk/resilient factors for development of PTSD (Brewin et al. 2000), and test the therapeutic efficacy of emerging candidates for clinical trials (Mithoefer et al. 2011, 2013; Oehen et al. 2013; Thomas et al. 2013). These methods will enable us to not only better characterize the development of PTSD, but to identify potential risk factors to distinguish those that will be more susceptible to developing PTSD. The military may make use of this information to assign tasks to their soldiers, based on what will maximize their potential and reduce their harm. For example, in animal models of PTSD, pre-exposing subjects to escapable stress can prevent the development of LH behaviors (Petty et al. 1992). A famous example of this was observed following the 1976 kidnaping of 26 children who were kidnaped and buried alive (Terr 1990). Long-term follow-ups of these children revealed a high incidence of PTSD. However, one of the children who facilitated their escape in the face of death was not as traumatized by the event as the other children (Levine and Frederick 1997). He did not associate the experience with a sense of helplessness. He took action and freed himself and the rest of the children from their would-be grave. In doing so, he was able to have a cathartic response to the experience as it was happening.

By identifying these types of factors in a patient's medical and social history, we may be able to develop a more accurate framework to test therapies for PTSD, and potentially to steer certain individuals toward a lifestyle that will not lead to the development of PTSD in the first place.

Plans to apply syndromics to investigate ayahuasca for PTSD. (1) Build a database of previously published PTSD clinical trials, using syndromics to characterize which treatments are targeting the different components of PTSD; (2) Enrich this database with data from studies involving candidate therapies for PTSD, either specifically used for PTSD (e.g., the MDMA trials, mining data from healing centers treating PTSD with ayahuasca), or for other disorders (ayahuasca and ibogaine for addiction, psilocybin and LSD for end of life anxiety, among others); and (3) Conduct an observational study looking at ayahuasca for PTSD in different ceremonial contexts, combined with mining subjects' medical history to identify risk/resilience factors.

Concluding Remarks

DMT, the major psychoactive and possibly therapeutic component of ayahuasca, is currently classified as a Schedule I drug in the United States. According to the 2011 edition of the Drug Enforcement Administration (DEAs) resource guide on drugs of abuse, this class of drugs must meet the following criteria to be considered Schedule I under the Controlled Substances Act (see 21 USC para. 812): 1. High potential for abuse, 2. No currently accepted medical use in the US, and 3. Lack of accepted safety guidelines for use under medical supervision (United States, and United States Drug Enforcement Administration, Office of Chief Counsel 1996; Drug Enforcement Administration 2011).

As more research into psychedelics and marijuana is conducted (all of which are currently classified as Schedule I), these drugs will need to be reclassified if and when accepted therapeutic uses and treatment protocols are identified. The most promising example of this to date is the ongoing clinical trials with MDMA-assisted psychotherapy for PTSD. This has been shown to be safe and effective under supervised medical conditions (Mithoefer et al. 2011, 2013), and additional trials have been set up and published from international sites (Bouso et al. 2008; Oehen et al. 2013), and there are several ongoing and planned studies (MAPS 2013). We propose the same may be possible for the treatment of PTSD with ayahuasca, and aim to assess, using the syndromics approach, whether substances such as DMT can be considered for reclassification into the appropriate schedule based on their newly identified and accepted therapeutic potential and treatment protocols.

References

American Psychological Association. (1994). *Diagnostic and statistical manual of mental disorders* (4th ed., text rev.). Washington, D.C.: Author.

Barker, S. A., McIlhenny, E. H., & Strassman, R. (2012). A critical review of reports of endogenous psychedelic N, N-dimethyltryptamines in humans: 1955–2010. *Drug Testing and Analysis, 4*(7–8), 617–635. doi:10.1002/dta.422.

Blaustein, M., Cook, A., Cloitre, M., DeRosa, R., Ford, J., Henderson, M., et al. (2003). Complex trauma in children and adolescents: White paper from the National Child Traumatic Stress Network Complex Trauma Task Force. Retrieved June 18, 2013 from from http://www.nctsn.org/sites/default/files/assets/pdfs/ComplexTrauma_All.pdf.

Bouso, J. C., Doblin, R., Farre, M., Alcazar, M. A., & Gomez-Jarabo, G. (2008). MDMA-assisted psychotherapy using low doses in a small sample of women with chronic post-traumatic stress disorder. *Journal of Psychoactive Drugs, 40*(3), 225–236.

Brewin, C. R., Andrews, B., & Valentine, J. D. (2000). Meta-analysis of risk factors for post-traumatic stress disorder in trauma-exposed adults. *Journal of Consulting and Clinical Psychology, 68*(5), 748–766.

Callaway, J. C., Airaksinen, M. M., McKenna, D. J., Brito, G. S., & Grob, C. S. (1994). Platelet serotonin uptake sites increased in drinkers of ayahuasca. *Psychopharmacology (Berl), 116*(3), 385–387.

Caudle, K. L., Brown, E. H., Shum-Siu, A., Burke, D. A., Magnuson, T. S., Voor, M. J., et al. (2011). Hindlimb immobilization in a wheelchair alters functional recovery following contusive spinal cord injury in the adult rat. *Neurorehabil Neural Repair, 25*(8), 729–739. doi:10.1177/1545968311407519.

Dao, J., & Lehren, A. W. (2013, May 15). Baffling rise in suicides plagues the U.S. military. *New York Times*. Retrieved from http://www.nytimes.com/2013/05/16/us/baffling-rise-in-suicides-plagues-us-military.html.

de Araujo, D. B., Ribeiro, S., Cecchi, G. A., Carvalho, F. M., Sanchez, T. A., Pinto, J. P., et al. (2012). Seeing with the eyes shut: Neural basis of enhanced imagery following ayahuasca ingestion. *Human Brain Mapping, 33*(11), 2550–2560. doi: 10.1002/hbm.21381.

Dharmshaktu, P., Tayal, V., & Kalra, B. S. (2012). Efficacy of antidepressants as analgesics: A review. *Journal of Clinical Pharmacology, 52*(1), 6–17. doi:10.1177/0091270010394852.

Dolan, E. W. (2011, May 16). Federal agency blocks FDA-approved marijuana research for veterans. Retrieved June 18, 2013 from http://www.rawstory.com/rs/2011/10/04/dept-of-health-and-human-services-blocks-fda-approved-marijuana-research-for-veterans/.

Dos Santos, R. G., Valle, M., Bouso, J. C., Nomdedeu, J. F., Rodriguez-Espinosa, J., McIlhenny, E. H., et al. (2011). Autonomic, neuroendocrine, and immunological effects of ayahuasca: A comparative study with d-amphetamine. *Journal of Clinical Psychopharmacology, 31*(6), 717–726. doi: 10.1097/JCP.0b013e31823607f6.

Drug Enforcement Administration. (2011). Drugs of abuse. Retrieved June 18, 2013 from http://www.justice.gov/dea/docs/drugs_of_abuse_2011.pdf.

Engel, G. L. (1977). The need for a new medical model: A challenge for biomedicine. *Science, 196* (4286), 129–136.

Erowid. (2012). Ayahuasca reports. Retrieved June 18, 2013 from http://www.erowid.org/experiences/subs/exp_Ayahuasca.shtml.

Erowid. (2013, 4/25/13). Ayahuasca fatalities/deaths. Retrieved June 18, 2013 from http://www.erowid.org/chemicals/ayahuasca/ayahuasca_death.shtml.

Feinberg, J. (2013). Wordle. Retrieved May 20, 2013 from http://www.wordle.net/.

Ferguson, A. R., Huie, J. R., Crown, E. D., Baumbauer, K. M., Hook, M. A., Garraway, S. M. et al. (2012a). Maladaptive spinal plasticity opposes spinal learning and recovery in spinal cord injury. *Frontiers in Physiology, 3*, 399. doi: 10.3389/fphys.2012.00399.

Ferguson, A. R., Huie, J. R., Crown, E. D., & Grau, J. W. (2012b). Central nociceptive sensitization vs. spinal cord training: Opposing forms of plasticity that dictate function after complete spinal cord injury. *Frontiers in Physiology*, 3, 396. doi: 10.3389/fphys.2012.00396.

Ferguson, A. R., Irvine, K. A., Gensel, J. C., Nielson, J. L., Lin, A., Ly, J., et al. (2013). Derivation of multivariate syndromic outcome metrics for consistent testing across multiple models of cervical spinal cord injury in rats. *PLoS One, 8*(3), e59712. doi: 10.1371/journal.pone.0059712.

Ferguson, A. R., Stuck, E. D., & Nielson, J. L. (2011). Syndromics: A bioinformatics approach for neurotrauma research. *Translational Stroke Research, 2*(4), 438–454.

Gould, M., Greenberg, N., & Hetherton, J. (2007). Stigma and the military: Evaluation of a PTSD psychoeducational program. *Journal of Traumatic Stress, 20*(4), 505–515. doi:10.1002/jts.20233.

Grau, J. W., Huie, J. R., Garraway, S. M., Hook, M. A., Crown, E. D., Baumbauer, K. M., et al. (2012). Impact of behavioral control on the processing of nociceptive stimulation. *Frontiers in Physiology, 3*, 262. doi: 10.3389/fphys.2012.00262.

Grau, J. W., Hyson, R. L., Maier, S. F., Madden, J. T., & Barchas, J. D. (1981). Long-term stress-induced analgesia and activation of the opiate system. *Science, 213*(4514), 1409–1411.

Hains, B. C., Everhart, A. W., Fullwood, S. D., & Hulsebosch, C. E. (2002). Changes in serotonin, serotonin transporter expression, and serotonin denervation supersensitivity: Involvement in chronic central pain after spinal hemisection in the rat. *Experimental Neurology, 175*(2), 347–362. doi:10.1006/exnr.2002.7892.

Johnson, S. L. (2009). *Therapist's guide to posttraumatic stress disorder intervention* (1st ed.). London: Academic Press.

Jones, T., & Moller, M. D. (2011). Implications of hypothalamic-pituitary-adrenal axis functioning in posttraumatic stress disorder. *Journal of the American Psychiatric Nurses Association, 17*(6), 393–403. doi:10.1177/1078390311420564.

Kaloupek, D. G., Chard, K. M., Freed, M. C., Peterson, A. L., Riggs, D. S., Stein, M. B., et al. (2010). Common data elements for posttraumatic stress disorder research. *Archives of Physical Medicine and Rehabilitation, 91*(11), 1684–1691. doi:10.1016/j.apmr.2010.06.032.

Leary, T. (1966). Programmed communication during experiences with DMT. *Psychedelic Review, 8*, 83–95.

Ledford, H. (2013). Psychiatry framework seeks to reform diagnostic doctrine. Advance online publication. *Nature.* doi: 10.1038/nature.2013.12972.

Levine, P. A., & Frederick, A. (1997). *Waking the tiger: Healing trauma*. Berkeley, CA: North Atlantic Books.

Lewis, T., Amini, F., & Lannon, R. (2000). *A general theory of love*. New York, NY: Vintage Books.

Longo, L. P., & Johnson, B. (2000). Addiction: Part I. Benzodiazepines—side effects, abuse risk, and alternatives. *American Family Physician, 61*(7), 2121–2128.

Longo, L. P., Parran, T, Jr, Johnson, B., & Kinsey, W. (2000). Addiction: Part II. Identification and management of the drug-seeking patient. *American Family Physician, 61*(8), 2401–2408.

Lyalka, V. F., Hsu, L. J., Karayannidou, A., Zelenin, P. V., Orlovsky, G. N., & Deliagina, T. G. (2011). Facilitation of postural limb reflexes in spinal rabbits by serotonergic agonist administration, epidural electrical stimulation, and postural training. *Journal of Neurophysiology, 106*(3), 1341–1354. doi:10.1152/jn.00115.2011.

McKay, K. M., Imel, Z. E., & Wampold, B. E. (2006). Psychiatrist effects in the psychopharmacological treatment of depression. *Journal of Affective Disorders, 92*(2–3), 287–290. doi:10.1016/j.jad.2006.01.020.

McKenna, D. J. (2004). Clinical investigations of the therapeutic potential of ayahuasca: Rationale and regulatory challenges. *Pharmacology & Therapeutics, 102*(2), 111–129. doi:10.1016/j.pharmthera.2004.03.002.

Mithoefer, M. C., Wagner, M. T., Mithoefer, A. T., Jerome, L., & Doblin, R. (2011). The safety and efficacy of {±}3,4-methylenedioxymethamphetamine-assisted psychotherapy in subjects with chronic, treatment-resistant post-traumatic stress disorder: The first randomized controlled pilot study. *Journal of Psychopharmacology,* 25(4), 439–452. doi:10.1177/0269881110378371.

Mithoefer, M. C., Wagner, M. T., Mithoefer, A. T., Jerome, L., Martin, S. F., Yazar-Klosinski, B., et al. (2013). Durability of improvement in post-traumatic stress disorder symptoms and absence of harmful effects or drug dependency after 3,4-methylenedioxymethamphetamine-assisted psychotherapy: A prospective long-term follow-up study. *Journal of Psychopharmacology*, 27(1), 28−39. doi: 10.1177/0269881112456611.

Multidisciplinary Association for Psychedelic Studies. (2013). MDMA-assisted psychotherapy. Research. Retrieved May 18, 2013 from http://www.maps.org/research/mdma/.

Murphy, S. E. (2010). Using functional neuroimaging to investigate the mechanisms of action of selective serotonin reuptake inhibitors (SSRIs). *Current Pharmaceutical Design, 16*(18), 1990–1997.

Murrough, J. W., Huang, Y., Hu, J., Henry, S., Williams, W., Gallezot, J. D., et al. (2011). Reduced amygdala serotonin transporter binding in post-traumatic stress disorder. *Biological Psychiatry, 70*(11), 1033−1038. doi: 10.1016/j.biopsych.2011.07.003.

National Institute of Mental Health. (2011). Research Domain Criteria (RDoC). Retrieved June 18, 2013 from http://www.nimh.nih.gov/research-funding/rdoc/nimh-research-domain-criteria-rdoc.shtml#toc_product.

Neumeister, A., Normandin, M. D., Pietrzak, R. H., Piomelli, D., Zheng, M. Q., Gujarro-Anton, A. (2013). Elevated brain cannabinoid CB1 receptor availability in post-traumatic stress disorder: A positron emission tomography study. Advance online publication. *Molecular Psychiatry.* doi: 10.1038/mp.2013.61.

Oehen, P., Traber, R., Widmer, V., & Schnyder, U. (2013). A randomized, controlled pilot study of MDMA (+/− 3,4-Methylenedioxymethamphetamine)-Assisted psychotherapy for treatment of resistant, chronic post-traumatic stress disorder (PTSD). *Journal of Psychopharmacology, 27*(1), 40–52. doi:10.1177/0269881112464827.

Petty, F., Kramer, G., & Wilson, L. (1992). Prevention of learned helplessness: In vivo correlation with cortical serotonin. *Pharmacology, Biochemistry and Behavior, 43*(2), 361–367.

Prigerson, H. G., Maciejewski, P. K., & Rosenheck, R. A. (2002). Population attributable fractions of psychiatric disorders and behavioral outcomes associated with combat exposure among US men. *American Journal of Public Health, 92*(1), 59–63.

Riba, J., Rodriguez-Fornells, A., & Barbanoj, M. J. (2002). Effects of ayahuasca on sensory and sensorimotor gating in humans as measured by P50 suppression and prepulse inhibition of the startle reflex, respectively. *Psychopharmacology (Berl), 165*(1), 18–28. doi:10.1007/s00213-002-1237-5.

Riba, J., Romero, S., Grasa, E., Mena, E., Carrio, I., & Barbanoj, M. J. (2006). Increased frontal and paralimbic activation following ayahuasca, the pan-Amazonian inebriant. *Psychopharmacology (Berl), 186*(1), 93–98. doi:10.1007/s00213-006-0358-7.

Saladin, M. E., Brady, K. T., Dansky, B. S., & Kilpatrick, D. G. (1995). Understanding comorbidity between PTSD and substance use disorders: Two preliminary investigations. *Addictive Behaviors, 20*(5), 643–655.

Shepherd, J. D., & Bear, M. F. (2011). New views of Arc, a master regulator of synaptic plasticity. *Nature Neuroscience, 14*(3), 279–284. doi:10.1038/nn.2708.

Stein, M. B., McQuaid, J. R., Pedrelli, P., Lenox, R., & McCahill, M. E. (2000). Post-traumatic stress disorder in the primary care medical setting. *General Hospital Psychiatry, 22*(4), 261.

Stickgold, R. (2002). EMDR: A putative neurobiological mechanism of action. *Journal of Clinical Psychology, 58*(1), 61–75.

Terr, L. (1990). *Too scared to cry: How trauma affects children and ultimately us all.* New York, NY: Basic Books.

Thomas, G., Lucas, P., Capler, N. R., Tupper, K. W., & Martin, G. (2013). Ayahuasca-assisted therapy for addiction: Results from a preliminary observational study in Canada. Advance online publication. *Current Drug Abuse Reviews. 6*(1):30–42

United States, & United States Drug Enforcement Administration, Office of Chief Counsel. (1996). *Controlled Substances Act as amended to February 15, 1996.* Washington, D. C.: U.S. Dept. of Justice, Drug Enforcement Administration, Office of Chief Counsel.

Ursano, R. J., Bell, C., Eth, S., Friedman, M., Norwood, A., Pfefferbaum, B. (2004). Practice guideline for the treatment of patients with acute stress disorder and post-traumatic stress disorder. *American Journal of Psychiatry, 161*(11 Suppl), 3−31.

van der Kolk, B., Greenberg, M., Boyd, H., & Krystal, J. (1985). Inescapable shock, neurotransmitters, and addiction to trauma: Toward a psychobiology of post-traumatic stress. *Biological Psychiatry, 20*(3), 314–325.

Wang, D., & Sun, T. (2011). Neural plasticity and functional recovery of human central nervous system with special reference to spinal cord injury. *Spinal Cord, 49*(4), 486–492. doi:10.1038/sc.2010.124.

Yehuda, R. (2002). Post-traumatic stress disorder. *New England Journal of Medicine, 346*(2), 108–114. doi:10.1056/NEJMra012941.

Zimmerman, M., & Mattia, J. I. (1999). Is post-traumatic stress disorder underdiagnosed in routine clinical settings? *The Journal of Nervous and Mental Disease, 187*(7), 420–428.

Chapter 4
Moments of Insight, Healing, and Transformation: A Cognitive Phenomenological Analysis

Benny Shanon

Abstract In this chapter, I examine instances of special significance in people's experience with ayahuasca. Specifically, I consider instances in which psychological insights are gained and personal transformation and/or healing take place. The analysis provides a structural typology of facets of the ayahuasca experience based on empirical data gathered in a broader study that presents a systematic charting of the phenomenology of the special state of mind induced by this brew. The analysis and discussion are from a phenomenological cognitive-psychological approach rather than a clinical-psychological or medical perspective.

Preliminary Remarks

This chapter examines instances of psychological insight, healing, and transformation as they occur within the special state of mind induced by ayahuasca. By way of defining the scope and orientation—both theoretical and methodological—of this discussion, let me open by introducing my professional stance and myself. I am a cognitive psychologist who has been investigating ayahuasca since the mid 1990s. My primary field of research concerns the phenomenology of human

This chapter is a translation and reduced version from the original Spanish version published in 2013 as, ''Momentos de Insight, Sanación y Tranformarción: Un análisis Fenomenológico Cognitivo,'' in B. C. Labate and J. C. Bouso, (Eds.), *Ayahuasca y Salud* (pp. 348–376). Barcelona: Los Libros de La Liebre de Marzo. I thank Michael Winkelman for editing the original and Clancy Cavnar for the revision.

B. Shanon (✉)
Department of Psychology, Hebrew University of Jerusalem, Mount Scopus, Jerusalem, Israel
e-mail: benny.shanon@mail.huji.ac.il

B. C. Labate and C. Cavnar (eds.), *The Therapeutic Use of Ayahuasca*,
DOI: 10.1007/978-3-642-40426-9_4, © Springer-Verlag Berlin Heidelberg 2014

consciousness. My goal is to chart the domain of the mental, to determine lawful regularities in it, and to attempt to conceptualize it within a cognitive-psychological theoretical framework. Pursuing this perspective, I have studied both ordinary and non-ordinary states of mind (for a general review, see Shanon 2008). My investigations of the former dealt with trains of verbal-like expressions that spontaneously pass through people's minds, with mental imagery, and with dreams. My study of non-ordinary states of mind focuses on ayahuasca and is summarized in my monograph *The Antipodes of the Mind* (Shanon 2002a) as well as in a series of articles, notably Shanon (1998a, 2001, 2002b, 2003a; for publications in Portuguese see Shanon 2003b, 2004). I apply the phenomenological approach to the ayahuasca experience.

My study of the ayahuasca experience is grounded in the assessment that there is a reciprocally beneficial relationship between ayahuasca and cognitive psychology. On the one hand, cognitive psychology offers a productive methodological and theoretical framework for the analysis of the ayahuasca experience, and on the other hand, the non-ordinary experiential phenomenology that ayahuasca induces unravels new facets of the human mind and offers new vistas for the study of human consciousness. As Huxley (1956) observed following his experimentation with mescaline, the non-ordinary phenomena encountered with powerful psychoactive substances may be likened to hidden, uncharted territories of the mind. He further suggested that the intellectual import of these substances is in allowing an expanded geography of the human psyche. I concur (see also James 1902/1929; and further discussion in Shanon 2003a).

My goal is to specify patterns in this experience in which moments of meaningful psychological impact tend to occur. The patterns I survey are neither mandatory nor exclusive, and it is not the case that each individual experiences all of them. Rather, taken in unison, these patterns define a heretofore not investigated aspect of the multifaceted domain which is the special state of mind that ayahuasca induces. My interest is the prototypical human being (as contrasted with any particular individual) established on the basis of data drawn from the experiences of a large number of people. The outcome of my research is a systematic portrayal of patterns that may be regarded as constituting a set of psychological possibilities.

On the personal level, let me note that many of the ayahuasca sessions in which I myself participated were healing sessions conducted in the Amazon by indigenous and mestizo ayahuasqueros. In these sessions, I both received treatment and observed other individuals as they underwent treatment. Like many other ayahuasca drinkers in the various contexts in which I have partaken of the brew, I too have experienced moments of self-healing and deep psychological insight. Obviously, all these have had great impact on my life. On a couple of occasions, patients were passed to me to treat them as well. This happened without prior planning or notification, in light of interpersonal developments within the session.

I do find it pertinent to clarify my stance with regard to the nature and status of ayahuasca visions and the experiences associated with them. As explained in Shanon (2002a), I do not believe in the paranormal. Specifically, I do not view the visions seen with ayahuasca as depictions of other, ontologically existing, realities.

Nor do I regard the insights gained in the course of the ayahuasca inebriation as messages conveyed from non-ordinary sources, whatever they might be. Moreover, I do not regard the items seen in ayahuasca visions as symbolic representations of something else. Rather, by my view, these items, like the things we encounter in the context of our ordinary life, are presentations of what they themselves are. Their meaning and psychological impact is not to be sought in the manner of classical psychoanalysis, by way of the interpretation of covert information they symbolize, conceal or replace, but rather through the experiential impact they have. I would say that the meaning of ayahuasca visions is to be conceived in a manner similar to that of works of art: paintings and pieces of music. Admittedly, some paintings are representational, but not all are, and usually the genius of masterpieces is not in their strict representational features. In general, it might be said that great paintings are instructive in that they make people look at the world and see it with a fresh perspective.

The case of music is even more poignant: Music is neither representational nor symbolic, yet it does convey meaning. This it does through placing listeners in moods and frames of mind, and dynamically carrying them from one mood or frame to another. Thus, music conveys hope and despair, joy and tragedy, serenity and also frivolity, and it can invoke the grand impetus of life, the broad perspective of "being" as well as the dimension of the sacred. All these, I find, hold for ayahuasca visions. In fact, it might be ventured that the more abstract ayahuasca visions could be regarded as music in the visual mode. Furthermore, ayahuasca may function in a manner similar to the theater (or psychodrama) in its putting people through powerful, non-ordinary experiences. Obviously, encountering a jaguar in a vision is not something that leaves one unmoved. The objective (that is, from a third-person point of view) fact that the apparition is a so-called "hallucinatory vision" does not in any way detract from its experiential impact by making it less frightening, less challenging, and so forth.

Given my phenomenological-experiential perspective, I believe that the healing and transformative power of ayahuasca is to be viewed neither as recourse to the paranormal (as is believed by almost all users of ayahuasca, both traditional and modern) nor in classical psychoanalytical or psychodynamic terms. Rather, I examine the phenomenology of the ayahuasca experience to define those moments, patterns, and configurations during the course of the inebriation in which meaningful psychological insight, personal change, and healing occur. Such an examination reveals a series of salient patterns; together, these define the typology that is the subject matter of this chapter.

Guided by the approach sketched above, I systematically charted the various facets of the ayahuasca experience. These include the general atmosphere that the brew induces, the bodily and affective responses it triggers: non-ordinary perceptions in all sensory modalities, personal and intellectual ideations and insights, patterns of creativity and overt performance, and mystical and religious experiences. My research project is based on the analysis of a large corpus of empirical data from my own experiences with ayahuasca and the interviews I have conducted with almost 200 individuals. My informants included indigenous shamans, indigenous and mestizo (mixed blood) lay persons, residents of South America who are members of various syncretic groups using ayahuasca, independent drinkers (that is, persons with extensive experience who are not members of any group), as well as Europeans and North Americans; some of my informants were first timers with no prior experience with the brew. A full, systematic account of this research is presented in Shanon (2002a), which is the basis for the following survey and analysis.

My stance with regards to the status of ayahuasca visions and their interpretation is grounded in a general theoretical (and non-orthodox) approach to psychology that is radically non-representational (for details, see Shanon 1993). Specifically, I do not maintain that the basis for cognitive activity and behavior are covert mental representations; instead of grounding psychological theory in symbolic representation, I focus on the systematic study of the experiential (hence conscious) articulations of human cognition, which I call presentations. By my approach, the task of scientific psychology is to study the lawful patterns and dynamics of these presentations.

A Phenomenological Survey

The following phenomenological survey examines the aspects of psychological insight, personal change, and healing as they occur in conjunction with different aspects of the ayahuasca experience. These aspects are: the physical dimension, general atmosphere and the affective dimension, the visions, enactment, interaction, mentation, the religious and spiritual dimension, experiences of light, and patterns of manifest behavior.

The Physical Dimension

Although the topic of our discussion is psychological, I would like to begin with the consideration of physical effects. Confronting bodily discomfort and dealing with it can have significant psychotherapeutic ramifications. Indeed, I would single out such confrontation as the most basic psychotherapeutic and healing aspect of the ayahuasca experience.

The first effects I shall mention have to do with the general flavor of the intoxication. Ayahuasca is notorious for the awful nausea and physical malaise it induces. Often (although definitely not always), these are accompanied by violent vomiting. This effect, and the brew itself, is called *purga*, purging. Vomiting, it is believed, cleanses one's body from impurities. Such bodily cleansing is a prior, first step toward psychological healing. For one thing, strong discomforting experiences, along with the anxiety associated with them, demand some sort of response. These force drinkers to engage in self-examination, to learn to be in touch with their bodies, to collect their resources, and to attempt to confront challenges and overcome them. Moreover, the very act of vomiting has various psychological aspects. Central among these is the recognition of one's weakness and the concomitant sentiment of humility. Often associated with this is the physical posture of bowing and lowering one's head that normally accompanies the act of vomiting. Asking my informants about the most significant moments they have had with ayahuasca, several replied with a description of the first powerful physical purge they experienced. The purge was extremely unpleasant, yet it also brought about radical personal changes; in some cases, the impact of these changes was life-long.

Dealing with the purge is just one, albeit the most common, case of dealing with bodily malaise. With the generally enhanced sensitivities that ayahuasca induces, people learn to listen to their bodies and be more attuned to them. On the one hand, they discover finer and finer gradations in their sensations; on the other hand, they learn to attend to these gradations and tenderly take care of the pains and discomforts associated with them. Many told me that under the intoxication, they realized they could enter their inner organs and even cells and carry out minute and extremely delicate operations, mending the system from within. The ability to manage difficult bodily sensations and the experience of self-healing usually serve as meaningful lessons from which one may profit later, outside the context of ayahuasca.

As an example of a non-ordinary handling of bodily discomfort, let me report one experience I myself had; it has to do with a chronic prostate problem I have which forces me to urinate frequently. Once during an ayahuasca session, I felt I had to relieve myself, but I was apprehensive about leaving the hall. What I did instead was concentrate on the liquid that accumulated in my bladder and directed it upward. In my visionary frame of being, I channeled the urine toward my head, and then it all came out from the top of my skull emerging as a wonderful multi-colored fountain. In doing this, I ceased to be bothered by my bodily needs.

Throughout my long-term experience with ayahuasca I have also come to manage vomiting by transforming it to another physical act, namely, singing. In other words, instead of pouring out vomit, I would emit song. I might note that overall, I have vomited in just about 5 % of the times I have partaken of the brew.

The physical dimension is not confined to only negative sensations. Obviously, people partake of ayahuasca because it also induces good feelings. Ayahuasca drinkers report that the brew connected (or re-connected) them to that energy which is the source of well being and health; and that, as a consequence, they were revitalized. In general, having overcome the negative effects of ayahuasca, drinkers feel invigorated and experience heightened stamina. They also feel joyful and happy. One external manifestation of this is the ability to engage in night-long dancing without fatigue. Another publicly observable manifestation is drinkers' countenance. Towards the end of ayahuasca sessions, drinkers usually appear to be remarkably relaxed—indeed, serene—and often they seem to be both rejuvenated and strikingly good-looking. Usually, such effects disappear when the effect of the brew is over about a day afterward. However, it seems to me that in itself the very taste of well being and bliss can have a significant, viable positive therapeutic effect.

Atmosphere and the Affective Dimension

The second dimension along which ayahuasca effectuates psychological change and healing has to do with the overall ambiance of the intoxication and the various affective reactions to it. Overall, ayahuasca induces an ambiance of otherworldliness, whereby people have the feeling of entering into another, heretofore unknown, reality. Often, this feeling is coupled with enchantment. Characteristic of these feelings is the appraisal that the world is more beautiful than it normally appears to be, and that everything is invested with deep meaning. Both effects—the esthetic and the semantic—often impart a feeling that the world is awash with a bounty of good. Together, all these experiences generate sentiments of wonder and marvel. Such positive reactions can, in themselves, have significant therapeutic and curative effects.

The recognition that there is bountiful goodness in the world and the acknowledgement that one is potentially privy to it can define a new perspective for the assessment of one's human condition. Invariably, this perspective is characterized as less egotistic, more optimistic, more harmonious, and laden with more meaning and responsibility. The bounty of good discovered in all of existence is often interpreted as a manifestation of grace and/or heavenly love. Typically, this entails sentiments of appreciation and gratitude. For many, the ayahuasca experience also brings forth profound spiritual and religious feelings, which, in some cases, result in radical changes in people's belief systems and the manner in which they conduct their lives.

Another feature of the general atmosphere induced by ayahuasca has to do with temporality. With ayahuasca, people often feel that they are privy to the dimension of eternity. The experience of atemporality, which may be associated with what is taken to be the realms of the gods, lends human existence a new perspective. With this, the problems and concerns that an individual faces during the course of his or her life may receive different proportions and the measure of what is significant for one may change. In particular, one learns to appreciate the good things in one's life, to modify the relative importance that one allots to whatever one has and whatever one lacks, and to adopt an overall perspective of appreciation and gratitude.

There are also negative reactions, notably ones of fear. Fear may, however, have significant constructive psychological effects. For one thing, it may force drinkers to confront their own smallness and weakness. Overcoming fear, drinkers invariably have a sense of accomplishment. This in itself has a major transformative effect.

Lastly, ayahuasca typically generates marked positive interpersonal feelings; notably, love, empathy, compassion, and forgiveness. Each of these has its own salutatory impact. Empathy and closeness are also experienced *vis à vis* animals, plants, and nature at large. In particular, the tie to nature makes people feel that they are connected to "positive energies" which can effectuate healing. Such sentiments, which I have heard from many of my informants and which I have also experienced myself, are at the heart of traditional ayahuasca medicinal practice.

The Impact of Visions

Ayahuasca is especially famous for the powerful visions it induces. In this regard, I would like to point out that many of the general effects discussed above are often experienced in conjunction with the visions and may be especially salient as part or along with the visual experience. This is particularly marked with regard to the esthetic dimension: Time and again, drinkers report that the beauty exhibited by the visions surpasses anything that they have ever seen or imagined. Often, the very encountering of such beauty induces all sorts of "good feelings" which can entail a new, positive attitude to life.

More specific is the instructive, informative impact of the visions. In the different contexts of ayahuasca usage, the visions are valued primarily for the teachings they impart. Indeed, in all contexts of ayahuasca usage the brew is regarded as the Master, the teacher (see Luna 1984, 1986). Usually, the visions impart their teaching by showing. A paradigmatic case is for the visions to present the drinker with past situation in his or her life. Looking at these as an observer, one can view one's life in new light. In particular, this is so with visions that consist of snapshots of the past. Inspecting a past situation as an observer, one may gain insights with respect to his or her personality and behavior. Especially remarkable are the compound structures I call "thematic serials"; these are series of visions pertaining to a common theme. For example, one of my informants saw a series of snapshots depicting various moments of her biography. The shots were not ordered chronologically, but rather juxtaposed thematically. The juxtaposition revealed some patterns in the drinker's personality and conduct of which she had not been previously aware.

Another type characterized by its instructive impact is what I call "metaphorical parables." Visions of this type are similar to parables in the Bible: An image is presented and the viewer draws a moral from it. In the data I have collected, almost all instances of this type involve personal psychological insights with ramifications on the drinker's conduct of his or her life. For instance, one woman told me that in her first ayahuasca session, she saw herself fully encased in a transparent plastic sheet. Whenever she moved, the cover moved with her. She realized that she had been leading her life separated from other people. Even though it seemed that she was in contact with other people, in essence she was insulated and had no direct contact with anyone. This realization made this person change her attitude regarding human interpersonal relations. Of this same type is a vision of a dilapidated building I have heard reported independently by two different individuals. Apparently, when originally constructed, the building was a nice one, but now it was shabby and in disrepair. Upon inspecting their visions, each of the two individuals recognized the building appearing in the vision as himself; this, in turn, made these individuals appreciate that they should make some drastic changes in their lives.

> The following vision is my own, experienced when I was suffering from malaria. I saw two snakes wrapped around each other. Seeing that, I realized that health and sickness are the two facets of one complex. Specifically, I reflected that if one engages with the snakes in one direction one is inflicted with disease, whereas in the other direction health and well being are gained. Indeed, both illness and good health are energy. The symptoms of the body—that is, the illness—are pertinent to the process of cure. First, they are signs that the body sends to one, and thus they have important informative value. Second, if they are channeled appropriately, they can direct the organism to a new state of well being. The key to healing is rooted in grasping the energy of the illness and transforming it into the energy of healing. It further occurred to me that this is analogous to the taking, in physics, of potential energy and transforming it into kinetic energy.

With this realization, I made the most significant step toward being cured from my illness.

Several informants told me about visions in which they were confronted with two possibilities between which they had to choose. In all cases, the choice was conceived as being between good and evil. For example, in one such vision, one informant saw a black panther on one side and a wise man on the other. He understood that he had to choose between the two, and that he should follow the course that is good.

More dramatic than the metaphorical parables is personification, such as that exemplified in the following narrative that is focally concerned with disease. It was reported to me by a middle-aged European man afflicted with HIV. In his vision, he saw a person in bad health, poorly taken care of, and with a rather repellent appearance. This person criticized the drinker for depleting him of his vital energies. Seeing him, the drinker had the insight that he was actually encountering his own virus. This made him make peace with the virus, and wish healthy co-existence for both. At the time of the report, about 2 years after the episode of the vision, the man told me he was in good health.

There are also cases in which the visualization depicts actual teaching. Specifically, a teacher or a guide appears in the vision and instructs the drinker and guides her or him. In some cases, this figure is conceived as a divine or angelic being who directs the drinker in the further conduct of his or her life. At times, it is one's own "inner" or "higher" self or voice who gives the instruction. Instruction by a guide is especially common in accounts of indigenous ayahuasqueros with regard to their learning how to heal. They note that ayahuasca instructs them both how to diagnose their patients and how to proceed in curing (see Siskind 1973; Chaumeil 1983; Payaguaje 1983; Luna 1984, 1986; Gebhart-Sayer 1986; Baer 1992; Langdon 1992; as well as Luna and Amaringo 1991). Similar claims were made by several of my non-indigenous informants, especially those associated with the health and helping professions. Personally, I felt this once when I treated a patient myself. As I have noted, I am neither a clinical psychologist nor a medical doctor, but on a couple of occasions I found myself attending to sick persons. This happened in the context of traditional healing sessions in the Amazon, in the midst of a session, without prior planning or notification. The following is an account of this episode:

> As is common in such practices, I placed my hands on my patient's head and blew on it. As I was doing this, I saw myself at the head of a long line of forest animals. The animals formed a long triangular column and one to one were passing energy and support forward. Eventually, it all converged in my hands and breath giving me the power to heal.

I might add that the treatment of this patient was successful.

Enactment

Usually, the relationship of the ayahuasca drinker to the visions that he or she experiences is that of a spectator. However, when visions are powerful, they may be most absorbing and involve the drinker as an active participant, immersed in the scene of the vision. What is experienced to happen in the vision may have a great impact on people and, consequently, have significant transformative and curative effects. Following work I have done on ordinary consciousness, I refer to the phenomenon of acting within the vision as "enactment" (see Shanon 1988, 1998b). This phenomenon is not specific to non-ordinary states of consciousness. Both empirical and theoretical research (see Shanon 1993, 1998b) has led me to conclude that one of the key functions of consciousness is for human beings to have a kind of virtual reality in which they can act. Acting is important because, by my non-representational, non-symbolic, approach to cognition, the basic capability of the human cognitive system is not the processing of information, but precisely this: acting in the world (This view follows Heidegger 1927/1962; see also Dreyfus 1990, Merleau-Ponty 1962; as well as Varela, Thompson and Rosch 1991, and their paradigm of enaction). But acting in the real world can be risky, dangerous, and even impossible. Having subjective experiences of hypothetical scenarios enables us to simulate action in the province of our minds even when such actions are not feasible in the real world. For example, we can rehearse an important conversation before we actually meet our interlocutor or examine different possible solutions to problems without actually making concrete changes in the physical world (see Johnson-Laird 1983 and his theory of "mental models"). Ayahuasca visions present people with extreme cases of virtual realities in the province of consciousness. Whereas the virtual realities people entertain in ordinary states of consciousness are, in general, similar to states of affairs they normally encounter in the external world, the states of affairs experienced with ayahuasca are usually most extraordinary.

As in life, so in the visions: Confronting challenges and managing hurdles, overcoming fear, collecting one's resources and findings solutions to difficult problems and situations—all these are learning experiences that invest ayahuasca drinkers with feelings of accomplishment and boost their sense of self-worth and self-esteem. All these can be of great therapeutic value.

An episode that was of great personal significance to me is the following one, which exemplifies what may be characterized as intra-vision achievement. The following example is my own:

> There were seven men in front of me, each holding a puma on a leash. At one instant, the pumas were freed and moved towards me. I knew I had to act fast. And then it happened: A brook appeared between me and the pumas and I placed beautiful water lilies in it. The pumas were attracted to the flowers and they came to the river and drank. Having done so, they forgot about me and they all turned back and went away.

After this session, I felt a deep satisfaction; it seemed to me that I had advanced a grade in the school of ayahuasca.

And again, as in life, there are also failures. Here is an example from my own experience:

> In my vision, I embark on a journey and followed a path. At one point, I passed by an old, apparently wise and benevolent, man who instructed me to follow a certain itinerary. Sometime afterwards, I encountered a beautiful mansion and I entered it. There I was greeted by a host of lovely maidens who invited me to a feast. I joined in and forgot the path that I was supposed to follow.

Reflecting upon the experience afterward made me learn something about myself.

A special kind of inner action that is specifically related to healing are visions in which the drinker experiences himself as seeing the cells and inner structures of her or his body, travels inside them and experiences them to be mended and put back in shape; there are cases in which this operation is conceived of as being applied to one's DNA (see, for instance, Topping 2002; for analogous indigenous reports, see Reichel-Dolmatoff 1981; as well as the discussion in Narby 1998). For some, this process is experienced as carried out by the brew itself, for others the actor is the drinker him or herself, inspired by the brew and invested and guided by special powers and sensitivities. Typically, in such cases drinkers also feel themselves gaining information about the structure and function of the body.

Interaction

Closely related to enactment are visions of interaction. Whereas in enactment, the person under the effect of ayahuasca is the main actor, in interaction, the action is a joint engagement in which both the drinker and other agents take part. There are also interactive visions in which, by and large, the drinker is passive, and other persons, beings, or creatures that appear in the vision undertake the bulk of action. A Brazilian man with extensive experience with the brew furnished the following narrative. The vision at hand took place after this person had (actually) been stung by two wasps. He was in agony and was served with ayahuasca, and then (in his own words): "I saw two beautiful women who sucked the wasp poison out of the two sides of my nose. They passed it to my mouth and told me to spit. I did this and was, in reality, cured."

Several of my informants and I have experienced what is conceived as a magical operation. In my own case, several figures surrounded me and a very fine veil was spread over me and I let myself be carried into the realms of enchantment. On another occasion in which I was not feeling well a helping being appeared and presented me with a vial containing a soothing balm. I have heard of similar reports from other persons.

A visionary experience that is bound to have great transformative impact is that of self-death and rebirth. In visions of this kind the person who has partaken of ayahuasca feels that he or she is going to die, or actually that he or she does undergo death. Either just before this happens, or perhaps when this does happen, the drinker experiences rebirth. The experience is usually exhilarating, and those who undergo it equate it with salvation. Following are two examples of grand visions whose theme is a process of death and rebirth that leads to salvation. A South American psychologist who partook of ayahuasca only once reported the first to me, in a session conducted in a private home; a European woman partaking of the brew with a traditional healer in the Peruvian Amazon reported the second:

> The scene was that of a grand Aztec ceremony. Human beings were being sacrificed and I was one of those thus designated. I first considered resisting, but soon I realized that this would be of no avail. Thus, I altered my attitude and willingly let the priests in charge carry me to the top of the pyramid. There I was placed on the altar and the priests were above me, to take my heart. Without any coercion, I was offering myself. With this, my entire feeling changed radically. From a terrifying scenario of torture and death it all turned into a wonderful process of rebirth and salvation.
>
> The scene was that of a religious Egyptian ritual in the course of which I saw myself being sacrificed. A priest bent over me with a knife and cut my breast. At first, I thought to resist, but then I gave up. Subsequently, I had an out-of-body experience in which I inspected myself from above, and saw my heart being taken out. In its place was the sun, which was giving light and life to everything. Realizing this, and in order not to blind the other people present, I fainted.

Interestingly, a very similar report is given in Wolf (1992), a book which my informants had not heard of.

Mentation

Very often, ayahuasca drinkers report that the brew endows them with remarkable mental lucidity and makes their minds run faster and in a more creative manner. As a result, drinkers feel that their power of ideation and understanding is greatly enhanced. With this, all sorts of new ideas come up through people's minds. Many of these have to do with the individual's own life. Thus, the ayahuasca experience presents people with what may be likened to a deep self-search and psychological analysis. I can attest that after the first time I partook of the brew, I felt that I had gained more insight than I had in several years of classical psychoanalysis. I have heard the same appraisal from several of my informants.

Often, ayahuasca makes people entertain metaphysical ideas (see Shanon 1998a). Typically, these are in line with what is known as "perennial philosophy" (Huxley 1944). In particular, the appreciation that all that exists is harmoniously interconnected is very common. As noted earlier, this often puts the drinker's own being in a new perspective. This involves putting things in proportion, modifying the magnitude and import one lends to one's problems and needs, and is usually ensued with sentiments of appreciation, humility, and gratitude. All this is likely to set the ground for psychological growth and change.

The Religious and Spiritual Dimension

As noted above, an important facet of the ayahuasca experience is the spiritual and religious dimension. In all traditional and institutionalized contexts of ayahuasca, the consumption of the brew is a sacrament: a sacred ritual. It is not for nothing that psychoactive plants have been called "plants of the gods" (Schultes and Hoffmann 1979) and that for many the term entheogen (i.e., "generating the god within"; see Ruck et al. 1979; Ott 1996) is currently replacing the older and, to some, pejorative terms "hallucinogenic" and "psychedelic" (for discussions of the spiritual dimensions in conjunction with ayahuasca healing, see Mabit, Giove and Vega 1996; Mercante 2006).

What the experience of encountering the divine means is a very private matter which each individual has to determine and settle alone. Whatever the manner and the mode of its interpretation, the experience is bound to have great impact on people. Often this impact is long lasting, resulting in radical changes in people's belief systems, attitudes, and behavior. Personally, if I were to pick the single most important effect of ayahuasca on my life (there were many and the choice of one is not at all easy), I would say that before my encounter with the brew I was an atheist. I used to define myself as a nineteenth century middle-European-like intellectual who is a devout atheist with a strong affinity to Jewish history and its scholarly tradition. Now, a decade and a half afterward, I am no longer one. Likewise, a significant number of informants I have interviewed indicated that the main lesson that they received from ayahuasca was religious or spiritual. "Ayahuasca showed me that God exists," "I have come to appreciate the place of the sacred in human life," "I have encountered the divine," are all statements I have heard more than one person say. There are many individuals who, as a direct consequence of their experience with ayahuasca, underwent a radical religious or spiritual conversion. Often, the transformative impact of ayahuasca is long lasting and its effects remain throughout the course of a person's entire life.

By way of marking the direct link between the religious and spiritual sentiments and the visions, let me cite an episode recounted to me by one of my informants when describing the greatest impact ayahuasca had on her life. The informant said that the most important thing she learned from her experiences with ayahuasca was appreciating that God exists. To my asking how this came about, she replied by telling me of her seeing, with open eyes, the trees in the garden being interlinked by a web of translucent lines of light. This web, she realized, interlinks everything and sustains all of existence. With this, her theistic credence was kindled. I shall note that the seeing, with open eyes, of such a web of lines of light is extremely common with ayahuasca (For similar descriptions in the context of the dealing with a severe medical condition, see Topping 1998, 1999).

Next, let me recount an episode of my own. The vision was among the most powerful I have had with ayahuasca, and had a long-term effect on me. It took place in a session held with indigenous people in the Putumayo region in southern Colombia. I was offered a large dosage of the brew and the effect came quickly: Immediately I felt I was thrown up into a realm high above the planet and found myself in the midst of what I interpreted to be a cosmic lottery. My understanding was that my entire existence, both physical and mental, was at stake: If I played it right, I would be saved, if not—I would lose everything and perish. In order to redeem myself, I began to sing. There was no reflection involved in this decision, nor any recourse to past experience with ayahuasca (as would be the case today). For 6 or 8 h I continuously sang the praises of God. The words that spontaneously came out of my mouth were (in Spanish) *Gloria a Dios* (in English, "Glory to God"); the melody was being composed as it was being sung. As I was singing, I found myself surrounded by an immense choir of angels; I was taking the leading role and they were accompanying me. The music was exceedingly beautiful. Every now and then the choir was joined by guest groups that came in, performed, and then left. One such group that especially impressed me was one of Black, very sensuous, players. The music they played was very different from that sung by the angels, but it all fit very well and the ultimate meaning and purpose of it all was one and the same: "Hallelujah," that is, the singing of God's praises. Since then, I have been singing; both when I partake of ayahuasca and on many occasions in the context of my regular life.

Light

Light permeates the ayahuasca experience. As explained in Shanon (2002a), light constitutes both the most rudimentary and the most powerful ayahuasca visualizations; light is also a common feature of the visions themselves. In fact, I have heard it said that in its very essence, the ayahuasca experience is an experience of light. A distinct and very powerful experience characteristic of ayahuasca is the seeing of what may be characterized as the "supreme light." By way of example, let me cite the report of a European woman furnished to me in response to my questioning about the most remarkable experience she had with ayahuasca:

> In front of me was a most brilliant source of light. Like a lantern of many, many facets. I knew that were I to look at it straight ahead, I would collapse and perhaps die. Thus, I turned my head. During this experience, I felt as if I was losing my sense of self and the faculty of memory.

Another example is that of a young European man who, following his first ayahuasca vision, in which I was present too, emotionally declared: "I saw God!" To my query as to what that meant, he replied:

> I was in a region which was pure and perfect, full of light and love, and I was healed.
>
> I looked at the skies up there and the heavens parted. There came a ray of light and it struck my heart. With this I was healed.

Overt Behavior

The ayahuasca experience is not confined to the inner provinces of the mind; it also has overt, publicly observable manifestations. The most notable of these is singing. As already noted above, singing can have great psychological and therapeutic impact. Indeed, singing is the primary tool of healing that the traditional ayahuasqueros use. Throughout the Amazonian region, it is being said: *el que canta, el que cura*, he who sings is he who heals. In the anthropological literature the focus is on the singing as it affects those who listen to it (see, for instance, Bellier 1986; Dobkin de Rios and Katz 1975; Hill 1992; and Luna 1992). However, no less powerful is the effect of singing on those who produce the music, whether they are healers or not. I know more than one person who vouched that ayahuasca made her or him sing and, consequently, introduced a most meaningful change in his or her life.

General Typological Summary

The following summary highlights the principles governing the moments of psychological and therapeutic significance during the course of the ayahuasca experience. In terms of organization, the following exposition is somewhat different from that of the preceding sections, which were ordered in terms of the different dimensions or domains of experience.

First is the affective impact. The very experiencing of physical and psychological well being and of positive affects may, in itself, have significant psychological and therapeutic impact on people. This is especially true for sentiments such as bliss and marvel and of attitudinal reactions such as appreciation and gratitude, as well as of rapture and spiritual uplifting. In addition, such affects and attitudinal reactions can entail changes in people's belief systems and outlook.

Second is the experiential level. As in ordinary life, so with ayahuasca: Going through powerful experiences can have great impact on people. The impact is especially forceful with difficult experiences. Confronting such experiences and overcoming the ordeals that they present constitute veritable tests and achievements. The experiences often force people to reevaluate what is really meaningful to them in their lives and they often reveal, trigger, or generate personal resources that can become permanent psychological assets.

An experiential effect to be singled out is that of being connected to that which is sensed to be the source of all vital energy, the ultimate *fons et origo* of all things. Regardless of how one conceptualizes this, the experience has a powerful, direct, and unmediated curative and transformative effect.

One thing the visions do is "showing." Looking at one's own life, past and present, as an observer, contemplating it and reflecting upon it is prone to be instructive. The visions can also instruct by actual teaching and guidance. Both in conjunction with the visions and apart from them, ayahuasca induces enhanced ideation, and hence reflection and insight. Through these, people can arrive at novel, meaningful understandings, both psychological and intellectual. Especially powerful are the spiritual and religious experiences that ayahuasca induces. These can effectuate radical changes in people's beliefs systems and their effects can be long lasting. Lastly, the manifest behaviors that ayahuasca facilitates—notably, singing—can have very significant psychological and transformative effects.

Closing, I would like to point out that none of the effects I have noted is automatic. It is not the case that ayahuasca, in and of itself, heals people, transforms them, and makes their lives better. The special experiences that ayahuasca induces present people with possibilities and potentials. It reveals to them sentiments, states of minds, situations, ideas, and patterns of behavior that they may have not encountered or thought of before. Whether all this will have an enduring effect depends on the individual drinker, not on ayahuasca. It is up to each person to gage what ayahuasca has shown to him or her, judge its value and significance, and act, or not act, upon it. Yes, ayahuasca is a great teacher and healer, but the ultimate responsibility for psychological growth and cure remains with each one of us.

References

Baer, G. (1992). The one intoxicated by tobacco: Matsigenka shamanism. In E. J. Langdon & G. Baer (Eds.), *Portals of power: Shamanism in South America* (pp. 79–102). Albuquerque, NM: University of New Mexico Press.

Bellier, I. (1986). Los cantos mai Huna del yajé (Amazonia Peruana). *America Indígena, 46*, 129–145.

Chaumeil, J. (1983). *Voir, savoir, pouvoir: Le chamanisme chez les Yagua du nord-est Péruvien*. Paris: Editions de l'Ecole des Hautes Etudes en Sciences Sociales.

Dobkin de Rios, M., & Katz, F. (1975). Some relationships between music and hallucinogenic ritual: The jungle gym in consciousness. *Ethos, 3*, 64–76.

Dreyfus, H. L. (1990). *Being-in-the-world*. Cambridge, MA: M.I.T. Press.

Gebhart-Sayer, A. (1986). Una terapia estetica: Los diseños visionarios del ayahuasca entre los Shipibo-Conibo. *America Indígena, 46*, 189–218.

Heidegger, M. (1927/1962). *Being and time*. New York, NY: Harper & Row.

Hill, J. (1992). A musical aesthetic of ritual curing in the northwest Amazon. In E. J. Langdon & G. Baer (Eds.), *Portals of power: Shamanism in South America* (pp. 175–210). Albuquerque: University of New Mexico Press.

Huxley, A. (1944). *The perennial philosophy*. New York, NY: Harper & Row.
Huxley, A. (1956). *Heaven and hell*. London: Chatto and Windus.
James, W. (1902/1929). *Varieties of religious experience*. New York, NY: Modern Library.
Johnson-Laird, P. N. (1983). *Mental models*. Cambridge, MA: Harvard University Press.
Langdon, E. J. (1992). Dau: Shamanic power in Siona religion and medicine. In E. J. Langdon & G. Baer (Eds.), *Portals of power: Shamanism in South America* (pp. 41–61). Albuquerque: University of New Mexico Press.
Luna, L. E. (1984). The concept of plants as teachers among four mestizo shamans of Iquitos, northeastern Peru. *Journal of Ethnopharmacology, 11*, 135–156.
Luna, L. E. (1986). *Vegetalismo shamanism among the mestizo population of the Peruvian Amazon*. Stockholm: Almqvist & Wiksell International.
Luna, L. E. (1992). Icaros: Magic melodies among the mestizo shamans of the Peruvian Amazon. In E. Langdon & G. Baer (Eds.), *Portals of power: Shamanism in South America* (pp. 231–252). Albuquerque: University of New Mexico Press.
Luna, L. E., & Amaringo, P. (1991). *Ayahuasca visions: The religious iconography of a Peruvian shaman*. Berkeley, CA: North Atlantic Books.
Mabit, J., Giove, R., & Vega, J. (1996). Takiwasi: The use of Amazonian shamanism to rehabilitate drug addicts. In M. Winkelman & W. Andritzky (Eds.), *Yearbook of cross-cultural medicine and psychotherapy, Zeitschrift for Ethnomedizin* (pp. 257–286). Berlin: VWB.
Mercante, M. (2006). *Images of healing: Spontaneous mental imagery and healing process of the Barquinha, a Brazilian ayahuasca religious system*. San Francisco, CA: Saybrook Graduate School and Research Center.
Merleau-Ponty, M. (1962). *Phenomenology of perception*. London: Routledge and Kegan Paul.
Narby, J. (1998). *The cosmic serpent: DNA and the origins of knowledge*. New York, NY: Jeremy P. Tarcher.
Ott, J. (1996). Entheogens II: On entheology and ethnobotany. *Journal of Psychoactive Drugs, 28*, 205–209.
Payaguaje, F. (1983). *El bebedor de yaje*. Quito: Libri Mundi.
Reichel-Dolmatoff, G. (1981). Brain and mind in Desana shamanism. *Journal of Latin American Lore, 7*, 73–98.
Ruck, C., Bigwood, J., Staples, R., Wasson, R., & Ott, J. (1979). Entheogens. *Journal of Psychedelic Drugs, 11*, 145–146.
Schultes, R. E., & Hoffmann, A. (1979). *Plants of the gods: Origins of hallucinogenic use*. London: McGraw-Hill.
Shanon, B. (1988). Channels of thought. *Discourse Processes, 11*, 221–242.
Shanon, B. (1993). *The representational and the presentational: An essay on cognition and the study of mind*. London: Harvester-Wheatsheaf.
Shanon, B. (1998a). Ideas and reflections associated with ayahuasca visions. *Bulletin of the Multidisciplinary Association for Psychedelic Studies, 8*, 18–21.
Shanon, B. (1998b). What is the function of consciousness? *Journal of Consciousness Studies, 5*, 295–308.
Shanon, B. (2001). Altered temporality. *Journal of Consciousness Studies, 8*, 35–58.
Shanon, B. (2002a). *The antipodes of the mind: Charting the phenomenology of the ayahuasca experience*. Oxford: Oxford University Press.
Shanon, B. (2002b). Ayahuasca visualizations: A structural typology. *Journal of Consciousness Studies, 9*, 3–30.
Shanon, B. (2003a). Altered states and the study of consciousness: The case of ayahuasca. *Journal of Mind and Behavior, 24*, 125–154.
Shanon, B. (2003b). Os conteúdos das visões da ayahuasca. *Mana: Estudos de Antropologia Social, 9*, 109-152.
Shanon, B. (2004). Ayahuasca and the study of mind. In B. C. Labate & W. S. Araújo (Eds.), *Uso Ritual da ayahuasca* (pp. 681–709). Campinas, Brazil: Editora Mercado de Letras.

Shanon, B. (2008). Towards a phenomenological psychology of the conscious. In J. Stewart, Gapenne (Eds.), *Enaction: Towards a new paradigm for cognitive science*. Cambridge, MA: M.I.T. Press.

Siskind, J. (1973). Visions and cures among the Sharanahua. In M. J. Harner (Ed.), *Hallucinogens and shamanism* (pp. 28–39). Oxford: Oxford University Press.

Topping, D. M. (1998). Ayahuasca and cancer: One man's experience. *Bulletin of the Multidisciplinary Association for Psychedelic Studies, 8*, 22–26.

Topping, D. M. (1999). Ayahuasca and cancer: A postscript. *Bulletin of the Multidisciplinary Association for Psychedelic Studies, 9*, 22–25.

Topping, D. M. (2002). Making friends with cancer and ayahuasca. In C. S. Grob (Ed.), *Hallucinogens: A reader* (pp. 138–155). New York, NY: Jeremy P. Tarcher/Putnam.

Varela, F. J., Thompson, J. E., & Rosch, E. (1991). *The embodied mind*. Cambridge, MA: M.I.T. Press.

Wolf, F. A. (1992). *The eagle's quest: A physicist's search for truth in the heart of the shamanic world*. New York, NY: Touchstone.

Chapter 5
Healing with Ayahuasca: Notes on Therapeutic Rituals and Effects in European Patients Treating Their Diseases

Janine Tatjana Schmid

Abstract Ayahuasca is commonly referred to as a "medicine" and is used for healing in traditional Amazonian societies as well as in recent Western rituals. This chapter will report on the results of 15 patients interviewed about their personal experience with the curative effects of ayahuasca. The "healing" the patients narrate was often not limited to the cure of physical and mental diseases, but was expanded to include spiritual problems or challenges concerning everyday life. The qualitative data analysis revealed a variety of positive effects, not only in regard to the curing of specific diseases, but also in regard to a better quality of life and well being in general. The therapeutic effects of ayahuasca in the treatment of various diseases, such as cancer tumors, chronic pain, hepatitis C, asthma, migraine, gastritis, tinnitus, depression, and alcohol abuse will be discussed. I will also point out implications for further therapeutic approaches.

Introduction

Ayahuasca is a Quechua word meaning "vine of the souls" or "vine of the dead." Ayahuasca is also known by different names like yagé, caapi, natem, mihi, dapa, Daime or hoasca. The psychoactive beverage has been used traditionally for medico-religious purposes in shamanic rituals by at least 72 indigenous groups of the Upper Amazon (Luna 1986). It is not only traditional indigenous cultures in the Amazon and Orinoco basin of South America that have used ayahuasca for divination and healing; from the beginning of the twentieth century, a number of religious (Santo Daime, União da Vegetal, Barquinha) and other cultural expressions have integrated this potion into different cultural settings, including

J. T. Schmid (✉)
Institute for Medical Psychology, University of Heidelberg, Bergheimer Straße 20, 69115 Heidelberg, Germany
e-mail: schamanismusforschung@web.de

B. C. Labate and C. Cavnar (eds.), *The Therapeutic Use of Ayahuasca*,
DOI: 10.1007/978-3-642-40426-9_5, © Springer-Verlag Berlin Heidelberg 2014

psychotherapeutic treatment. "Healing" is one of the most prominent concepts and motives present in all kinds of different uses of ayahuasca. Participants considered nearly all kinds of ayahuasca rituals to be "healing rituals" (Winkelman 2005; Fotiou 2012; Schmid et al. 2010). Ayahuasca is said to have healing powers and is seen as a kind of medicine, for some even as a panacea.

Ayahuasca is made of a vine (*Banisteriopsis caapi*), an monoamino-oxidase inhibitor (MAOI), which is usually cooked together with a dimethyltryptamine (DMT) containing plant (*Psychotria viridis* or *Diplopterys cabrerana*). In few cases (as I have observed in Europe), ayahuasca is also available without a DMT-containing substance.

From 2002 to 2010, I studied healing experiences and therapeutic effects of ayahuasca in Europe. This included Germany, The Netherlands, Austria, and Switzerland. I conducted two semi-structured qualitative interviews with 15 people who had been diagnosed with a disorder by a medical professional, about therapeutic effects of ayahuasca regarding their personal experience. These 15 patients related 25 different complaints, and spoke of their first-hand experience attending diverse ayahuasca rituals. Three major settings of ayahuasca rituals in Europe could be found:

Most common are Santo Daime rituals from the Centro Eclético de Fluente Luz Universal Raimundo Irineu Serra (CEFLURIS) branch. Santo Daime was founded in the Brazilian Amazonian state of Acre in the 1930s and became a small but worldwide movement in the 1990s. Santo Daime is a syncretic spiritual practice that incorporates elements of different religious or spiritual traditions, such as folk Catholicism, Kardecist Spiritism, African religiosity, and South American shamanism. Santo Daime rituals are usually held in churches and are strongly influenced by Catholic representations. Classical Santo Daime practice features three main kinds of rituals: *Hinários* (hymnals), *concentrações* (concentrations) and *curas* (healing). Participants drink Daime (ayahuasca) as a sacrament in all types of rituals. Ceremonies, which are called *trabalhos* (works), typically last for several hours. Hinários involve dancing with special formalized dances called *bailados*, and singing hymns. Those rituals may last up to 12 h. Concentrações are silent, seated meditations, which include periods where sequences of hymns are also sung. Although, according to the group itself, all Santo Daime rituals have "healing effects," the curas are particularly devoted to healing. In these rituals, participants sit in chairs while singing special hymns for healing. These rituals sometimes include healing mediumship sessions or the use of other special healing practices.

Neoshamanic ayahuasca ceremonies with a great variety of indigenous elements (including sweat lodges) are also very common. Rituals in Europe usually take place either in a tent, a yurt or in private homes, hotel rooms, or yoga studios. Participants sit in semi-darkness at night. At times they rest on blankets or sleeping bags or they sit on the floor or on chairs depending on instructions of the guide and the location of the ritual. Sometimes a "real" shaman from South America guides these rituals, other times these are conducted by European apprentices of a "traditional" shaman or by a self-proclaimed European shaman or designated "shamanic practitioners."

Individual "ritual experiments," described as "do-it-yourself rituals" by A-delaars (2006), were also observed in Europe. For the purpose of this study, I classify a wide category of activities under this label. "Self-made" rituals are rituals that an individual or a very small group of users created on their own. Such "rituals" are very diversified; they do not have a firm shape or delineated philosophical commitments. Sometimes these activities are intended as "no rituals," which actively seek to have no formal rules and norms. In very few cases people cook their own brew, for example, buying "ayahuasca kits" from online markets.

Although the spiritual or religious orientation of these rituals is very different, "healing experiences" could occur within all three settings. This study did not intend to do a statistical analyses or scientific pharmaceutical tests of the effectiveness of ayahuasca in treating special diseases. It was designed as a qualitative analysis of subjective reports of (self-) treatment with ayahuasca in diverse forms of "healing rituals." Before describing the therapeutic effects of ayahuasca to different diseases, I want to clarify some concepts and terms about healing and curing.

Cultural and Individual Conceptualizations of Healing

Although everybody uses the word "healing," it is often not really clear what is meant by it. Scientifically, there is no consistent definition of healing, since there are a lot of divergent concepts in the different disciplines, varying from strict medical definitions (curing and health) to religious ideas of healing and salvation. The word "healing" is used in very different contexts. In medical or psychological contexts the term "healing" is usually avoided because of its ambivalent and sometimes religious nature. In the context of ayahuasca rituals, healing does not only mean convalescence but also coping in general. This means not only coping with the illness itself, but coping with all kind of difficulties and challenges in life (such as lack of money, an unsatisfying job, personal relationships, etc.). Often the term "healing" is used to describe a kind of problem solving, including awareness or sudden revelations or insights. For many participants in ayahuasca rituals, healing is not a state, but is understood as a process of learning about coping with life in general and becoming psychologically, or even spiritually, mature. It is believed that many diseases in the West come from a spiritual disconnect from other human beings or from nature in general. These findings are similar to those of Fotiou (2012).

In accord with Csordas (2002), I define four healing categories: (a) healing as solving problems or curing symptoms of a disease, (b) healing as salvation, (c) healing as a process of inner growth or psychological maturation, and (d) healing as enlightenment or perception of the truth. This is a much broader view of healing than the strictly scientific one. This can also lead to cases such as that of one patient who firmly believed that he was healed from his disease in a spiritual way in an ayahuasca ritual, but indeed died a few weeks later because of his age.

Medicine, Salutogenesis and Placebo Effects

> In many European ayahuasca rituals, the ayahuasca tea is called "medicine." In the tribal societies where these plants and plant preparations are used, they are regarded as embodiments of conscious intelligent beings that only become visible in special states of consciousness, and who can function as spiritual teachers and sources of healing power and knowledge. The plants are referred to as "medicines," a term that means more than a drug: something like a healing power or energy that can be associated with a plant, a person, an animal, even a place. They are also referred to as "plant teachers" and there are still extant traditions of many-years-long initiations and trainings in the use of these medicines (Metzner et al. 1999, 2006, p. 3).

For many people in Europe, ayahuasca is such a medicine, even "the greatest medicine on Earth" (Adelaars et al. 2006). These ideas fit in conceptualizations of "salutogenesis" (Antonovsky 1987). Salutogenesis can be translated as "the development of health." It describes an approach focusing on factors that support human health and well being, rather than on factors that cause disease (pathogenesis). More specifically, the salutogenic approach is concerned with the relationship between health, stress, and coping. Many scientific studies have since worked out the salutogenic perspective. This approach is, in my opinion, the best way of dealing with successful outcomes of ayahuasca use or therapeutic effects of ayahuasca.

In the context of healing and therapy, many aspects of the performance of an ayahuasca ritual, or even some properties of the substance, may induce positive placebo effects. Many people regard placebo effects as the absence of effects. This is not true. Placebo effect can lead to real biochemical changes in the body and brain. Moerman (2002) calls this effect "meaning response": a bodily response to meaning. A healer or a healing ritual may initiate this effect. Meaning response is defined as the physiological or psychological effect of meaning attribution in the treatment of an illness. This placebo response is based on the release of various chemicals by the brain in response to human expectations, having a positive outcome on a disease (Moerman 2002, p. 14ff).

Description of Study Participants

Seven patients were members of the Santo Daime church, seven consumed ayahuasca mostly in shamanic rituals, and one person had made a do-it-yourself ritual at home. The frequency of rituals attended extended from one time to over a hundred times. The occurrence of a healing experience was not related to the frequency of rituals. The study comprised eight women and seven men; ages ranged from 27 to 61 (mean average 44.5 years).

Ayahuasca rituals were sought by nine persons as an alternative to treat their illness; they were looking for a more holistic or spiritual kind of approach ("combining body, mind, and soul"), often due to a lack of confidence in conventional biomedicine. Alternative methods such as homeopathy, diets, acupuncture, or even spiritual treatments by healers or psychics were used by 80 % of the sample. There were four people who declared that they had given up biomedicine after having exhausted all available treatments, and who considered ayahuasca therapy to be their "last chance." The other six persons had already been in contact with ayahuasca before they became ill (mostly Santo Daime members). More details about the sample are described in Table 5.1.

Table 5.1 Profession, age, context and reported diagnosis in the sample $N = 15$

	Pseudonym	Profession	Age	Frequency	Context[a]	Diagnosis
1	Claudia Dahm	Cook	43	>100	Daime	Stomach cancer
2	Ingrid Delf	Social educationalist	52	>100	Daime	Herniated vertebral disk gastritis
3	Annemarie Müller	Book seller	55	>50	Daime	Acute hearing loss, tinnitus pyelitis
4	Nicole Braun	Dentist (disabled)	36	15–20	Ayahuasca	Benign uterus tumors (myoma) borreliosis/pain
5	Andreas Weller	Agronomist	39	>100	Daime	Alcohol abuse, aggressiveness pain on the knee
6	Patricia Klaase	Physiotherapist, body therapist	40	>20	Ayahuasca + daime	Detached retina shoulder-arm syndrome
7	Georg Steinfeld	Employee (middle management)	59	10	Ayahuasca	Prostate cancer glaucoma
8	Friedrich Blum	Public employee	37	10–15	Ayahuasca	Depression
9	Simon Virnen	Employee	26	1–2	Ayahuasca	Inflammation/pain in the shoulder joint
10	Tobias Doradi	Geriatric nurse, steward	30	3	Daime	Allergic asthma
11	Werner Harken	Police officer, social scientist	43	>100	Daime	Hepatitis C migraine
12	Carla Boogen	Geriatric nurse (pension)	54	10	Ayahuasca	Depression chronic pain (fibromyalgia)
13	Isabell Maier	Artist therapist	53	10–15	Ayahuasca	Allergy, food incompatibility
14	Egon Dauner	Psychologist, psychotherapist	61	>100	Daime	Asthma influenza
15	Sandra List	Healer, shaman	40	>100	Ayahuasca	Uterine tumor

[a] Daime = Santo Daime rituals
Ayahuasca = neoshamanic rituals (with indigenous healers or self-made ayahuasca rituals)

Table 5.2 Frequency of reported illnesses in the sample of $N = 15$

Disease	Quantity
Chronic pain	7
Cancer/tumors	4
Asthma	3
Depression/alcohol abuse	3
Eye problems (detached retina, glaucoma)	2
Inflammations	2
Hepatitis C	1
Tinnitus	1
Influenza	1

Therapeutic Effects of Ayahuasca

All participants of the study declared that ayahuasca had positive effects on them. None of them regarded ayahuasca rituals as worthless, negative or harmful. The healing effects of ayahuasca were not attributed to the pharmacological nature of the substance, but to its spiritual nature and the role of ritual, including songs, aromatherapy, and the performances of the healers. I found patients using ayahuasca to treat all kinds of different diseases (as listed in Table 5.2).

To evaluate therapeutic effects, I have used medical terms like recovery or remission. It should be noted that this study represented a qualitative analysis of subjective statements, and not of objective tests.

All complaints resolved for five people who said that they were completely recovered. Six people made reports of lasting decline of their observed symptoms. Temporary remission of the symptoms of two people was reported for about a week, and ayahuasca therapy seemed to have no effect on six complaints. One case was hard to appraise because the person reported a "remission," but had never been to a doctor to confirm this.

Case Studies

In the following section, I will give a short description of the complaints and the changes attributed to ayahuasca as shown in Table 5.3.

1. *Cured, complete recovery*. Werner Harken suffered from a hepatitis C he had got while experimenting with different drugs, including heroin. For years he had visited his doctor routinely, once or twice a year. Two weeks after an ayahuasca healing ritual in which he had intensively focused on the curing of his hepatitis, the doctor told him he could not find any signs of this disease in his tests. So the doctor tested him again and again over a period of 3 years until he came to the conclusion that he had had a spontaneous remission and was

Table 5.3 Course of illness and subjective experienced effects of ayahuasca on state of health

	Dimension	Result	Quantity
1	Complete recovery (restutio ad integrum)	Hepatitis C, detached retina, shoulder arm syndrome, (benign) tumors, slipped disk, gastritis, influenza	7
2	Lasting decline of symptoms	Inflammation in the shoulder, depression, tinnitus, alcohol abuse, food incompatibility	5
3	Remission	Asthma	2
4	Worse state of health	Benign tumors, borreliosis	2
5	No effect	Migraine, cancer (prostate), glaucoma, pyreliosis, Fibromyalgia, chronic pain	6
6	Not able to be evaulated	Cancer (stomach)	1

cured. Werner H. said he does not really know what happened, but he thinks it is an "interesting" coincidence because he had never experienced such an intensive healing ritual (Santo Daime) before or after.

Patricia Klaase had a healing experience while doing a neo-shamanic ayahuasca ritual. She "saw" the spirit of a spider showing her how to "weave" her detached retina. Before this ritual, Patricia K. had laser surgeries almost every year, but since then she never again needed one. Also, in another ritual, when she had pain in her shoulder (shoulder-arm-syndrome) and "worked with the energies," she recognized that the problem was gone and did not return afterwards.

Sandra List told me that she was diagnosed with a tumor. She then took ayahuasca regularly and intensively and, after 4 or 5 months, the tumor was not found anymore. The scheduled surgery was not necessary any more and she was told she had a spontaneous remission.

Ingrid Delf had heard the sentence "you are healed" during a Santo Daime work. She explained that in her opinion, when this happened initially, her soul was healed on a spiritual dimension. She said that it took about 6 months for her physical body to follow. Therefore, it was about half a year after the ritual that she was completely pain-free.

Egon Dauner's symptoms were completely gone after taking ayahuasca and since then he always takes a little bit to cure such symptoms.

2. *Lasting decline of symptoms*. Simon Virnen was an athletic person who complained about a pain in his shoulder for several weeks. Despite a few visits to his doctor, nothing seemed to give him long-term relief. After a few days, the pain always returned. After a healing ritual with ayahuasca, the pain in his shoulder was completely gone. He still suffered from stiffness in his shoulder, but this did not bother him to a great degree.

   Isabell Maier had seen the ghost of a deceased relative who told her what to eat to avoid food incompatibility. While doing this diet, she did not have allergic reactions any more.

   Andreas Weller recognized in a ritual that he had lived the alcoholism of his dead father. He realized that he had unconsciously imitated his fathers drinking

and his aggression. Since then, he says he is able to drink alcohol in a controlled way, much less than before and without having symptoms of craving.
Annemarie Müller's traumatic tinnitus declined after a Santo Daime healing ritual. The tinnitus was so distressing before that she nearly committed suicide. She still suffers from a hearing loss, but the sound effects were gone.

3. *Remission.* Egon Dauner and Tobias Doradi had remission of their asthmatic complaints for about 7 days. The week following a ritual, they did not need to take their usual medications.
4. *No effect.* Werner Harken said that in some rituals, he had a feeling that ayahuasca opened his crown chakra and relieved his headaches. However, sometimes the headaches came back right after the ritual. He often experienced an overall positive effect, but this effect seems not to be predictable. The migraine still exists, but there have been some positive changes, at least during a ritual.
Georg Steinfeld had the feeling that the deficits in his visual fields decreased, but a perimeter test did not find any significant changes. The same goes for his PSA (prostate cancer indicator). It slightly got better, but was not statistically significant.
Annemarie Müller did not notice any change of her pyelitis.
Carla Boogen said ayahuasca did not change any symptoms of her fibromyalgia (chronic pain syndrome), but the rituals had helped her overcome problems concerning her psychotherapy. Psychotherapy helped her to cope with her illness, but she had a time when she was not willing to do psychotherapy; ayahuasca rituals helped her overcome these blocks.
Andreas Wellers suffered from chronic pain in his knees. He confirmed Santo Daime had minimized the pain, but in the second interview, a year later, he said he had needed surgery. The surgery went better than expected and there were no complications.
5. *Worse state of health.* Nicole Braun was diagnosed having myomas (benign tumors in the uterus). She came in contact with Sandra List who talked about how she healed similar problems with ayahuasca. While doing these rituals, Nicole B. still went for gynecological tests. First, the tumor shrunk, but then a second and a third one grew, increasing in size. This resulted in intense pain. She thought that she should not combine the opiates she was taking with ayahuasca. Sitting in one ceremony (without taking ayahuasca) she heard the "voice of ayahuasca" telling her to have a hysterectomy, because that would be the only way for her to live. She proceeded to have the operation, and recovered rapidly. She thought this fast recovery was due to the influence of ayahuasca.
6. *Not rateable.* Claudia Dahm told about thinking and feeling that she had a remission of her tumors. She "saw" them shrinking and she felt better. But, because she did not want to go to a doctor, no one was able to confirm this.

Analysis of the Therapeutic Effects

The case studies show that there are interesting therapeutic effects in nearly all reported cases. In most cases, there is at least a minimal positive influence of ayahuasca. This does not mean that all people taking ayahuasca are cured; however, ayahuasca seems to affect the way of coping with a disease in a positive way. Coping includes all kinds of aspects of handling a disease: acceptance, positive way of life, relaxing, etc.

In addition, there is a tendency for people to use ayahuasca *before* an illness manifests itself in the body, for preventive purposes. Participants insisted on the idea that before problems manifest on the "material dimension," they already exist on a "spiritual dimension." Ayahuasca is a medium to work in these dimensions. By ingesting ayahuasca one can reach an emotional-spiritual dimension in which the "true" cause of an illness can be discovered and influenced, and the self-healing of the body can be activated. Many patients think illnesses emerge from stress; for example, repetitive negative thoughts. Negative thoughts (fear, anger, etc.) are seen as a magnet for "energy," causing a chemical stress reaction in the body that can lead to diseases. This could lead to a homeostatic imbalance or an imbalance between body and soul. These aspects are often considered to be the true cause of an illness.

Participants perceive that ayahuasca use had an overall positive effect on their conduct of life and their well being in general. These profound and life-changing effects of ayahuasca were not related to specific diseases. They include:

1. a change in health behaviors, including diets, and restraining from alcohol or cigarettes;
2. enhanced clarity, recognition and sensibility;
3. increased physical well being;
4. energy, power, and strength;
5. better coping with problems and daily hassles;
6. confidence and tranquility;
7. a renewed sense of happiness, love, and joy;
8. a change of life orientation, sometimes including striving for non materialistic values; and
9. improved social competencies, including emotions like gratitude, forgiveness, and humility.

Discussing Therapeutic Effects in General

It is not that easy to scientifically evaluate the specific therapeutic effects of ayahuasca. There are various aspects to be considered, including: the pharmacological effects of the substance and its impact on the human body and mind (Riba and Barbanoj 1998, 2005; Riba et al. 2002, 2006); outcomes of the "setting variables," credited to the circumstances of the ritual; and effects of the "set variables," credited to the attitudes and beliefs and "inner work" of the individual. There are many factors contributing to the general outcome.

We also have to discuss the concept of spontaneous remission. Many medical conditions involve a natural course of better and worse periods, and this can make it difficult to recognize if a health upswing should be attributed to a drug effect or to the effect of a healing ceremony. Moreover, there are indeed spontaneous remissions due to factors we do not yet know. There are also problems differentiating ayahuasca effects from placebo effects. Calling a ritual a "healing ceremony" can activate "meaning responses." Belief in the effectiveness of a treatment can have a positive influence on recovery as well. People do benefit from their belief to become cured by the ritual in itself or through the help of God, energies or spirits from another world. Also, we should not forget, subjective reports can be incorrect. Nearly all healing experiences of the participants happened in the past (from months to several years before the interviews) and therefore there could be false memory effects. Remembering is an active process of reconstructing, and thus the effects of healing rituals may have been falsely attributed; for example, they may have been overestimated or underestimated.

Last, but not least, there is the problem of scientific tests and statistical analyses not fitting so easily into the field of various ayahuasca experiences. Personal subjective reports, as shown in the case reports, sometimes speak languages other than "objective" scientific ones. What do we make of these persons having surgery, doing psychotherapy, and so on because ayahuasca told them to do so? Of course, an operation solves the problem; but should this effect only be credited to medicine? What would have happed if the patients had not been "told" in rituals to go to the doctors? Weeks later, they may have been in much worse condition and maybe then the operations would not have been so successful. As a psychologist, I am convinced that patients' own ideas and theories are as relevant for their recovery from an illness as the "hard facts" provided by science. These subjective theories can be an essential contribution to the understanding of people‘s thoughts and actions (Groeben and Scheele 2001; Currer and Stacey 1986). In the following section, I will discuss some selected theories regarding the curative power of ayahuasca.

Individual Understanding of Ayahuasca

All 15 participants regarded ayahuasca as a therapeutic tool or as a medicine in general. Only three persons reported a pharmacological understanding of ayahuasca's effects, but in line with other often more spiritual concepts.

Unpleasant effects, like intense vomiting and diarrhea, were quite frequently interpreted as perceptible signs of a "healing process." Hence, the experience of vomiting can be an important contribution to healing. It should be noted that subjective beliefs commonly are more salient for the individual than "objective" facts. The majority of participants believed that vomiting contributed to or initiated a healing process through "cleansing the body and soul" while supporting physical, emotional or spiritual healing.

Even in diverse European contexts, dietary rules were almost always associated with the use of ayahuasca. These taboos were perceived to not only avoid harm or risks, but were also a tool to intensify and benefit most from the experience.

One-third of the persons interviewed expressed a religious or spiritual understanding of ayahuasca related to different Christian and non-Christian discourses. They consider ayahuasca to be a "sacrament." Another third of the participants expressed a magical or shamanic understanding of their ayahuasca experiences. The ingredients of the psychoactive tea were described as "spiritual healing plants" or "power plants." Ayahuasca was referred to as the "mother of all plants" and as a "teacher." Despite the cultural difference, an animistic worldview, quite common in traditional indigenous South American cultures, has been imported to European circles in a reinvented manner. This perspective was fully adopted by five participants, who considered ayahuasca a "spiritual being" with its own "personality"; others were ambivalently torn between science and shamanistic thinking.

It is common to call ayahuasca ceremonies not "rituals," but "works." Apart from expressing the origins of people in a society based on the concept of "work," the term "works" here refers to the idea that the experience is not always fun, but often a hard and demanding experience. For these reasons, I propose adopting the term "transhedonistic understanding," with "transhedonistic" signifying that ayahuasca may involve some kind of "having fun," but also incorporates many rules, norms, and personal challenges. One participant made up the term "Gottesdienst-Arbeits-Party" that can be translated to "service-work-party." These aspects are regularly linked to serious and often demanding topics, making it hard to compare this to the hedonistic use common with psychoactives like alcohol and cannabis. None of the participants reported using ayahuasca for recreational purposes only.

Beliefs About Etiology of Disease

I will refer to one interesting aspect of etiology: No one believes they succumb to a disease by chance. All of these 15 patients discovered personal reasons for having their diseases (internal attribution). They could refer to biomedical theories (infections, genetic dispositions, etc.) or psychosomatic theories (stress, traumas, and relationship between psyche and body) or environmental influences. Often, these known categories—that I will not consider further in this chapter—are mixed with other ideas, for example, "balance" or "energy" theories (five persons). To summarize the statements: "Being out of balance makes you sick"; "If body, mind, and soul are unbalanced, it is only a matter of time before you will fall ill"; "If your energy is blocked, you might get an ailment"; "Disturbances in the flow of energy might result in severe diseases." Participants insisted on the idea that, before problems manifest on the material level, they already exist on a spiritual level. Being "out of balance" (not only physically but psychically and spiritually) is considered as a source of illness. The disease you might get appeared to be undetermined, but it seemed just a matter of time before you would get a disease. This belief is often combined with complex theories about the energy flow of the body. This could also include a lack of spirituality, or not being connected with Mother Nature. It is also said that constant repetition of negative thoughts or affirmations will not only make one unbalanced, but cause chemical reactions of the body that could make one sick. Therefore, people frequently tried to use ayahuasca *before* "an illness manifests itself in the body" (primary prevention).

About one-third of them had either magical ideas (six persons) or shamanic ideas (four persons). One idea presented was that if you had once the strong wish to die, you would get cancer; or, if you have problems with your sexuality, you might get a prostate cancer; or, if you "swallow" your anger or your negative emotions in general, you will get cancer in your stomach. There are also ideas of spirits sucking energy that might result in depression, or the loss of one's soul, which also might precipitate depression.

Most of the persons interviewed also had the idea that their disease teaches them important things and gives them deep insights into their conduct in life, or that it is an initiation process. Not only can ayahuasca be a "teacher," but also, so may the disease itself. Ayahuasca often helped "translating" the intent of an illness to the sick person. This means that the disease may not be purely negative, and may even be helpful; for example, to get a rest or timeout.

Beliefs About the Healing Mechanisms of Ayahuasca

Chemical or pharmacological effects only play a minor role in peoples' understanding of the healing mechanisms of ayahuasca. Only four participants mentioned pharmacological effects. They related to their knowledge of MAOIs and their antidepressant effect, or brought up the idea of MAOIs having an antiallergenic effect, with DMT potentiating these effects.

The most important healing mechanism in the cleaning of body, mind, and soul is the purgative effects of ayahuasca. Although purging is not a necessary part of all rituals, it is sometimes instigated with the use of liquid tobacco, and people are encouraged to get rid of negative things through this kind of "cleansing process." Most patients experienced not only cleansing the body (physical healing) but also an emotional cleansing (emotional healing) or spiritual cleansing ("healing of the soul"). This purification was regarded as fundamental for the improvement of health.

All participants expressed the idea that ayahuasca helped them by activating or stimulating their self-healing powers. This idea is often connected with the concept of an "inner healer." This is based on the belief that everybody has the wisdom and the power to heal any illness without the need of invasive procedures or the introduction of pharmaceutical drugs. People having this idea did not consider themselves as passive patients but as actively contributing to their healing process. Subjects were also convinced of the possibility that ayahuasca itself maintained a "spiritual level of consciousness." The plant itself was seen as a spiritual being. One participant stated that psychoactive plants had a "constructive intelligence" of their own. She thought that the "spirit" of the plant would be able to "communicate with every cell of a person and repair the DNA of a person." Participants commonly perceived "vibrations" felt under the influence of ayahuasca as a "communication between plant and body."

Insights and realization of "the truth" were also important for all of the subjects. These insights can affect not only the disease, but also life in general, often leading to changes in mind. After becoming aware of the "true reason" for a problem, people were able to change things in their lives that might have caused the illness.

Almost all subjects thought that a transpersonal experience could be curative in itself by changing their way of thinking or acting. Transpersonal experience included religious, spiritual, animistic or indigenous-shamanic aspects and episodes such as out-of-body experiences and similar moments in which people lose their fear of death. Fourteen people referred to such transpersonal experiences.

There is also another aspect that should not be ignored: Some people experienced getting help from other entities. These entities, or spirits, helped them in various ways: performing spiritual operations, extractions, providing insights, and in other ways. Sometimes such entities took the form of negative spirits that could also be the source of an illness, as in cases of spiritual possession.

Comparing ayahuasca therapy to professional biomedicine, participants regarded ayahuasca as the medium that gave them the possibility of healing on a spiritual level. They believed such spiritual principles would not be seriously regarded within the "materialistic" concepts of biomedicine. In contrast to biomedicine, there is plenty of space for spiritual concepts in the ayahuasca rituals. Additionally, people perceived a "holistic dimension" in ayahuasca experience that they considered to be essential.

Types of Ayahuasca Users

Based on the comparative analysis of the main motivational orientation, I could identify seven types of ayahuasca users (Schmid 2010):

1. Only loosely connected to an ayahuasca network or church, the "event type" uses ayahuasca only occasionally (e.g., often by attending in workshop-like settings or within an organized trip to South America). Often, they only attend a few rituals a year or have only one trip to a "healing camp."
2. The "therapy type" is either searching for an alternative cure for a specific medical disease as a complement to scientific medical treatment or for

"psycholytic therapy," as a complement to classical psychotherapy. Ayahuasca is considered a therapeutic device for all kinds of maladies. When the intended curative effects fail to occur, the therapy types often transform into a spiritual or religious type. Remarkably, when people become more spiritual, they also become healthier.
3. The "seeker type" is an individual searching for a philosophy, concepts of identity, or an affirmation of his or her reality. This frequently unresolved search is not limited to psychoactives, but may also include meditation, yoga, Buddhism, and many other schools of thought. Often a seeker is a postmodern rationalist.
4. The "healer type" is often a "gifted" person who thinks of him or herself as having the power and mission to cure or help other people by facilitating ayahuasca sessions for them. This usually happens after they have had a healing experience with ayahuasca or had revelations about their future as a "healer."
5. The "spiritual type" is on a search for individual transpersonal or spiritual experiences. The religious type differs from the spiritual one by using ayahuasca within a stable committed community of ayahuasca users, like a church, and is therefore often more willing to accept dogmatic world views.
6. The "substance user type" is often experienced with a large number of psychoactive drugs. He consumes ayahuasca in a way that is very similar to his or her use of other kinds of psychoactive substances (LSD, magic mushrooms, etc.). He may be driven by recreational motives or sheer curiosity.
7. Being different is part of the "alternative type," a category that is often an expression of ecological orientation sometimes combined with non-conformist personalities. Often these persons are engaged in activities like saving the rainforest or fighting for the rights of indigenous people.

This typology constitutes qualitatively grounded prototypes. These could be used for further research to substantiate them into statistically grounded empirical types. The seven types are useful for describing diverse ayahuasca users. Also, being grounded in a study of healing experiences, this typology is not limited to those in search of healing or improvement of disease. The typology acknowledges the possibility that an individual could switch between different types over the course of time. For example, an individual may at first be categorized as a "substance user" and later as a "spiritual type," or even a "healer."

Some Personal Notes on the Different Diseases

These are my concluding remarks on some of the main diseases I came across in my 10 years of working in the field.

Cancer. I came across various stories about curing cancer with ayahuasca. Not all of them seem to be reliable, and only parts of them can be checked to some extent. There are so many different kinds of cancer, and even if you have the same group of cancer (prostate, breast or uterus) there are all kind of stages (size, deepness, lymph nodes affected or metastasis) that are responsible for positive or negative outcomes. As described, I met people who tried to cure themselves with ayahuasca and who found themselves going to hospitals for surgery because the spirit of ayahuasca told them to do so. On the other hand, I met people who were given up on by biomedicine and who still are alive or who have lived for many years. One of these was Geraldine Fijneman, a leader of Santo Daime in the Netherlands, who had an inoperable brain tumor (see: http://www.santodaime.org/archives/midia/geraldine.htm). In my personal view, it would be inexcusable not to recognize and utilize this progress in science.

Depression and burnout. From a psychological point of view, ayahuasca is a good tool in the treatment of depressions and burnout. Ayahuasca rituals can change moods which is a good support in overcoming depression. If joy, love, and other positive feelings are experienced, the body's own chemicals may change, having the same effects as an antidepressant pill. Additionally, the brain changes because of these experiences: thinking may be altered, and therefore behavior. Furthermore, people may realize what caused their depression, for example, bad relationships, unsatisfying jobs, traumatic events, etc., and learn a better relationship with themselves. These insights can help to solve these problems; for example, getting a satisfying new job might alleviate depression. Of course, though not every bad mood is a depression, ayahuasca might be of some assistance. There are also interesting aspects in the topic of burnout. Many of the unspecific effects patients experience with ayahuasca (awareness, tranquility, tending toward a non-materialistic way of life, etc.) are essential steps in overcoming burnout or depression in general.

Cigarettes, alcohol, and drug abuse. As a result of ayahuasca use, many people seem to have given up some of their bad habits, or have achieved a controlled way of consumption of drugs like cigarettes and alcohol. An exception is marijuana ("Santa Maria") that was a sacrament in some Santo Daime groups and was therefore often used in the rituals. Ayahuasca seems to be really effective in the treatment of drug abuse (see chapters by Bouso and Riba; Loizaga-Velder & Loizaga Pazzi; and Labate, this volume).

Pain (chronic back pain, headaches and migraine). Several participants remarked on the painkilling effects of ayahuasca. It is important to know that pain is often aggravated by anxiety. There are some studies showing ayahuasca diminishes anxiety (Santos et al. 2007), which may result in less pain. There is a vicious circle of pain—tension—feeling. Fear, anxiety, and bad moods aggravate pain and tension. Being in high spirits results in better coping with pain.

Some people have overcome their migraines, or at least dramatically reduced the amount of migraine attacks; on the other hand, I have met a lot of ayahuasca users still suffering from them. One reason for this might be that stress can be a concern when attending rituals. Stress is a main factor in headaches and can trigger migraines. Stressors are mostly not in the ritual itself and its effect, but in the surroundings. In Europe, people often have to travel a long way to get to ayahuasca rituals. Driving several hours by car, and other demands, can be nerve-wracking. In my opinion, ayahuasca can be helpful in the treatment of migraines, but it is essential to care for oneself and to respect one's own limits. Also, we must face the problem that in many countries in Europe, ayahuasca is illegal. A lot of people have been in trouble with the police or have even been arrested. So, people are often afraid of being discovered, persecuted, or legally charged. Even in the Netherlands, where the Santo Daime holds some level of legal recognition, the police often make their presence known and cause the participants to feel uncomfortable, or may even disturb rituals without any reason. Many rituals, both of Santo Daime and neoshamanic practitioners in Europe, are underground and kept secret. These are not the best conditions for building strong communities and establishing solid informal, social, and cultural means of control.

Conclusions

Healing effects occurred in all these different kinds of ayahuasca rituals but, of course, all these rituals are intended for healing. "Healing" is not limited to the cure of physical and mental diseases, but is expanded to a variety of psychological and even spiritual problems. Most Westerners employ ayahuasca almost exclusively for spiritual purposes, in line with traditional usage, neo-shamanic ceremonies, organized churches, and workshop-like settings. There is growing evidence from natural science and psychology that drinking ayahuasca can be a very rewarding experience (Schmid 2010; Grob et al. 1996).

Its users regard ayahuasca as an important aid in solving problems and in coping with diseases. However, it seems to be a Westerners' view to consider ayahuasca strictly as a healing medium. Instead, in traditional cultures, ayahuasca can also be used for sorcery and can even be used to harm others. In traditional medicine, ayahuasca is understood as a plant that can heal or can harm depending on the person who uses it or the purpose for which it is used.

It is very important not to give the impression that ayahuasca is a panacea that cures all kind of diseases in all of their stages. Sometimes, other therapies are crucial; for example, surgeries, and it is important for patients to know this. It should come as no surprise that an indigenous healer may give advice to go to a Western doctor or that a patient may get an insight that surgery really is necessary. As with other complementary treatments, there should be a way to combine both methods.

References

Adelaars, A., Rätsch, C., & Müller-Ebeling, C. (2006). *Ayahuasca rituale, zaubertränke und visionäre kunst aus amazonien*. Baden: AT Verlag.

Antonovsky, A. (1987). *Unraveling the mystery of health: How people manage stress and stay well*. San Francisco, CA: Jossey Bass.

Csordas, T. J. (2002). *Body/meaning/healing (contemporary anthropology of religion)*. New York, NY: Palgrave Macmillan.

Currer, C., & Stacey, M. (1986). *Concepts of health, illness and disease: A comparative perspective*. Oxford, UK: Berg Publishers.

Fotiou, E. (2012). Working with "La Medicina": Elements of healing in contemporary ayahuasca rituals. *Anthropology of Consciousness, 23*(1), 6–27.

Grob, C. S., McKenna, D. J., Callaway, J. C., Brito, G. S., Neves, E. S., Oberlender, G., et al. (1996). Human psychopharmacology of hoasca, a plant hallucinogen used in ritual context in Brazil. *The Journal of Nervous and Mental Disease, 184*(2), 86–94.

Groeben, N., & Scheele, B. (2001). Dialogue-Hermeneutic method and the "research program subjective theories." *Qualitative Social Research: Forum Qualitative Sozialforschung, 2*(1), Art. 10. http://nbn-resolving.de/urn:nbn:de:0114-fqs0002105. Retrieved 27 May 2013.

Labate, B. C., dos Santos, R. G., Strassman, R., Anderson, B., & Mizumoto, S. Effect of Santo Daime Membership on Substance Dependence. In this volume.

Loizaga-Velder, A., & Loizaga Pazzi, A. Therapist and patient perspectives on ayahuasca-assisted treatment for substance dependence. In this volume.

Luna, L. E. (1986). *Vegetalismo: Shamanism among the mestizo population of the Peruvian Amazon*. Stockholm: Almqvist & Wiksell International.

Metzner, R. (1999). *Ayahuasca: Hallucinogens, consciousness and the spirit of nature*. New York, NY: Thunder's Mouth Press.

Metzner, R. (2006). *Ayahuasca: Sacred vine of spirits*. Rochester, NY: Park Street Press.

Moerman, D. (2002). *Meaning, medicine, and the "placebo effect."* Cambridge: Cambridge University Press.

Riba, J., & Barbanoj, M. J. (1998). A pharmacological study of ayahuasca in healthy volunteers. *Bulletin of Multidisciplinary Association for Psychedelic Studies, 8*(3), 12–15.

Riba, J., Anderer, P., Morte, A., Urbano, G., Jane, F., Saletu, B., et al. (2002). Topographic pharmaco-EEG mapping of the effects of the South American psychoactive beverage ayahuasca in healthy volunteers. *Clinical Pharmacology, 53*, 613–628.

Riba, J., & Barbanoj, M. (2005). Bringing ayahuasca to the clinical research laboratory. *Journal of Psychoactive Drugs, 37*(2), 219–230.

Riba, J., Romero, S., Grasa, E., Mena, E., Carrio, I., & Barbanoj, M. (2006). Increased frontal and paralimbic activation following ayahuasca, the pan-Amazonian inebriant. *Psychopharmacology, 186*, 93–98.

Santos, R. G., Landeira-Fernandez, J., Strassman, R. J., Motta, V., & Cruz, A. P. (2007). Effects of ayahuasca on psychometric measures of anxiety, panic-like and hopelessness in Santo Daime members. *Journal of Ethnopharmacology, 112*(3), 507–513.

Schmid, J. T. (2010). Selbst-Behandlungsversuche mit der psychoaktiven Substanz Ayahuasca: Eine qualitative Studie über subjektive Theorien zu Krankheit, Gesundheit und Heilung. (Doctoral dissertation). Südwestdeutscher Verlag für Hochschulschriften (SVH). Saarbrücken, Germany.

Schmid, J. T., Jungaberle, H., & Verres, R. (2010). Subjective theories about (self-) treatment with ayahuasca. *Anthropology of Consciousness, 21*(2), 188–205.

Winkelman, M. (2005). Drug tourism or spiritual healing: Ayahuasca seekers in Amazonia. *Journal of Psychoactive Drugs, 37*(2), 209–218.

Chapter 6
Ayahuasca and the Treatment of Drug Addiction

José Carlos Bouso and Jordi Riba

Abstract The public health impact of addiction, with its high relapse rates and the limited efficacy of available treatments, has prompted the search for alternative therapeutic approaches. In recent times, there has been renewed interest in the anti-addictive potential of psychedelics. Consumption of ayahuasca, the N,N-dimethyltryptamine-containing Amazonian plant tea, is experiencing unprecedented expansion. The ritual use of this brew, obtained from *Banisteriopsis caapi* and *Psychotria viridis,* in shamanistic and religious contexts is now popular in Europe and North America. Studies of long-term ayahuasca-church members in Brazil have recorded discontinuation of drug use after starting ayahuasca use. Furthermore, several centers that offer therapies based on ayahuasca as a means to treat addictive behavior claim higher success rates than more traditional approaches. In this chapter, we review the pharmacology of ayahuasca and the data available concerning its efficacy in the treatment of drug addiction. Although the therapeutic potential of ayahuasca, based on the evidence examined, is promising, the lack of systematic studies precludes firm conclusions. Ideally, research methodology should be improved, with future studies implementing well-planned clinical protocols with adequate controls, end-points, and follow-up.

J. C. Bouso (✉)
Institut Hospital del Mar d'Investigacions Mèdiques de Barcelona (IMIM), International Center for Ethnobotanical Education, Research and Service (ICEERS), C/Sants 168, 3° 1ª 08028 Barcelona, Spain
e-mail: jcbouso@iceers.org
URL: http://www.iceers.org

J. Riba
Departament de Farmacologia i Terapèutica, Universitat Autònoma de Barcelona and Centre d'Investigació de Medicaments, Hospital de la Santa Creu i Sant Pau, C/Sant Antoni María Claret, 167 08025 Barcelona, Spain
e-mail: jriba@santpau.cat

B. C. Labate and C. Cavnar (eds.), *The Therapeutic Use of Ayahuasca*,
DOI: 10.1007/978-3-642-40426-9_6,

What is Ayahuasca and Who Takes it?

Ayahuasca is a psychotropic brew widely used throughout the Amazon Basin by the indigenous and *mestizo* peoples in their magical, ritual, and medicinal practices (Schultes and Hofmann 1979). In its most common form, ayahuasca is obtained by brewing the stems of *Banisteriopsis caapi*, a vine containing the β-carboline alkaloids harmine, harmaline, and tetrahydroharmine, together with the leaves of the bush *Psychotria viridis* or the leaves of the vine *Diplopterys cabrerana*, depending on the ecological area. Both plants are rich in the psychedelic compound N,N-dimethyltryptamine (DMT). In reality, however, the Amazonian ayahuasca mixtures are much more complex regarding their plant content, and the only ingredient that all mixtures necessarily contain is *Banisteriopsis caapi*. Whatever the combination, *B. caapi* is usually boiled and then, depending on the specific indigenous group, and even on the particular shaman, other plants are generally added. According to Ott (1994), around 100 plant species from 39 different families are known to be used as ayahuasca additives. Several of these admixture plants have medicinal properties and some contain stimulant and visionary compounds (for a comprehensive list of the different admixture plants used, see Ott 1994). Each Amazonian ayahuasca brew may therefore have its own idiosyncratic effects that are unique to that particular preparation. The Amazonian peoples' tremendously rich knowledge of plants is perfectly illustrated in the quote: "Every time one of the old shamans dies, it's as if a library has burned to the ground" (Plotkin 1994).

The narrow Western conception of considering ayahuasca as the mixture of *B. caapi* and *P. viridis* or, from a pharmacological perspective, as the combination of a monoamine oxidase inhibitor (MAOI) and DMT, is perhaps the consequence of the popularity and worldwide expansion of the so-called "ayahuasca religions" (Labate et al. 2008). Ayahuasca religions originated in Brazil and they all share the syncretism between Christian beliefs and Amazonian cosmovision. For most Amazonian cultures, ayahuasca is the tool that allows entry into the spiritual, *real* world, where the entities that rule the forces of the world and nature live. By entering this world and invoking the spiritual entities, ayahuasca can be used for whatever purpose one desires: for healing, for sorcery, for finding lost objects and persons, or just to know and understand the nature of reality. In sum, an Amazonian perspective according to which ayahuasca is considered an entity or spiritual being seems to be universal to all the classes of Amazonian *ayahuasqueros*, such as shamans, *vegetalistas*, and ayahuasca religion practitioners. (For a recent, updated and comprehensive review of the Amazonian cosmovision of ayahuasca, see Beyer 2009; see also McRae 1992, for the history and evolution of the Santo Daime church).

In the particular case of the Brazilian ayahuasca religions, Amazonian shamanic cosmological elements are combined with Christian mythologies in a kind of syncretism. Each concrete religion has its own influences, offering a fascinating diversity of rituals, syncretisms, and belief systems. The two most popular and most widespread ayahuasca religions are the Santo Daime church and the União do Vegetal (UDV). Barquinha is another important ayahuasca religion, but unlike Santo Daime and the UDV, it has not spread internationally. With the exception of the UDV, which is rather rigid and pyramidal, Brazilian ayahuasca religions are dynamic and flexible. Religious groups are constantly dissolving and new groups are created, adopting new names and variations in the doctrine. It is therefore almost impossible to know how many different religious groups really exist. What they all have in common, however, is that they consider that the ayahuasca beverage is the mixture of *B. caapi* and *P. viridis*, and there are rarely any other plants added to their beverages. Even those religious groups that used different ayahuasca formulas in their origins—as was the case of the UDV (Labate et al. 2011)—do not currently accept any plants other than *B. caapi* and *P. viridis* in their ayahuasca.

With the international expansion of the ayahuasca churches, and because of the Internet and globalization, foreigners are becoming familiar with the world around ayahuasca. At the same time, traditional healers, shamans, all kinds of medicine men, and vegetalistas are offering ayahuasca ceremonies outside of their natural ecosystems, and traveling to different parts of the world. There is also a very intense "ayahuasca tourism" (Winkelman 2005), consisting of foreigners traveling to South America just to spend a few days in some jungle location where shamans administer ayahuasca. In the large cities of some countries such as Peru or Ecuador, it is also quite common to encounter travel agencies that offer the occasional short tourist trip to visit a shaman and participate in an ayahuasca session.

In sum, most people belonging to the "ayahuasca culture," independently of whether they are members of an ayahuasca church or followers of a specific shaman, medicine man or practitioner, share the use of ayahuasca not as a drug where people find some kind of psychoactive effect or new experience, but as a kind of therapy or healing process, which they sincerely believe is specific and unique to ayahuasca. It is no surprise then, that they, the ayahuasqueros (the people who use ayahuasca), refer to the beverage as *la medicina* ("the medicine").

Neuropsychopharmacology and Long-Term Effects of Ayahuasca

The visionary effects of ayahuasca are thought to be caused essentially by DMT, which can access the brain thanks to the action of the β-carbolines present in the tea. DMT is not active orally because the MAO in the gastrointestinal tract and liver destroys it in a first-pass effect. (For a recent, exhaustive review of the pharmacology of DMT and MAOIs, see dos Santos 2011). In the recent and distant past, Amazonian peoples developed methods of administering DMT to experience its psychoactive effects, circumventing gastrointestinal metabolism. Inhalation of DMT in snuffs and ingestion in combination with MAOIs in ayahuasca are the most commonly used strategies.

In an attempt to understand its pharmacology, and to characterize its subjective effects and its impact on human physiology, we administered ayahuasca in laboratory conditions. We developed a series of experiments in which ayahuasca was given to healthy volunteers to study the above-mentioned objectives. We used Brazilian ayahuasca prepared from *B. caapi* and *P. viridis* in all our experiments. The ayahuasca was lyophilized and the powder was quantified for alkaloid contents and encapsulated. The ayahuasca thus administered in our laboratory had the same characteristics as "natural" ayahuasca, but lacked the water. The advantage of this form of ayahuasca is that, by administering it in a capsule, we could standardize doses and control for the participants' and experimenters' expectations using placebos and blind designs.

In the studies performed to date, we administered doses ranging between 0.5 and 1 mg of DMT per kilogram of body weight. To characterize the subjective effects, we used the Hallucinogen Rating Scale (HRS) (Riba, Rodríguez-Fornells, Strassmann, and Barbanoj 2001a), the Addiction Research Center Inventory (ARCI) (Lamas, Farré, Llorente, and Camí 1994), and visual analog scales (VAS). Using these instruments, a characteristic pattern of effects emerged. VAS items, which were administered repeatedly throughout an experimental session to study the time course of effects, were significantly increased even at the 0.5 dose compared to placebo. Doses of 0.75 and 1 mg/kg of DMT also increased scores on various subscales of the HRS and the ARCI. It was interesting to note that there were no differences between the various doses administered and placebo in the "volition" subscale of the HRS, a measure of the degree of incapacitation experienced by the participant, which means that volunteers were able to interact with the environment without apparent impairment (Riba et al. 2001b). These psychological effects were replicated in subsequent studies assessing physiological variables and the potential development of tolerance or sensitization (Riba et al. 2003; dos Santos et al. 2011, 2012). An interesting finding in this series of experiments was that the intensity of psychological effects of ayahuasca appeared to be dose-dependent. This dose-response relationship is not typically observed in field conditions when expectation is not controlled carefully.

In our pharmacological studies we also found that following ayahuasca administration, the maximum intensity of the subjective and physiological effects coincided with the peak of DMT plasma concentrations. Another interesting pharmacokinetic finding was the unexpectedly low levels of harmine present in the plasma samples of most participants. This suggests intense metabolism and is also indicative that, at least in some people, harmine contributes little to the central effects of ayahuasca (Riba et al. 2003). Ayahuasca also induced cardiovascular effects, which were less intense than expected, basically consisting of moderate elevations of diastolic blood pressure (Riba et al. 2003; dos Santos et al. 2011, 2012). Furthermore, it promoted the liberation of prolactin and cortisol, but not growth hormone (dos Santos et al. 2011, 2012), and induced time-dependent modifications in the distribution of circulating immune cells. The study of lymphocyte subpopulations showed that the percentages of CD4 and CD3 cells decreased during the acute effects of ayahuasca, while the percentages of natural killer cells increased. All physiological parameters returned to baseline in the 24 h after administration. In a recent study where two different doses of ayahuasca were administered 4 h apart, we observed a trend to tolerance for cardiovascular measures but not for subjective effects (dos Santos et al. 2012). No studies have yet assessed the possible impact of repeated ayahuasca intake on immunity and health in long-term ayahuasca users.

At the neurophysiological level, ayahuasca induces significant effects on the spontaneous electrical activity of the brain, shifting the energy distribution in the electroencephalogram (EEG) toward the higher end of the power spectrum. This shift toward the so-called faster frequencies of the EEG can be measured as an increase in the relative power of the EEG beta band (Riba et al. 2002). While this effect can be interpreted as reflecting enhanced central nervous system (CNS) activity, this activation is different from that induced by traditional psychostimulants, as we demonstrated in a study where ayahuasca was compared with *d*-amphetamine (dos Santos et al. 2011). Another interesting finding from the clinical trials mentioned is the identification of areas the brain where activity is modified under the acute effects of ayahuasca. As discussed below in more detail, at the peak of the ayahuasca experience, activation is observed in cortical and paralimbic areas of the brain involved in cognitive control, emotion, and memory (Riba et al. 2006). The impact of ayahuasca intake on brain activity was also evidenced studying sleep architecture. Daytime consumption of the tea many hours before sleep time effectively inhibited rapid eye movement (REM) sleep, decreasing its duration both in absolute values and as a percentage of total sleep time (Barbanoj et al. 2008).

Regarding long-term effects of ayahuasca, our group also published one of the few longitudinal studies conducted to date. The study included acceptable sample sizes and assessed mental health and cognitive performance in long-term ayahuasca users (Fábregas et al. 2010; Bouso et al. 2012). A group of 127 ayahuasca users who were members of various Brazilian ayahuasca churches and had been using ayahuasca for at least 15 years were compared with a control group in a series of measures of personality, psychopathology, life attitudes, and neuropsychological performance at baseline and 1 year later. No evidence was found regarding psychological maladjustment, mental health deterioration, or cognitive impairment in the ayahuasca-using group. What is more, ayahuasca users scored better than controls in most measures. These results are in line with previous studies with more limited sample sizes where short- (Barbosa et al. 2005; Santos et al. 2007), mid- (Barbosa et al. 2009; Doering-Silveira et al. 2005a; Da Silveria et al. 2005) and long-term (Grob et al. 1996; Halpern et al. 2008) effects of ayahuasca use were assessed. Although the published studies tend to conclude that ayahuasca use can be regarded as reasonably safe, in some case reports, ayahuasca appears to have precipitated serious mental health problems requiring psychiatric treatment (Santos and Strassman 2008; Lima et al. 2002). The reason for this discrepancy in findings may be some kind of bias in the selection of subjects in the cited studies. For example, in the pharmacological studies by our group, subjects had to pass a psychiatric interview and to have sufficient previous experience with psychedelics.

Another requirement was that they had not suffered serious adverse consequences. Another possible bias is that in the mid- and long-term studies, participants were all frequent ayahuasca users. It is therefore possible that people who took ayahuasca and had intense bad experiences or psychiatric complications as a consequence of ayahuasca intake had stopped using ayahuasca altogether and were therefore not available for examination. Future research into the mental health consequences of ayahuasca use should follow individuals or people who begin to use ayahuasca and become involved in its regular use, but decide to stop it suddenly for some reason (Bouso et al. 2012; Bouso and Riba 2012; Barbosa et al. 2012).

Ayahuasca and the Treatment of Drug Addiction

Although ayahuasca has become popular among the psychedelic community as a kind of medicine to treat drug abuse and addiction (there are nearly 150,000 citations in Google for the words "ayahuasca drug addiction"), evidence is weak, fragmentary, and disperse. Its fame as a potential anti-addiction treatment is supported mainly by claims from former drug users who recovered after joining an ayahuasca religion and also by reports from several clinics treating drug addicts with ayahuasca, such as Takiwasi ("the house that sings" in Quechua) in Peru, where patients have been treated using ayahuasca and other traditional plants and healing techniques for over 20 years. Takiwasi is therefore the world pioneer center using this kind of treatment. Other centers in Peru and in other parts of the world also offer patients treatments with ayahuasca, but few have published any assessment of their interventions. Here we review all the fragmentary evidence obtained from the medico-anthropological literature and the reports of various treatment centers regarding the effectiveness of ayahuasca in the treatment of drug addiction. It is important to note that, as no peer reviewed studies have yet been published on this topic, the information discussed can only be considered as anecdotal.

In their preliminary report regarding the long-term effects of ayahuasca assessing personality, psychiatric status, and neuropsychology, Grob et al. (1996) compared a sample of 15 subjects from the UDV church with 15 non-ayahuasca users. They found that although none of the UDV members had a current psychiatric diagnosis, five had previously met criteria for alcohol abuse according to DSM-III-R and ICD-10. Furthermore, in the life story interviews, the investigators also recorded that 11 subjects had a history of moderate to severe alcohol use prior to joining the UDV, with five of them reporting episodes of binging associated with violent behavior. Two had been jailed because of their violence. Four subjects also related prior involvement with other drugs of abuse, including cocaine and amphetamine. Eight of the 11 subjects with prior histories of alcohol and other drug use and misuse were addicted to nicotine at the time of their first encounter with the UDV and ritual ayahuasca use. The authors said, "A common theme was the perceived belief while in the induced altered state of consciousness that they were on a self-destructive path that would inevitably lead to their ruin and even demise unless they radically changed their personal conduct and orientation." A more recent study, conducted by Halpern et al. (2008), assessed 32 regular ayahuasca users, all members of the Santo Daime church in Oregon in the USA. The study found that 24 subjects met criteria for drug/alcohol abuse or dependence in the past, and one met criteria for marijuana dependence, but was in remission at the moment of the assessment. Of the 24 who had alcohol problems in the past, six described church participation as the key turning point in their recovery.

On our part, we have conducted informal interviews with several patients diagnosed with drug dependence and ayahuasca providers such as psychotherapists and neoshamans who use ayahuasca to treat drug abuse. Information from our informants suggested that the therapeutic potential of ayahuasca came from the visions that patients experience when they are under the psychoactive effects. This coincides with findings by Grob et al. (1996), as quoted in the paragraph above. The somatic component of ayahuasca (known in shamanistic jargon as *purga* or purge, a kind of internal cleansing as a result of vomiting) is also very important throughout the therapeutic process. The purga, however, seems to be more useful in terms of body detoxification and the visions seem to be more useful in terms of psychological healing. For many of the ayahuasca providers, however, the purga and the visions are important effects throughout the therapeutic process: Patients undergoing purga not only excrete toxins from their bodies, but also seem to "expel" morbid mental contents. The visions induced by ayahuasca may transfer patients to the past and bring back repressed memories that they can work through, restructure thoughts on how they are conducting their lives, and establish plans where life without drugs is a real possibility. At the same time, ayahuasca intoxication has a physical impact on the body and one of its manifestations is precisely the purga. In this way, the simultaneous experience of physical malaise, visions, and reflections on their life-path help them begin to give up toxic habits. In effect, it is not uncommon that individuals begin to take care more regarding their nutrition and health after they begin to participate in ayahuasca ceremonies (Harris and Gurel 2012).

Recent neuroimaging studies may explain the process underlying the therapeutic schema that both ayahuasca providers and patients report. Using the neuroimaging technique SPECT (single photon emission tomography), Riba et al. (2006) found that acute ayahuasca administration influences regional cerebral blood flow in specific brain areas. Ayahuasca increases the activity of the anterior insula bilaterally, with greater intensity in the right hemisphere. It also hyperactivates the anterior cingulate/frontomedial cortex of the right hemisphere, areas previously known to be implicated in somatic awareness, subjective feeling states, the processing of emotional information, and emotional arousal. Additional increases were observed in the left amygdala/parahippocampal gyrus, structures also involved in emotional arousal and the processing of memories. It might be speculated that ayahuasca helps to bring to consciousness memories from the past, to re-experience associated emotions, and to reprocess them in order to make plans for the future. The reason why these processes may help people reshape their life attitudes may be explained by another recent neuroimaging study. This study, carried out by a Brazilian group using fMRI (functional magnetic resonance), found that while subjects were under the effects of ayahuasca remembering a picture they had been previously shown, the same visual areas in the occipital cortex were activated as when subjects saw the same picture under normal conditions. According to the authors of this fMRI study, their results "indicate that ayahuasca seeings stem from the activation of an extensive network generally involved with vision, memory, and intention. By boosting the intensity of recalled images to the same level of natural image, ayahuasca lends a status of reality to inner experiences" (de Araujo et al. 2011). In other words, patients feel that the visions and emotions that emerge under the effects of ayahuasca are "real," and, if they are real, then one can work therapeutically toward "real" new behaviors in the future.

One might argue that drug-dependent patients starting ayahuasca use are simply substituting one psychoactive substance for another. However, in our longitudinal study, long-term ayahuasca users showed no differences from nonusers in Novelty Seeking and Impulsiveness (Pedrero-Pérez and Mota 2008). Since high scores in these measures have been associated with drug use (Pedrero-Pérez and Rojo Mota 2008; Verdejo-García et al. 2008), the mere search for new experiences may not be the reason underlying their involvement with ayahuasca. On the contrary, members of the ayahuasca religions reported that the experiences transcend the merely perceptual or recreational aspects of psychoactive drug effects.

In a study performed on a group of adolescents from the UDV with a median of 50 ayahuasca experiences each and at least 2 years of continuous ayahuasca intake, the authors could not find differences in the patterns of drug use between UDV members and their controls, but there was a nonsignificant reduction in alcohol use in the ayahuasca group (Doering-Silveira et al. 2005b). In one of our 1-year longitudinal studies with a large group of members from Brazilian ayahuasca churches (Fábregas et al. 2010), ayahuasca users also showed significantly lower scores than controls on the alcohol use and psychiatric status subscales included in the Addiction Severity Index (ASI) , a semi-structured interview designed to assess the impact of drug use in a multi-dimensional fashion (Medical Status, Employment/Support, Drug and Alcohol Use, Legal Status, Family/Social Relationships, and Psychiatric Status). We concluded, "The ritual use of ayahuasca, as assessed with the ASI in currently active users, does not seem to be associated with the psychosocial problems that other drugs of abuse typically cause." Ayahuasca does not therefore appear to be associated with the deleterious psychosocial effects typically caused by other drugs of abuse. Even more, according to our longitudinal study, ayahuasca users take fewer drugs than controls, but have a longer history of drug use before their involvement in their ritual use of ayahuasca.

Some anthropological research has shown how ayahuasca can be useful when it is taken in a religious context. Field research by Ricciardi (2008) and Labigalini (1998), interviewing informants from the UDV who were recovering from drug addiction after their enrollment in the UDV, found that an "existential vacuum" was a common primary reason for subjects to use drugs compulsively. Ayahuasca served to put them into contact with the "sacred," and having an experience of transcendence allowed them to re-orient their behavior in order to give up drugs. Obviously, the doctrine also played a major role in the abstinence process, as did support from the group, which serves as a factor of social cohesion and increases confidence in the recovery. Again, in our longitudinal study, we found that religious ayahuasca users had lower scores in Self-Directiveness (Fabregas et al. 2010), a personality trait that is socioculturally mediated (Cloninger et al. 1993). This might suggest that the doctrine is more relevant than individuality in the self-direction of the initiates. The vacuum reported by Ricciardi's (2008) informants may be filled by the combination of the doctrine and the ayahuasca experience.

Only one study has published quantitative data on the rates of prior and present drug dependence problems related to the moment subjects joined an ayahuasca church. A total of 83 individuals (41 men and 42 women, aged between 18 and 40 years old) participated in this research (Labate et al. this volume). Thirty-six (44 %) participants had been members of the church for at least 3 years. They filled in a self-administered questionnaire that had two parts. The first part was a list of drugs, and the second part was a series of seven items based on DSM-IV criteria. In the list of drugs, the subjects had to mark which drug or drugs they had used in the past and which ones they were currently using. They next had to score the seven items, first from the point of view of their past situation, and then from their present situation at the moment of the survey. If subjects scored five items (of seven) positively, they were considered drug dependent according to DSM-IV criteria. The criterion for remission was not to be presently using that drug. The results showed that 38 (46 %) subjects did not meet criteria for a history of drug dependence. Of 41 subjects that met criteria for dependence in the past, 37 (90 %) had stopped taking drugs, while only 4 (10 %) remained dependent. Nineteen percent of the 41 had recovered from tobacco dependence, 27 % from alcohol dependence, 24 % from cocaine dependence, 8 % from crack dependence, and 5 % from other substance dependence (MDMA, solvents, LSD, and heroin). Though these are quite spectacular results, it is difficult to know if abstinence was achieved thanks to the potential anti-addictive properties of ayahuasca, or thanks to their involvement with a formal religious group. Taking all these data into account, however, it seems clear that involvement with an ayahuasca religion may provide a useful alternative for many people wishing to overcome drug dependence.

In his pioneering book, *The Varieties of Religious Experience,* written one century ago, James (1902/1992) stated: "The only radical remedy I know for dipsomania is religiomania." Although it is quite difficult to isolate the components (such as group cohesion, ayahuasca, and doctrine) that mediate positive outcomes, in our longitudinal study we obtained some indicators that may be in consonance with James' famous quote: Ayahuasca users scored significantly higher than controls in Self-Transcendence, a personality trait that is believed to be socioculturally mediated (Cloninger et al. 1993). Subjects also scored higher in the Spiritual Orientation Inventory (a measure of spirituality) and in Purpose of Life (Bouso et al. 2012). For certain drug-dependent subjects, therefore, belonging to a religious group may be a positive step toward quitting an addiction, and ayahuasca probably strengthens this benefit, potentiating group cohesion while taken under the context of a doctrinal purpose. Whether or not this is so, it is interesting to note that in the study mentioned, ayahuasca users and nonusers did not differ in the personality trait Cooperativeness, so only the fact of ingesting ayahuasca, even in the context of a religious setting, does not seem to make somebody a "better person," if the trait of Cooperativeness (and its subdimensions, Social Acceptance, Empathy, Helpfulness, Compassion, and Pure-Hearted Conscience) are an indicator of "goodness."

The other context where ayahuasca is used in the treatment of drug addiction is in ayahuasca clinics. Usually, an ayahuasca clinic is a center located somewhere in the forest where the tea is administered in the context of ceremonies and retreats, and where Western medicine and shamanistic knowledge are usually integrated. Takiwasi is the most famous center of this kind in the world. It is located in Tarapoto, Peru. Local ayahuasqueros work alongside psychologists and physicians, integrating shamanistic and Western knowledge. The Peruvian authorities recognize Takiwasi's therapeutic method. Takiwasi also provides treatments using other plants and different kinds of traditional Amazonian medicines and practices. Because of the international fame and reputation that Takiwasi has achieved over the last 20 years, other centers in the Tarapoto area also offer ayahuasca retreats to treat addictions. Besides clinics of this type in Peru, underground therapists and centers that use ayahuasca in the treatment of drug addiction problems are scattered throughout the world.

Despite the popularity of ayahuasca as a potential medicine to treat drug addiction (there are even some documentary films about ayahuasca as an anti-addictive medicine; see for example, *The Jungle Prescription* [http://flavors.me/ayahuasca]), and the increasing number of centers where ayahuasca is administered as a treatment for addiction, data regarding real efficacy are lacking. One classic report, which also explains the therapeutic method developed in Takiwasi, offers some data regarding the patients treated in the center from 1992 to 1998 (Mabit 2002). More than 380 patients were admitted between these dates but just 211 initiated treatment. At Takiwasi, treatment is considered to start after 1 month of acclimatization. It is then that the first ayahuasca ceremony takes place. The duration of the stay in Takiwasi is 9 months and there are follow-ups over the next 2 years. Of these 211 patients, 175 were first-time patients and 36 were returning patients; 28 % reached the 6th month of treatment, and 23.4 % finished the entire treatment. Sixty-six percent of the patients were cocaine-paste users; 80 % consumed alcohol alone or in addition to other drugs. Fifty-five percent had already tried treatment, and 33 % had resorted to mental health services. The average age was 30 years and the average duration of substance use at the time of admission was 12.5 years. However, the percentage of those receiving a medical discharge was at most moderate. Most discharges were voluntary; 52 % compared to 23 % medical discharges, 23 % runaways, and 3 % expulsions. Based on the outcome, patient progression during their stay was classified as "good" (favorable development, problems apparently resolved thanks to a true structural change manifested upon several life levels), "better" (some improvement, with evident structural changes, but vestiges of the original problem still present), and "same or bad" (relapse of consumption of substances, although often more discrete, no convincing structural change, frequent abandonment of substances for alcohol). Out of the total, 31 % were classified as "good" and 23 % as "better" while 23 % were classified as "same or bad" and 23 % "unknown." According to Mabit (2002): "With hindsight, we can affirm that about 35 % of those who have lost contact with the Center are, in the end, 'good' or 'better' (that's 8 % of the total), which means that about 62 % of the patients have, in the end, positively benefited of the model proposed at the Takiwasi Center. When one only takes into account the subgroup of the patients receiving a medical discharge (those who have completed the entire program), the positive results rise to 67 %."

Finally, promising results on the efficacy of ayahuasca in the treatment of drug addiction have been reported from IDEAA ("Instituto de Etnopsicología Amazónica Aplicada"), a former treatment center located in the Brazilian Amazon. Because ayahuasca use is legal for religious but not therapeutic purposes in Brazil (CONAD 2010), IDEAA has now ceased its activities. IDEAA was a center of integrative psychotherapy that mainly combined transpersonal psychotherapy, several Oriental techniques of meditation, such as Yoga and Tai Chi, and ayahuasca rituals following Western and Amazonian traditions, such as those taken from the Santo Daime church. For a detailed explanation of IDEAA's therapeutic method, see Fernández and Fábregas (in this volume) and Villaescusa (2008).

Although psychosocial status and evolution was recorded in IDEAA, and follow-ups were conducted for most patients, no data on follow-up has been published to date. To our knowledge, IDEAA was the only ayahuasca center using a standardized protocol of data collection. The protocol included the administration of psychometric rating scales, such as the Temperament and Character Inventory-Revised (Cloninger et al. 1993), to assess personality; the SCL-90-R (Derogatis 2001) to assess psychopathology; the SOI (Elkins et al. 1988); the PLT (Crumbaugh and Maholick 1976) to assess spirituality and purpose in life; and the Frontal Systems Behavior Scale (FrSBe) (Grace and Malloy 2001) to assess executive function deficits. Neuropsychological performance tests such as the Stroop Test (Golden 1994) and some memory subtests from the Wechsler Adult Intelligence Scale-III (Wechsler 1997) were also administered. Assessments were made before and after treatment. In a preliminary study that analyzed data from 13 subjects who underwent treatment for cocaine addiction at IDEAA, positive outcomes were found in all the variables assessed. There was a positive change in the "Self-Directedness" dimension of the TCI-R, a result that is related to good therapeutic outcome. Also, there was a reduction in the "Impulsivity" subscale of the TCI-R, and an improvement in some psychopathological dimensions, reflected as decreases in some subscales of the SCL-90-R, such as Obsession-Compulsion and Anxiety. Moderate decreases were also observed in the Paranoia, Psychosis, Phobia, and Hostility subscales. Several neuropsychological functions also improved, as was reflected in both the FrSBe, a neuropsychological behavioral rating scale, and the tests of performance Fernández et al. (in this volume). Again, these data can only be considered anecdotal. There was no control group, the sample size was small, and some changes may simply be related to the fact that recovery can perhaps be reached simply with the mere passing of time while living in a beautiful jungle setting.

To our knowledge, the data presented above amounts to all the scientific information available to date regarding efficacy of ayahuasca in the treatment of drug addiction.

Conclusions and Future Research

Ayahuasca is a traditional plant preparation that is receiving increasing attention as a potential treatment for drug abuse and addictive disorders. Many private centers around the world offer rehabilitation stays with ayahuasca to treat addictive behaviors. Almost all of these centers combine traditional medicine and ceremonies with Western psychotherapy and medicines. Although the pharmacology of ayahuasca is relatively well characterized, and studies on the consequences for mental health of the long-term use of ayahuasca are increasing, evidence on the efficacy of ayahuasca to treat drug addiction is scarce. It seems that in the context of a highly ritualized setting where intense social forces are at work, ayahuasca can be useful for drug-dependent patients. Future studies should investigate the different factors involved in the potential therapeutic effects of ayahuasca.

Since ayahuasca treatments for drug addiction have a long tradition in South American countries, where the combination of traditional medicines with Western psychotherapy is common, it would be ideal if these centers could record information in a systematic way in order to address the question of efficacy. Ideally, clinical trials should be conducted and protocols should be elaborated for data collection before, during, and after discharge. Ayahuasca providers should also gather information on potential hazards both in the short and the long term. Ideally too, clinical trials should be designed and their outcomes compared with results from naturalistic settings. Only in this way will the question be answered as to whether ayahuasca should be included in the therapeutic arsenal as a treatment for drug addiction.

References

Barbanoj, M. J., Riba, J., Clos, S., Giménez, S., Grasa, E., & Romero, S. (2008). Daytime ayahuasca administration modulates REM and slow-wave sleep in healthy volunteers. *Psychopharmacology (Berl), 196*(2), 315–326.

Barbosa, P. C., Giglio, J. S., & Dalgalarrondo, P. (2005). Altered states of consciousness and short-term psychological after-effects induced by the first time ritual use of ayahuasca in an urban context in Brazil. *Journal of Psychoactive Drugs, 37*(2), 193–201.

Barbosa, P. C., Cazorla, I. M., Giglio, J. S., & Strassman, R. (2009). A six-month prospective evaluation of personality traits, psychiatric symptoms and quality of life in ayahuasca-naïve subjects. *Journal of Psychoactive Drugs, 41*(3), 205–212.

Barbosa, P. C., Mizumoto, S., Bogenschutz, M. P., & Strassman, R. J. (2012). Health status of ayahuasca users. *Drug Test Analysis*, *4*(7–8), 601–609. doi:10.1002/dta.1383.

Beyer, Stephan. V. (2009). Singing to the plants: A guide to mestizo shamanism in the upper Amazon. Albuquerque: University of New Mexico Press.

Bouso, J. C., & Riba, J. (2011). An overview of the pharmacology and neuropsychiatric effects of long term use of ayahuasca. In R. G. Santos (Ed.), *The ethnopharmacology of ayahuasca* (pp. 55–63). Kerala, India: Transworld Research Network. Ebook retrieved June 30, 2012 from http://www.trnres.com/ebook/uploads/rafael/T_12998350813%20Rafael.pdf.

Bouso, J. C., González, D., Fondevila, S., Cutchet, M., Fernández, X., Ribeiro Barbosa, P. C. et al. (2012). Personality, psychopathology, life attitudes and neuropsychological performance among ritual users of ayahuasca: A longitudinal study. *PLoS ONE, 7*(8), e42421. DOI: 10.1371/journal.pone.0042421.

Cloninger, C. R., Svrakic, D. M., & Przybeck, T. R. (1993). A psychobiological model of temperament and character. *Archives of General Psychiatry, 50*(12), 975–990.

CONAD. (2010). Resolução n° 01 do Conad, de 25 de janeiro de 2010. Retrieved June 30, 2012 from: http://portal.mj.gov.br/services/DocumentManagement/FileDownload.EZTSvc.asp?DocumentID={B233B4FE-F67B-4D44-911B-962329DA3D47}&ServiceInstUID={74624DEB-0C14-4B3A-B8F3-CD26DEF53FC1}.

Crumbaugh, J. C., & Maholick, L. T. (1976). *The purpose in life test*. Murfreesboro, TN: Psychometric Affiliates.

Da Silveira, D. X., Grob, C. S., de Rios, M. D., Lopez, E., Alonso, L. K., Tacla, C., et al. (2005). Ayahuasca in adolescence: A preliminary psychiatric assessment. *Journal of Psychoactive Drugs, 37*(2), 129–133.

de Araujo, D. B., Ribeiro, S., Cecchi, G. A., Carvalho, F. M., Sanchez, T. A., Pinto, J. P., et al. (2011). Seeing with the eyes shut: Neural basis of enhanced imagery following ayahuasca ingestion. *Human Brain Mapping, 33*(11), 2550–2560. DOI: 10.1002/hbm.21381.

Derogatis, L. R. (2001). *Cuestionario de 90 síntomas (SCL-90-R)*. Madrid: TEA Ediciones, S.A.

Doering-Silveira, E., Lopez, E., Grob, C. S., de Rios, M. D., Alonso, L. K., Tacla, C., et al. (2005a). Ayahuasca in adolescence: A preliminary psychiatric assessment. *Journal Psychoactive Drugs, 37*(2), 123–128.

Doering-Silveira, E., Grob, C. S., de Rios, M. D., Lopez, E., Alonso, L. K., Tacla, C., et al. (2005b). Report on psychoactive drug use among adolescents using ayahuasca within a religious context. *Journal of Psychoactive Drugs, 37*(2), 141–144.

dos Santos, R. G. (2011). Ayahuasca: Physiological and subjective effects, comparison with d-amphetamine, and repeated dose assessment (Doctoral dissertation). Universitat Autònoma de Barcelona - UAB, Dep. Farmacologia, Terapèutica i Toxicologia, Barcelona. Retrieved June 30, 2012 from https://www.educacion.gob.es/teseo/mostrarRef.do?ref=959049.

dos Santos, R. G., Grasa, E., Valle, M., Ballester, M. R., Bouso, J. C., Nomdedéu, J. F., et al. (2012). Pharmacology of ayahuasca administered in two repeated doses. *Psychopharmacology (Berl), 219*(4). 1039–1053.

dos Santos, R. G., Valle, M., Bouso, J. C., Nomdedéu, J. F., Rodriguez-Espinosa, J., McIlhenny, E. H., et al. (2011). Autonomic, neuroendocrine, and immunological effects of ayahuasca: A comparative study with d-amphetamine. *Journal of Clinical Psychopharmacology, 31*(6), 717–726.

Elkins, D. N., Hedstrom, L. J., Hughes, L. L., Leaf, J. A., & Saunders, C. (1988). Toward phenomenological spirituality: Definition, description, and measurement. *The Journal of Humanistic Psychology, 28*(4), 5–18.

Fábregas, J. M., González, D., Fondevila, S., Cutchet, M., Fernández X., Barbosa, P. C., et al. (2010). Assessment of addiction severity among ritual users of ayahuasca. *Drug and Alcohol Dependency, 111*(3), 257–261.

Fernández, X., & Fábregas, J. M. Experience of treatment with ayahuasca for drug addiction in the Brazilian Amazon. In this volume.

Fernández, X., dos Santos, R. G., Cutchet, M., Fondevila, S., González, D., Alcázar, M. A., et al. Assessment of the psychotherapeutic effects of ritual ayahuasca use on drug dependency: A pilot study. In this volume.

Golden, C. J. (1994). *Stroop, test de colores y palabras*. Madrid: TEA Ediciones, S.A.

Grace, J., & Malloy, P. F. (2001). *Frontal Systems Behavior Scale: Professional manual*. Lutz, FL: Psychological Assessment Resources, Inc.

Grob, C. S., McKenna, D. J., Callaway, J. C., Brito, J. S., Neves, E. S., Oberlaender, G., et al. (1996). Human psychopharmacology of hoasca, a plant hallucinogen used in ritual context in Brazil. *Journal of Nervous and Mental Disease, 184*(2), 86–94.

Halpern, J. H., Sherwood, A. R., Passie, T., Blackwell, K. C., & Ruttenber, K. J. (2008). Evidence of health and safety in American members of a religion who use a hallucinogenic sacrament. *Medical Science Monitor, 14*(8), SR15–22.

Harris, R., & Gurel, L. (2012). A study of ayahuasca use in North America. *Journal of Psychoactive Drugs, 44*(3), 209–215.

James, W. (1902/1992). *The varieties of religious experience: A study on human nature*. London: Longmans, Green, & Co. Retrieved June 30, 2012 from: http://imagomundi.com.br/espiritualidade/james_varieties.pdf.

Labate, B. C., Rose, I. S., & dos Santos, R. G. (2008a). *Ayahuasca religions: A comprehensive bibliography and critical essays*. Santa Cruz, CA: MAPS.

Labate, B. C., Camurça, D. M., Brissac, S., & Ott, J. (2011). Hoasca ethnomedicine: Traditional use of "Nove Vegetais" ("Nine Herbs") by the União do Vegetal. In B. C. Labate & H. Jungaberle (Eds.), *The internationalization of ayahuasca* (pp. 49–70). Zürich: LIT Verlag.

Labate, B. C., dos Santos, R. G., Strassman, R., Anderson, B., & Mizumoto, S. Effect of Santo Daime Membership on Substance Dependence. In this volume.

Labigalini, E. (1998). *O uso de ayahuasca em um contexto religioso por ex-dependientes de alcohol: Um estudo qualitativo*. Master's thesis, Universidade Federal de São Paulo, Escuela Paulista de Medicina, São Paulo, Brazil. Retrieved June 30, 2012 from http://www.psiquiatriainfantil.com.br/artigo.asp?codigo=141. Accessed 2012 June 30.

Lamas, X., Farré, M., Llorente, M., & Camí, J. (1994). Spanish version of the 49-item short form of the Addiction Research Center Inventory (ARCI). *Drug and Alcohol Dependence, 35*(3), 203–209.

Lima, F., Naves, M., Migueli, J. C., Motta, J. M. C., & Brito, G. S. (2002). Sistema de monitoramento psiquiátrico em usuários do chá hoasca. *Revista Brasileria de Psiquiatria, 24* (Suppl 2). Retrieved June 30, 2012 from: http://dx.doi.org/10.1590/S1516-4446200200 0600014.

Mabit, J. (2002). Blending traditions: Using indigenous medicinal knowledge to treat drug addiction. *MAPS Bulletin, 7*(2), 25–32. Retrieved June 30, 2012 from: http://maps.org/news-letters/v12n2/12225mab.pdf.

MacRae, E. (1992). Guided by the moon: Shamanism and the ritual use of ayahuasca in the Santo Daime religion in Brazil. São Paulo: Editora Brasiliense. Ebook retrieved June 30, 2012 from: http://www.neip.info/downloads/edward/acks.htm.

Ott, J. (1994). Ayahuasca analogues: Pangean entheogens. Kennewick, WA: Natural Products Co.

Plotkin, M. J. (1994). *Tales of a shaman's apprentice: An ethnobotanist searches for new medicines in the Amazon rain forest*. New York, NY: Penguin Books.

Pedrero-Pérez, E. J., & Rojo Mota, G. (2008). Diferencias de personalidad entre adictos a sustancias y población general: Estudio con el TCI-R de casos clínicos con controles emparejados. *Adicciones, 20*(3), 251–262.

Riba, J., Rodríguez-Fornells, A., Strassman, R. J., & Barbanoj, M. J. (2001a). Psychometric assessment of the Hallucinogen Rating Scale. *Drug and Alcohol Dependence, 62*(3), 215–223.

Riba, J., Rodríguez-Fornells, A., Urbano, G., Morte, A., Antonijoan, R., Montero, M. et al. (2001b). Subjective effects and tolerability of the South American psychoactive beverage ayahuasca in healthy volunteers. *Psychopharmacology (Berl), 154*, 85–95.

Riba, J., Anderer, P., Morte, A., Urbano, G., Jane, F., Saletu, B., et al. (2002). Topographic pharmaco-EEG mapping of the effects of the South American psychoactive beverage ayahuasca in healthy volunteers. *British Journal of Clinical Pharmacology, 53*, 613–628.

Riba, J., Valle, M., Urbano, G., Yritia, M., Morte, A., & Barbanoj, M. J. (2003). Human pharmacology of ayahuasca: subjective and cardiovascular effects, monoamine metabolite excretion, and pharmacokinetics. *Journal of Pharmacology and Experimental Therapeutics, 306*(1), 73–83.

Riba, J., Romero, S., Grasa, E., Mena, E., Carrió, J., & Barbanoj, M. J. (2006). Increased frontal and paralimbic activation following ayahuasca, the Pan-Amazonian inebriant. *Psychopharmacology (Berl), 186*(1), 93–98.

Ricciardi, G. S. (2008). O Uso da Ayahuasca e a experiência de "transformação" de ex-usuários de drogas no contexto religioso da União do Vegetal. 26ª Reunião Brasileira de Antropologia, Porto Seguro, Brasilia, June 1–4, 2008. Retrieved June 30, 2012 from http://www.neip.info/html/objects/_downloadblob.php?cod_blob=709.

Santos, R. G., & Strassman, R. J. (2008). Ayahuasca and psychosis. *British Journal of Psychiatry* (Online), 3 December. Retrieved June 30, 2012 from http://bjp.rcpsych.org/content/190/1/81.2/reply#bjrcpsych_el_22556.

Santos, R. G., Landeira-Fernandez, J., Strassman, R. J., Motta, V., & Cruz, A. P. (2007). Effects of ayahuasca on psychometric measures of anxiety, panic-like, and hopelessness in Santo Daime members. *Journal of Ethnopharmacology, 112*(3), 507–513.

Schultes, R. E., & Hofmann, A. (1979). *Plants of the gods: Origins of hallucinogenic use*. New York, NY: McGraw-Hill.

Villaescusa M. (2008). Proyecto IDEAA: Terapia integrativa de sustancias visionarias y disciplinas psicoespirituales en el tratamiento de toxicomanías. NEIP 2008. Retrieved June 30, 2012 from: http://www.neip.info/html/objects/_downloadblob.php?cod_blob=714.

Verdejo-García, A., Lawrence, A. J., & Clark, L. (2008). Impulsivity as a vulnerability marker for substance-use disorders: Review of findings from high-risk research, problem gamblers and genetic association studies. *Neuroscience and Biobehavioral Reviews, 32*(4), 777–810.

Wechsler, D. (1997). *Wechsler Adult Intelligence Scale* (3rd ed.). San Antonio, TX: The Psychological Corporation.

Winkelman, M. (2005). Drug tourism or spiritual healing? Ayahuasca seekers in Amazonia. *Journal of Psychoactive Drugs, 37*(2), 209–218.

Chapter 7
Hypotheses Regarding Ayahuasca's Potential Mechanisms of Action in the Treatment of Addiction

James I. Prickett and Mitchell B. Liester

Abstract Drug addiction is an epidemic problem affecting millions worldwide with high rates of morbidity and mortality. Although the number of pharmacological options available to treat addiction has increased, these treatments demonstrate only modest efficacy. New treatments with improved efficacy rates and favorable side effect profiles are needed. Ayahuasca is a medicine that is increasingly being utilized to treat addictions. However, despite its growing popularity, the mechanisms underlying ayahuasca's effectiveness as a treatment for addictions remain unknown. We propose biochemical, physiological, psychological, and transcendent hypotheses to explain how ayahuasca treats addictions.

Keywords Ayahuasca · Mesolimbic pathway · Harmine · Addiction · Dopamine · Serotonin · Dual deficit hypothesis · Neuroplasticity · Psycholytic therapy · Psychedelic therapy

Addiction: A Global Problem

Substance abuse and drug addiction are enormous global problems, with health and social costs exceeding $500 billion annually (United Nations Office of Drugs and Crime 2012). Each year more than 200,000 people die from abusing cocaine, heroin, and other drugs. In the United States, more than 22.6 million individuals

J. I. Prickett
Department of Psychiatry, The University of Arizona, Tucson, AZ, USA
e-mail: james.i.prickett@gmail.com

M. B. Liester (✉)
PO Box 302, Monument, CO 80132, USA
e-mail: liester@aol.com

B. C. Labate and C. Cavnar (eds.), *The Therapeutic Use of Ayahuasca*,
DOI: 10.1007/978-3-642-40426-9_7,

had a substance abuse or dependence problem in 2010 (Substance Abuse and Mental Health Services Administration 2012). Nearly 15,000 people died from overdoses of prescription pain medications in 2008, and almost half a million emergency room visits resulted from misuse of prescription narcotics in 2009. In 2010, approximately 12 million people reported nonmedical use of prescription narcotics in the previous year (Center for Disease Control 2011).

Existing pharmacological treatments demonstrate only modest efficacy (Anton et al. 2006; Hughes and Cook 2006; Marsch 2002) and are associated with non-compliance (Fuller et al. 1986) and misuse (Yokell et al. 2011). Given the high morbidity and mortality rates, as well as the lack of effective treatments, new therapeutic options for drug addiction are desperately needed.

One potential treatment is a medicine known as ayahuasca. Created from plants indigenous to the Amazon rain forest, ayahuasca is utilized by indigenous healers in South America for a variety of purposes (Schultes et al. 1998). Recently, ayahuasca has gained notoriety as a treatment for addictions (Fabregas et al. 2010; Halpern et al. 2008). Centers utilizing ayahuasca to treat addictions have arisen in Peru, Brazil, Argentina, Uruguay, and Chile. Despite this medicine's increasing popularity, the mechanisms by which ayahuasca treats addictions remain unclear. We propose biochemical, physiological, psychological, and transcendent hypotheses to explain ayahuasca's effectiveness as a treatment for addictions.

Biochemistry of Ayahuasca

Ayahuasca is a medicinal tea that is prepared by boiling two plants together for several hours until only a thick liquid remains. The plants most commonly utilized are *Banisteriopsis caapi* and *Psychotria viridis*. *Banisteriopsis caapi* is a vine of the Malpighiaceae family. The bark and vine of this plant contain the beta-carboline alkaloids harmine, harmaline, and tetrahydroharmine (see Figs. 7.1, 7.2, 7.3), which function as monoamine oxidase inhibitors (MAOIs) (Metzner 1999).

Monoamines are a family of chemically related molecules that serve as neurotransmitters in the human nervous system. Monoamines include catecholamines (e.g., dopamine, norepinephrine, and epinephrine) and tryptamines (e.g., serotonin, melatonin, and DMT). When ingested orally, monoamines are degraded by enzymes in the gastrointestinal tract known as monoamine oxidases (MAOs). MAOIs are chemicals that block these enzymes (McKenna et al. 1984). In addition to their function as MAOIs, beta-carboline alkaloids also stimulate the release of

Fig. 7.1 Harmine

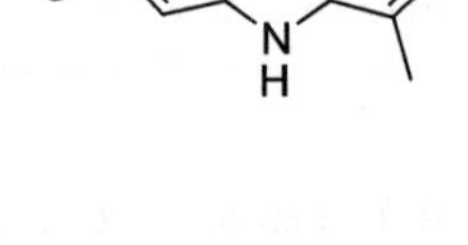

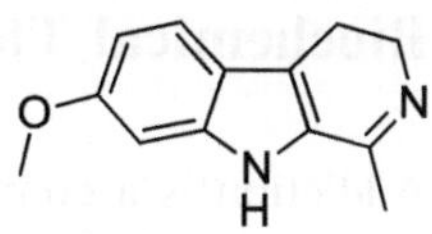

Fig. 7.2 Harmaline

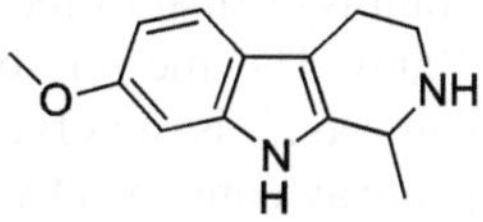

Fig. 7.3 Tetrahydroharmine

dopamine from presynaptic neurons in the mesolimbic pathway of the brain (Brierley and Davidson 2012). This dopamine releasing effect may play a key role in the anti-addictive properties of ayahuasca.

Psychotria viridis is a shrub from the coffee family that contains N,N-dimethyltryptamine, or DMT. DMT is a naturally occurring tryptamine alkaloid that has been isolated from numerous animal and plant sources, including human cerebrospinal fluid. When smoked or snorted, DMT causes a rapid alteration in consciousness (Strassman 2001). DMT is structurally similar to serotonin (5-HT) (see Figs. 7.4, 7.5) and demonstrates an affinity for most serotonergic receptors (Keiser et al. 2009). DMT acts as an agonist at 5-HT1a, 5-HT2a, and 5-HT2c receptors (Dart 2004; Deliganis et al. 1991; Smith et al. 1998; Stahl 2008; Strassman et al. 1994). When ingested orally, DMT is broken down by MAOs in the gastrointestinal tract (McKenna et al. 1984; Shulgin and Shulgin 1997). However, when ingested simultaneously with the beta-carbolines present in *Banisteriopsis caapi*, the DMT from *Psychotria viridis* remains orally active (Mabit 2007). The beta-carbolines, acting as MAOIs, block the enzymatic degradation of DMT, allowing it to remain intact through the gut, into the blood, and then into the brain.

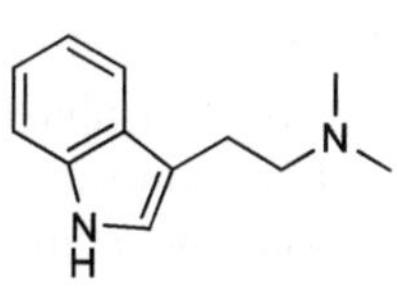

Fig. 7.4 *N,N-dimethyltryptamine*

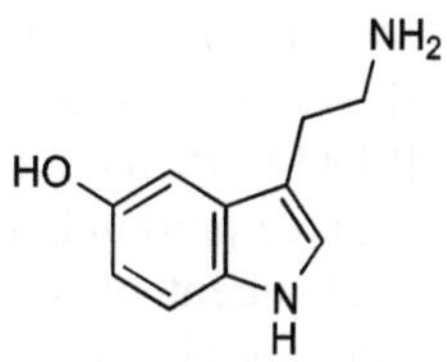

Fig. 7.5 Serotonin

Biochemical Theory of Addiction

Addiction is a complex phenomenon that results from multiple, interrelated factors. On a biochemical level, dopamine (DA) in the mesolimbic pathway of the brain is critical to the development and reinforcement of addictions (Hyman et al. 2006). The mesolimbic dopamine pathway (MDP), also known as the "reward pathway," is involved in motivation, pleasure, and reward (Stahl 2008). This pathway contains DA neurons whose cell bodies are found in the ventral tegmental area (VTA) in the midbrain. These neurons send axonal projections to areas of the limbic system including the amygdala, hippocampus, and medial prefrontal cortex, both directly and indirectly via the nucleus accumbens (Moore and Bloom 1978; Pierce and Kumaresan 2006; Ungerstedt 1971).

Pleasurable stimuli such as food, sex, and video games lead to DA release in the MDP. Dopamine then binds to DA receptors, which are a class of G-coupled protein receptors. Five types of DA receptors have been identified, known as D1, D2, D3, D4, and D5. Dopamine receptors are generally divided into two subtypes, "D1-like receptors" (D1 and D5) and "D2-like receptors" (D2, D3, and D4) (Camí and Farre 2003).

Genetic factors, such as variations in the D2 receptor gene, are estimated to account for 40–60 % of a person's risk of becoming addicted (Blum et al. 2012). Two alleles of the D2 receptor (DRD2) gene exist. Known as A1 and A2, these alleles exist in pairs. This results in three variants of the D2 receptors: A1/A1, A1/A2, and A2/A2. The A2 form of the DRD2 gene is found in two-thirds of the U.S. population, whereas the A1 form is found in one-third. Individuals with the A1 gene have 30–40 % fewer D2 receptors.

The presence of the A1 form of the gene has been associated with "reward deficiency syndrome" or "RDS," a term coined by Blum to describe the reduced dopaminergic state which predisposes individuals to addictions (Blum et al. 1996). Individuals with low DA levels or fewer DA receptors will attempt to raise their DA levels by seeking out substances or activities that increase DA (Blum et al. 2012).

Drugs of abuse (DOA) trigger DA release in the MDP (Adinoff 2004; Pierce and Kumaresan 2006). In fact, they release 2 to 10 times more DA than other pleasurable stimuli (Blum et al. 2012). DA release is believed to be the biochemical basis for the "high" or "rush" associated with the use of DOA and leads to their positive reinforcing effects (Adinoff 2004). Repeated self-administration of DA releasing drugs leads to addiction. Researchers have suggested dopamine release in the MDP may be the final common pathway for the reinforcing effect of all DOA (Pierce and Kumaresan 2006).

Three predominant hypotheses have been proposed to explain DA's role in the development of addictions. These are hedonia, learning, and incentive salience (Anton et al. 2006; Berridge 2007).

The hedonia hypothesis, also known as the "dopamine depletion hypothesis," proposes that DA acts as a "pleasure neurotransmitter" in the nucleus accumbens

(Wise 1980). The release of DA is associated with pleasure, whereas DA depletion is associated with anhedonia, or a lack of pleasure. According to this model, DOA initially trigger an elevation in DA resulting in pleasure. However, chronic administration leads to DA depletion, resulting in anhedonia and craving.

The learning hypothesis suggests DA acts to modulate synaptic plasticity, resulting in the reinforcement of reward-related learning (Kelley 2004). This hypothesis will be explored in the next section on the physiological theory of addiction.

The final hypothesis involves "incentive salience." This hypothesis lists three independent components of reward: liking, learning, and wanting. Dopamine is hypothesized to be responsible for the "wanting" component, also referred to as "incentive salience" (Berridge 2007). Regardless of the model one chooses, the current consensus is that DA release in the MDP is intimately linked with addiction (Adinoff 2004).

Paralleling the dopaminergic neurons in the MDP are neurons that release 5-hydroxytryptamine, also known as 5-HT or serotonin. These serotonergic neurons originate in the midbrain raphe nuclei and send axonal projections to the VTA, nucleus accumbens, and the prefrontal cortex (Molliver 1987; Steinbusch 1981). DOA cause the release of not only DA, but also 5-HT in the MDP. Chronic administration eventually leads to depletion of these neurotransmitters from presynaptic neurons (Dackis and Gold 1985; Morton 1999).

In the 1990s, Baumann and Rothman at the National Institute of Drug Abuse proposed a "dual deficit model" of addictions based upon these chemical changes. This model theorizes that the repeated self-administration of DOA results in decreased levels of DA and 5-HT. This neurotransmitter deficit is thought to be responsible for the symptoms of withdrawal that occur upon discontinuation of these drugs. Reduced DA levels are hypothesized to contribute to anhedonia and psychomotor slowing, whereas lowered 5-HT levels are believed to contribute to depressed mood, obsessive thoughts, and lack of impulse control. Together, decreased levels of DA and 5-HT are believed to contribute to withdrawal symptoms, drug craving, and relapse (Rothman et al. 2006, 2008).

Biochemical Treatments for Addictions

The MDP is being investigated as a potential target for the treatment of addictions. Two competing models have been proposed to explain how interventions at the level of the MDP might treat addictions. These are known as "antagonist" and "agonist" theories.

The "antagonist model" proposes medicines that block DA release in the MDP will reduce the self-administration of DOA. While antagonist theories are appealing, DA blocking agents have not been demonstrated to be effective in the treatment of addictions (Grabowski et al. 2000, 2004a, b; Kampman et al. 2003).

In fact, DA antagonists, including typical neuroleptics, may actually increase the self-administration of DOA (Carvalho et al. 2009; Matthews et al. 2011).

One possible explanation for this increased use of DOA by individuals who are taking DA blocking medications is a phenomenon known as mesolimbic dopaminergic supersensitivity, or MDS. MDS is thought to be the result of compensatory hypersensitization to dopamine via receptor upregulation following dopamine inhibition or blockade. For example, typical neuroleptics, which exhibit potent D2 blockade, may produce increased sensitivity to dopaminergic stimulation (Carvalho et al. 2009). Medicines that block DA receptors to a lesser degree, such as atypical neuroleptics, have been shown to prevent the development of MDS and are not associated with increased addictive behaviors (Carvalho et al. 2009).

The "agonist model" suggests that medicines which increase DA release in the MDP will reduce craving and withdrawal effects associated with the discontinuation of DOA, thereby reducing repeated self-administration (Rothman et al. 2008). This model employs medications that are less potent and less addictive than cocaine, methamphetamine, and other DOA to reduce the potential for abuse (Gorelick 1998). Rothman and Baumann refer to this method as "neurochemical normalization therapy" (NNT) (Rothman and Baumann 2003). Evidence supporting NNT comes from a 2005 study (Rothman et al. 2008) in which a nonamphetamine DA/5-HT releasing agent known as PAL-287 was tested to determine its effects on self-administration of cocaine. The researchers found PAL-287 suppressed self-administration of cocaine in Rhesus monkeys (Rothman et al. 2005). Additional support for the agonist model comes from the finding that low doses of DA-releasing medicines, such as amphetamine and phentermine, decrease the self-administration of cocaine (Glowa 1995; Grabowski et al. 2004b; Negus and Mello 2003a, b; Wojnicki et al. 1999). The dopamine agonist bromocryptine has also been shown to reduce craving for cocaine (Dackis and Gold 1985). NNT has been demonstrated to be an effective form of treatment for nicotine dependence (Henningfield 1995; Rollema et al. 2007), opioid dependence (Ling 1994), and alcohol dependence (Gual and Lehert 2001; Overman et al. 2003).

A major challenge associated with the agonist model is that DA agonists can themselves become addictive due to their activation of mesolimbic dopaminergic neurons (Grabowski 2004a; Rothman et al. 2008). High levels of DA are reinforcing. Thus, in order to be an effective treatment for addictions, an agonist must release enough DA to normalize levels, but not so much that it creates reinforcement leading to addiction. One method suggested to reduce the abuse liability of DA agonists is to add a medication with 5-HT agonist properties. Some 5-HT neurons have an inhibitory effect on the release of DA in the MDP and thus attenuate the reward associated with DA agonists (Rothman and Baumann 2006). Evidence supporting the concept that 5-HT agonists counteract the reinforcing effects of DA in the MDP includes the finding that the 5-HT precursor, L-tryptophan, decreases self-administration of cocaine and amphetamine (McGregor et al. 1993; Smith et al. 1986). Also, medications that broadly activate 5-HT systems in the brain reduce self-administration of stimulants and other DOA (Higgins and Fletcher 2003).

Table 7.1 5-HT receptors and their effects upon DA release

Receptor site	Agonist/ antagonist	Effect on DA in the MDP	Reference
5-HT1a	Agonist	Increases release	Stahl (2008), Li et al. (2004), Ichikawa et al. (2001), Alex and Pehek (2007)
5-HT2a	Agonist	Decreases release	Stahl (2008)
5-HT2a	Antagonist	Increases release	Stahl (2008)
5-HT2c	Agonist	Decreases release	Millan et al. (1998), Smith et al. (1998), Alex and Pehek (2007)
5-HT2c	Antagonist	Increases release	Millan et al. (1998), Alex and Pehek (2007)

Although activation of 5-HT neurons generally reduces DA release, 5-HT agonists exhibit mixed effects on the DA system. 5-HT agonism can either increase or decrease DA release, depending upon the 5-HT receptors involved (see Table 7.1).

Ayahuasca as a Biochemical Treatment for Addiction

Given our understanding of the biochemistry of addiction, an ideal biochemical treatment would provide the following:

- an increase in global serotonin levels
- normalization/stabilization of dopamine in the MDP.

Ayahuasca affects 5-HT in several ways. First, the beta-carbolines in ayahuasca would theoretically raise 5-HT levels via their inhibition of MAO enzymes. Second, as a result of its structural similarity to 5-HT, DMT binds with most, if not all, 5-HT receptors. The actions of DMT on particular 5-HT receptors may play a key role in ayahuasca's effects on DA as well.

As discussed above, dopaminergic surges associated with addictive behavior are thought to underlie, at least in part, the biochemical initiation and reinforcement of a particular reward. In contrast, a relative DA deficit is thought to support addictive behavior, especially the chronic self-administration of DOA. An ideal treatment would normalize and stabilize DA levels in the MDP between the extremes of withdrawal and reinforcement. It would provide levels of DA high enough to attenuate withdrawal, but low enough to avoid further reinforcement of addiction. We propose ayahuasca may achieve this therapeutic biochemical window via multiple opposing mechanisms in what we are dubbing a "tug-of-war" effect. Ayahuasca's effects on DA can be broken down into a dichotomy: mechanisms that raise DA and mechanisms that lower DA in the MDP.

Similar to their effects on 5-HT, the beta carbolines in ayahuasca block the enzymatic metabolism of catecholamines, which raise global DA levels. In addition to this generalized global increase, harmine has been shown to independently release DA in the nucleus accumbens shell (Brierley and Davidson 2012). Harmine has also been shown to block DA reuptake into neurons via the DA transporter (DAT) on synaptic membranes (Drucker et al. 1990). Beyond the beta carbolines, DMT's affinity for 5-HT receptors provides a mechanism for DA elevation in the MDP. DMT increases DA release via agonism at 5-HT1a receptors. Additionally, DMT has recently been found to be an agonist at the trace amine receptor TAAR1. TAAR1 receptors have been shown to modulate dopamine transporters (DAT), blocking the reuptake of DA into neurons, thereby increasing synaptic DA levels (Zhihua and Miller 2007).

DMT's affinity for 5-HT receptors also results in mechanisms that lower DA in the MDP. Its agonist actions at 5-HT2a and 5-HT2c receptors inhibit DA release. Additionally, DMT has been found to be a sigma-1 receptor agonist. Though the sigma-1 receptor is not well characterized, it is found throughout the limbic system and there is evidence that sigma-1 receptor agonism results in inhibition of DA release (Debonnel 1993; Fontanilla et al. 2009; Navarro et al. 2013). We propose that the net result of these opposing forces on DA efflux in the MDP is the achievement of a therapeutic window between withdrawal and reinforcement. Ayahuasca is thus proposed to have a "normalizing effect" on DA levels in the MDP. These effects of ayahuasca on the DA and 5-HT systems are consistent with other medications that have been explored as potential treatments for addictions based upon NNT.

Biochemical Hypothesis

Ayahuasca exerts anti-addictive properties via its direct and indirect actions on dopaminergic and serotonergic neurons in the mesolimbic pathway. Ayahuasca raises global 5-HT levels attenuating withdrawal effects and mitigating against potential dopaminergic excess when utilizing DA agonists. Ayahuasca balances DA in the MDP between the low levels associated with withdrawal and the elevated levels associated with initiation and reinforcement of addictive behavior. This therapeutic biochemical window is achieved via multiple opposing "tug-of-war" effects on DA.

Physiological Hypothesis of Addictions

The physiologic hypothesis of addictions is based upon a concept known as "neuroplasticity." Neuroplasticity refers to the ability of neurons to alter their synaptic connections. Such alterations may occur via the formation of new synapses, the elimination of existing synapses, or the remodeling of dendrites and axons (Chklovskii et al. 2004). Addictive drugs have been demonstrated to reorganize neural circuits. Cocaine and amphetamine, for example, have been demonstrated to produce morphological alterations in dendrites within the nucleus accumbens and prefrontal cortex (Li et al. 2003; Robinson and Kolb 1999). The mechanism responsible for these changes is believed to be altered gene expression in neurons.

Two types of gene regulation are hypothesized to contribute to the development of addictions. These are: (a) up or down regulation of the expression of a gene and (b) a brief burst of gene expression or protein translation. Both types of altered gene expression patterns have been observed in response to the administration of DOA (Berke et al. 1998; Hope et al. 1994).

By triggering the release of DA, DOA activate D1 receptors, which in turn activate cAMP leading to CREB activation (Berke et al. 1998). CREB (cyclic AMP response-element binding protein) is a cellular transcription factor that binds to DNA sequences known as "cyclic AMP response elements" or "CRE." This binding causes an increase or decrease in the translation of numerous genes and alters production of their downstream products including: c-fos, BDNF (Brain-derived neurotrophic factor), tyrosine hydroxylase, and numerous neuropeptides (e.g., somatostatin, endephalin, and corticotropin-releasing hormone) (Purves et al. 2011). DOA influence numerous genes. In fact, chronic cocaine administration has been found to induce more than 100 different genes (Zhang et al. 2005).

Stimulation of the D1 receptor-CREB pathway has been linked to tolerance and dependence with DOA (Hyman et al. 2006). Cocaine and amphetamine stimulate D1 receptors in the nucleus accumbens, which leads to CREB phosphorylation and activation of prodynorphin gene expression (Cole et al. 1995). The dynorphin peptides are then transported to axons of striatal neurons where they inhibit release of DA from terminals of midbrain DA neurons, thus reducing the responsiveness of DA systems (Spanagel et al. 1992; Steiner and Gerfen 1996). D1 receptor-mediated increases in dynorphin can thus be understood as a response to excessive DA in the nucleus accumbens. This increase in dynorphin feeds back to the nucleus accumbens, further reducing DA release (Steiner and Gerfen 1996). Overexpression of CREB in the nucleus accumbens increases prodynorphin gene expression and decreases the rewarding effect of cocaine (Carlezon et al. 1998). Thus, the induction of dynorphin appears to play a role in dependence and withdrawal via a reduction in the responsiveness of DA systems (Koob and Le Moal 1997; Steiner and Gerfen 1996).

In addition to DA, several other neurochemicals are known to influence neuroplastic changes in the context of addiction. BDNF, which is known to play a significant role in neuroplastic changes generally, is thought to play a significant role (Bramham and Messaoudi 2005; Thomas et al. 2009). Glutamate and gamma amino butyric acid (GABA) also play significant roles in the neuroplastic changes associated with addiction (Kalivas 2004).

In the context of addiction, neuroplasticity is thought to underlie what researchers have called "pathological learning" or "diabolical learning." These terms refer to maladaptive learning that occurs when neural mechanisms supporting learning and memory are usurped or "hijacked" by the addiction process.

The hijacked neural learning leads to associations and patterns of behavior that result in repeated self-administration of DOA (Hyman et al. 2006; Stahl 2008).

This maladaptive learning, though pathological in addicts, stems from the evolutionarily advantageous reward-based learning rooted in the biological drive for survival and reproduction. This drive leads individuals to search for natural resources and that are necessary for survival and reproduction such as food, shelter, and sex. The behaviors leading to the procurement of these resources are positively reinforced (i.e., they are rewarded) by the release of dopamine in the MDP. This positive reinforcement leads to these behaviors being learned (i.e., they persist and increase over time). With time and repetition, these behaviors become automatized.

As previously stated, DOA trigger DA release in the MDP. However, there is a quantitative difference in the intensity and longevity of dopaminergic activity with DOA relative to natural rewards. DOA release DA in much greater amounts and for longer periods of time than most natural stimuli (Hyman et al. 2006). This accentuated release of DA in the "reward pathway" has been proposed to reinforce behaviors designed to obtain more addictive drugs (Koob and Bloom 1998). Thus, the biochemical effects of DOA result in the transformation of an important beneficial brain circuit into a dysfunctional, maladaptive one.

The automatized reinforcement of addictive behavior with DOA can also lead to sensitization of the MDP to formerly neutral stimuli. These stimuli, once conditioned, reinforced, and "learned," become sources of dopaminergic elevations that may lead to drug use, relapse, and craving. For example, a heroin addict will learn to associate a particular street corner, spoons, needles, the color of a couch, or a particular time of day with his drug use. Exposure to these stimuli results in elevations in DA that prime the MDP and associated neurological processes, leading to further addictive behavior and reinforcement. Thus, the system has been "hijacked."

While early theories suggested that pleasure or reward associated with the release of DA in the MDP was responsible for the repeated use of DOA, subsequent studies have revealed the role of DA in the MDP to be significantly more complex and nuanced (Adinioff 2004). As noted earlier, there are multiple competing hypotheses. Rather than merely acting as a hedonic (i.e., pleasure producing) signal, DA has been suggested to promote reward-related learning as well (Hyman et al. 2006).

Physiological Effects of Ayahuasca

Ayahuasca acts on many neurochemicals known to be associated with brain plasticity. By acting on these chemicals and their associated pathways, cascades, and related processes, ayahuasca may facilitate adaptive neural architectural changes. These changes may then facilitate the breakdown of pathological associations, triggers, cues, and patterns of behavior associated with addiction.

Neurophysiologic changes can thus facilitate a "rewiring" of the "hijacked" reward pathway within the brain.

Harmine, the predominant beta carboline in ayahuasca, stimulates DA release in the nucleus accumbens (Brierley and Davidson 2012). DMT acts as an agonist at several 5-HT sub receptor types, which also triggers DA release. Harmine also increases levels of BDNF (Osorio et al. 2011). Though not yet well understood, ayahuasca also has effects on gabaminergic and glutamaturgic systems, both of which are heavily implicated in neuroplastic changes (Ciranna 2006; Li et al. 2011). These biochemical effects trigger alterations in the expression of genes that revise the communicative architecture between neurons. These neuroplastic changes are thought to correlate with changes in learned behavior. Thus, old maladaptive circuits may be altered under the influence of ayahuasca to new adaptive circuits, where pathological associations no longer control behavior.

Physiological Hypothesis

Ayahuasca triggers the release of DA in the nucleus accumbens, which stimulates D1 receptors leading to altered gene expression. The products resulting from these altered gene expression patterns trigger neuroplastic changes that reduce self-administration of addictive drugs. In addition to DA, ayahuasca exerts effects on other neurochemicals that have been implicated in neuroplastic changes in the context of addiction, including glutamate, GABA, and BDNF.

Psychological Theory of Addiction

A psychological model of addictions is based upon the finding from the 1950s and 1960s that the administration of lysergic acid diethylamide (LSD) decreased alcohol consumption in chronic alcoholics. Initially, researchers investigated LSD's purported ability to produce psychosis, a concept known as the "model psychosis" concept (Hoffer and Osmond 1967; Hoffman 2009). Subsequently, however, researchers theorized LSD's effects were more similar to alcohol withdrawal symptoms than psychosis, leading them to postulate LSD might produce an experience similar to delirium tremens. They hoped LSD would induce a "hitting bottom experience," thereby deterring alcoholics from drinking (Hoffer and Osmond 1967).

In 1953, Osmond and Hoffer conducted a study examining LSD's potential benefits as a treatment for alcoholism. They selected 24 alcoholics from the inpatient unit at the University Hospital in Saskatoon, Canada. These individuals, who had failed every available treatment and were viewed as having a very poor prognosis by their therapists, were administered a single dose of LSD. The results demonstrated 12 (50 %) subjects were "unchanged," 6 (25 %) were "improved," and 6 (25 %) were "much improved" (Smith 1958).

The positive findings of this study generated interest among other researchers who set out to explore LSD as a potential treatment for alcoholism. Results from early studies were so encouraging that by the late 1960s, six alcoholism treatment programs in North America were employing LSD in their treatment model (Ruck et al. 1979). Eventually, two distinct types of therapy evolved utilizing LSD as a treatment for addictions. These were known as "psycholytic therapy" and "psychedelic therapy."

Psycholytic therapy grew out of researchers' observations that LSD's effects were often very different from those predicted by the "model psychosis" concept. Rather than becoming paranoid or guarded during LSD sessions, subjects were noted to talk more freely about their problems. They also exhibited increased insight into the emotional meaning of symptoms, improvements in depression, reduced anxiety, reduced compulsions, increased sense of well being, and increased access to previously repressed memories (Hoffer and Osmond 1967; Hoffman 2009). These discoveries generated interest in the possibility of integrating LSD into psychotherapy.

The term "psycholytic" comes from the Greek roots psyche meaning "soul" or "personality" and lysis, meaning "dissolution" (Merriam-Webster, n. d.). Psycholytic therapy was reported to dissolve psychic conflicts and release emotional tension (Grof 2009). Utilized more frequently in Europe than North America, this method involved the administration of relatively low doses of LSD at one- to two-week intervals for 15–100 sessions.

Psychological Effects of Ayahuasca

Similar to psychedelic medicines such as LSD, the effects of ayahuasca are highly dependent upon the set and setting in which it is used. The term "set" refers to "the attitude of the person at the time of use, including his personality structure" whereas "setting" refers to "the influence of the physical and social setting within which the use occurs" (Zinberg 1984). Despite the highly variable set and setting in which ayahuasca is being used today, certain common features of the ayahuasca experience have been observed.

Psychologist Shanon (2002), who performed one of the most in-depth studies of ayahuasca's effects, described the following changes following ingestion of ayahuasca:

1. Alterations in thinking: Changes in concentration, attention, memory, judgment, and reflective awareness.
2. Altered sense of time: The rate by which time passes may appear to accelerate or decelerate. The duration of time may be experienced as infinite or infinitesimal. Feelings of timelessness or existing outside time may be experienced as well.
3. Fear of loss of control: A fear of losing control of reality. If cultural conditioning has resulted in positive expectations and a clear understanding of the experience, mystical, and transcendent states may ensue.

4. Changes in emotional expression: Heightened emotional reactivity may range from ecstasy to despair.
5. Changes in body image: Boundaries between the self and others may dissolve including feelings of depersonalization, derealization, and cosmic unity.
6. Perceptual alterations: Visual imagery and hallucinations are prominent and hyper-acuteness of sensory perception may occur. Individual and cultural expectations may influence the content of perceptual alterations.
7. Changes in meaning or significance: Feelings of heightened insight or profound meaning.
8. Sense of the Ineffable: The experience may be difficult or impossible to communicate to others.
9. Feelings of rejuvenation: A sense of hope, rejuvenation, or rebirth.
10. Hypersuggestibility: Increased susceptibility to verbal and nonverbal cues is characteristic of the altered state experience. The ordinary filtering mechanisms that allow individuals to discriminate between various forms of input may be temporarily suspended.

Grob at Harbor-UCLA Medical Center reported these same 10 characteristics are "virtually universal" to altered states of consciousness (2006). Shanon reported these changes might produce psychological benefits resulting from the experience of positive affects and enhanced reflection and insight (see Shanon, this volume). Grob et al. (1996) studied the effects of ayahuasca in members of a Brazilian ayahuasca religion, the União do Vegetal (UDV), who regularly ingest ayahuasca as part of their religious ceremony. He found these individuals scored higher on neuropsychological testing than controls who had never drank ayahuasca. Grob concluded, "the long-term consumption of ayahuasca within the structured UDV ceremonial setting does not appear to exert a deleterious effect on neuropsychological function" (p. 93).

Reports pertaining to ayahuasca's psychological and neuropsychological effects suggest two possible explanations that may help explain ayahuasca's psychological benefits in the treatment of addictions. One explanation suggests ayahuasca facilitates access to important conscious and unconscious memories, allowing the release of repressed emotions and catalyzing the healing of unresolved traumas. This results in individuals being freed from habitual, dysfunctional patterns of addiction. This explanation is based upon the psychodynamic model, which is similar to the psycholytic theory of addiction treatment.

A second explanation suggests ayahuasca allows individuals to observe and experience the past, present, and potential future outcomes of their choices. By witnessing the outcomes of the continued use of addictive substances as well as the outcomes of abstinence from these substances, individuals acquire a more complete understanding of the consequences of their decisions. This allows them to make better choices and to stop using addictive drugs (R. Yamberla, personal communication, March 25, 2013). These two explanations are not mutually exclusive, but in fact may be complementary.

Psychological Hypothesis

Ayahuasca treats addictions by facilitating access to important conscious and unconscious memories, allowing for the release of repressed emotions, and catalyzing the healing of unresolved traumas. Ayahuasca also provides increased insight and understanding of the past, present, and future outcomes of choices that contribute to addictive behaviors. This perspective allows for improved decision making. These effects result in psychological freedom from the habitual, dysfunctional patterns associated with addiction.

Transcendent Theory of Addictions

An alternative to the psycholytic model was the "psychedelic model" of treatment. Hoffer and Osmond developed this model during their research exploring LSD's potential as a treatment for alcoholism. "Psychedelic therapy" involved the administration of relatively high doses of LSD over one to three sessions (Hoffer and Osmond 1967). The goal of this type of therapy was to induce a "psychedelic peak experience," a concept modeled after Maslow's "peak experience" (Grinspoon and Bakalar 1997).

Grof (2008) defined a "psychedelic peak experience" as:

> An ecstatic state, characterized by the loss of boundaries between the subject and the objective world, with ensuing feelings of unity with other people, nature, the entire Universe, and God. In most instances this experience is contentless and is accompanied by visions of brilliant white or golden light, rainbow spectra or elaborate designs resembling peacock feathers. It can, however, be associated with archetypal figurative visions of deities or divine personages from various cultural frameworks.

Harvard professor Grinspoon (1997) explained the primary goal of psychedelic therapy was the induction of a mystical experience that would change the way individuals see themselves and the world. Researchers viewed psychedelic peak experiences as profound experiences that catalyzed recovery from addictions.

In a study published in 1970, Pahnke investigated whether alcoholic patients who experienced a "psychedelic-peak experience" improved more than patients who did not. He found a statistically significant ($p < 0.05$) improvement at 6-month follow-up in individuals who had a peak experience compared with individuals who did not.

Further evidence supporting the notion that transcendent experiences catalyze improvements in addictions comes from anecdotal sources. For example, William Griffith Wilson described a transcendent experience that turned the tide in his struggle with alcoholism. While hospitalized, Wilson hit bottom. As he later explained, what happened next would change his life forever:

> Lying there in conflict, I dropped into black depression. Momentarily my prideful obstinacy was crushed. I cried out, "Now I'm ready to do anything… If there be a God, will he

> show himself!" The result was instant, electric, beyond description. The place lit up, blinding white. I knew only ecstasy and seemed on a mountain. A great wind blew, enveloping and permeating me. It was not of air, but of Spirit. Blazing, came the tremendous thought, "You are a free man!" Then ecstasy subsided. Still on the bed, I was now in another world of consciousness, which was suffused by a Presence. One with the Universe, a great peace stole over me and I thought, "So this is the God of the preachers, this is the Great Reality." But reason returned, my modern education took over. Obviously I had gone crazy. I became terribly frightened (W. W. 1994).

After this experience, Wilson never drank alcohol again. Based upon his own personal experience, he believed the key to overcoming addictions was to have a spiritual or transcendent experience (W. W. 1994). Today, the founder of Alcoholics Anonymous is better known as Bill W.

Transcendent Effects of Ayahuasca

Similar to LSD, psilocybin, and other psychedelics, ayahuasca has been reported to induce transcendent, mystical, or peak experiences (Shanon 2002). Stace (1961) described the following seven characteristics of mystical experiences:

1. Unity: Feelings of oneness behind the multiplicity in the world or a dissipation of one's boundaries resulting in feelings of becoming one with an existence larger than one's self
2. Transcendence of time and space
3. Noesis: Direct, intuitive knowledge
4. Positive feelings of blessedness, joy, peace, and happiness
5. A sense of sacredness
6. Paradoxicality: Seeming dualities are transcended such that a unitive whole is experienced
7. Ineffability: Experiences cannot be defined with words.

Each of these characteristics has been reported to occur in association with ayahuasca use (Shanon 2002).

Ayahuasca has also been reported by others to produce transcendent experiences. Kjellgren et al. (2009) obtained questionnaires from 25 northern Europeans who had ingested ayahuasca between 1 and 70 times each. These individuals described six themes related to their ayahuasca experiences. One of these themes involved a shift from a frightening state to a state that is "limitless, omnipotent, and indescribable" (p. 312). A second theme involved reports of transpersonal experiences including encounters with a spirit world, changes in time and space, and experiences of their own death. A third theme involved changes in worldview, personal development, interests, and healing effects. These included greater self-awareness and a sense of being more present. Subjects also described feeling more love toward others and themselves. Negative psychological patterns were reported to decrease or stop (p. 313).

Trichter et al. examined changes in spirituality among 49 individuals who participated in ayahuasca ceremonies for the first time (2009). Utilizing the Peak Experience Profile (PEP), the Spiritual Well Being (SWB) scale, and Hood's Mysticism Scale (M Scale), they found more than 75 % of participants reported their ayahuasca experience impacted their spiritual beliefs, and over 75 % reported an increased interest in spiritual practices following their ayahuasca experience (p. 131).

Transcendent Hypothesis

Ayahuasca treats addictions by facilitating transcendent or peak experiences. These experiences produce changes in belief systems, personal values, and worldviews that reduce the use of addictive substances.

Summary

Drug addiction is a worldwide problem with high rates of morbidity and mortality, enormous social ramifications, and tremendous negative economic impacts. Existing pharmacological treatments offer only modest improvements in abstinence and remission rates, leaving a great need for new medicines that can more effectively treat addictions.

Ayahuasca is a plant-derived medicine with an extensive history of therapeutic use among indigenous cultures throughout the Amazon River Basin. Ayahuasca's potential benefits as a medicine and as a treatment for addictions remain largely uninvestigated by Western-trained physicians and scientists. Recently, studies have been initiated examining ayahuasca's effectiveness as a treatment for addictions. However, the mechanisms by which ayahuasca exerts its anti-addictive properties remain unknown.

We have proposed four unique yet interrelated hypotheses regarding ayahuasca's potential mechanisms of action in the treatment for addictions. We strongly encourage the reader to view these four hypotheses as distinct yet interdependent. Rather than focusing solely on one level, we believe it is important to recognize and utilize multiple levels of understanding and intervention in order to more fully comprehend the effectiveness of this medicine and to develop more effective treatments for addictions.

Previous studies indicate that ayahuasca can be safe and effective when used in a therapeutic setting. Additional research is needed to better understand and maximize ayahuasca's effectiveness as a treatment for addictions. Researchers will need to take into account the importance of set and setting when carrying out research studies. The belief system of the researcher as well as the individual utilizing ayahuasca may influence the experience resulting from ayahuasca ingestion. Furthermore, the physical and social context in which ayahuasca is utilized may effect the outcomes of ayahuasca use.

It is our hope that future research will involve collaboration with indigenous healers whose extensive experience and knowledge of ayahuasca may add significantly to our understanding of this medicine. Such collaboration has been woefully lacking in the past due to a variety of factors including: (a) cultural and language differences, (b) mistrust of outsiders due to a history of persecution for utilizing traditional healing methodologies, and (c) discounting the value of what indigenous healers have to offer. We must learn to appreciate and value the knowledge and experience of indigenous healers if we ever hope to learn from them. Acknowledging the experience and knowledge possessed by indigenous healers may help us to better understand the benefits of ayahuasca, as well as open doors to yet-unknown treatments for addictions.

References

Adinoff, B. (2004). Neurobiologic processes in drug reward and addiction. *Harvard Review of Psychiatry, 12*(6), 305–320.

Alex, K. D., & Pehek, E. A. (2007). Pharmacologic mechanisms of serotonergic regulation of dopamine neurotransmission. *Pharmacology & Therapeutics, 113*(2), 296–320.

Anton, R. F., O'Malley, S. S., Ciraulo, D. A., Cisler, R. A., Couper, D., Donovan, D. M., et al. (2006). Combined pharmacotherapies and behavioral interventions for alcohol dependence: The COMBINE study: A randomized controlled trial. *JAMA, 295*(17), 2003–2017. doi:10.1001/jama.295.17.2003.

Berke, J. D., Paletzki, R. F., Aronson, G. J., Hyman, S. E., & Gerfen, C. R. (1998). A complex program of striatal gene expression induced by dopaminergic stimulation. *Journal of Neuroscience, 18*, 5301–5310.

Berridge, K. C. (2007). The debate over dopamine's role in reward: The case for incentive salience. *Psychopharmacology (Berl), 191*, 391–431.

Blum, K., Sheridan, P. J., Wood, R. C., Braverman, E. R., Chen, T. J., Cull, J. G., et al. (1996). The D2 dopamine receptor gene as a determinant of Reward Deficiency Syndrome. *Journal of the Royal Society of Medicine, 89*(7), 396–400.

Blum, K., Werner, T., Carnes, S., Carnes, P., Bowirrat, A., Giordano, J., et al. (2012). Sex, drugs, and rock 'n' roll: Hypothesizing common mesolimbic activation as a function of reward gene polymorphisms. *Journal of Psychoactive Drugs, 44*(1), 38–55. doi:10.1080/02791072.2012.662112.

Bramham, C. R., & Messaoudi, E. (2005). BDNF function in adult synaptic plasticity: the synaptic consolidation hypothesis. *Progress in Neurobiology, 76*(2), 99–125.

Brierley, D. I., & Davidson, C. (2012). Harmine augments electrically evoked dopamine efflux in the nucleus accumbens shell. *Journal of Psychopharmacology, 27*(3), 98–108. doi:10.1177/0269881112463125.

Camí, J., & Farre, M. (2003). Drug addiction. *New England Journal of Medicine, 349*, 975–986.

Carlezon, W. A., Thome, J., Olson, V. G., Lane-Ladd, S. B., Brodkin, E. S., Hiroi, N., et al. (1998). Regulation of cocaine reward by CREB. *Science, 282*, 2272–2275.

Carvalho, R. C., Fukushiro, D. F., Helfer, D. C., Callegaro-Filho, D., Trombin, T. F., Zanlorenci, L. H., et al. (2009). Long-term haloperidol treatment (but not risperidone) enhances addiction-related behaviors in mice: Role of dopamine D2 receptors. *Addiction Biology, 14*(3), 283–293.

Center for Disease Control. (2011). Prescription painkiller overdoses in the US. *Vital Signs*, November 2011. Retrieved June 21, 2013 from http://www.cdc.gov/vitalsigns/painkilleroverdoses/.

Chklovskii, D. B., Mel, B. W., & Svoboda, K. (2004). Cortical rewiring and information storage. *Nature, 431*, 782–788.

Ciranna, L. (2006). Serotonin as a modulator of glutamate- and GABA-mediated neurotransmission: Implications in physiological functions and in pathology. *Current Neuropharmacology, 4*(2), 101–114.

Cole, R. L., Konradi, C., Douglass, J., & Hyman, S. E. (1995). Neuronal adaptation to amphetamine and dopamine: Molecular mechanisms of prodynorphin gene regulation in rat striatum. *Neuron, 14*, 813–823.

Dackis, C. A., & Gold, M. S. (1985). New concepts in cocaine addiction: The dopamine depletion hypothesis. *Neuroscience and Biobehavioral Reviews, 9*, 469–477. doi:10.1016/0149-7634(85)90022-3.

Dart, R. C. (Ed.). (2004) *Medical toxicology*, (3rd ed.) Philadelphia: Lippincott, Williams, and Wilkins.

Debonnel, G. (1993). Current hypotheses on sigma receptors and their physiological role: Possible implications in psychiatry. *Journal of Psychiatry and Neuroscience, 18*(4), 157–172.

Deliganis, A. V., Pierce, P. A., & Peroutka, S. J. (1991). Differential interactions of dimethyltryptamine (DMT) with 5-HT_{1A} and 5-HT_2 receptors. *Biochemical Pharmacology, 41*, 1739–1744.

Drucker, G., Raikkoff, K., Neafsey, E. J., & Collins, M. A. (1990). Dopamine uptake inhibitory capacities of beta-carboline and 3,4-dihydro-beta-carboline analogs of N-methyl-4-phenyl-1,2,3,6-tetrahydropyridine (MPTP) oxidation products. *Brain Research, 509*(1), 125–133.

Fabregas, J. M., Gonzalez, D., Fondevila, S., Cutchet, M., Fernandez, X., & Barbosa, P. C. (2010). Assessment of addiction severity among ritual users of ayahuasca. *Drug and Alcohol Dependence, 111*(3), 257–326.

Fontanilla, D., Johannessen, M., Hajipour, A. R., Cozzi, N., Jackson, M. B., & Ruoho, A. E. (2009). The hallucinogen N,N-Dimethyltryptamine (DMT) is an endogenous sigma-1 receptor regulator. *Science, 323*(5916), 934–937.

Fuller, R. K., Branchey, L., Brightwell, D. R., Derman, R. M., Emrick, C. D., Iber, F. L., et al. (1986). Disulfiram treatment of alcoholism: A Veterans Administration cooperative study. *JAMA, 256*(11), 1449–1455. doi:10.1046/j.1360-0443.1998.9345157.x.

Gorelick, D. A. (1998). The rate hypothesis and agonist substitution approaches to cocaine abuse treatment. *Advances in Pharmacology, 42*, 995–997.

Grabowski, J., Rhoades, H., Silverman, P., Schmitz, J. M., Stotts, A., Creson, D., et al. (2000). Risperdone for the treatment of cocaine dependence: Randomized, double-blind trial. *Journal of Clinical Psychopharmacology, 20*(3), 305–310.

Grabowski, J., Shearer, J., Merrill, J., & Negus, S. S. (2004a). Agonist-like replacement pharmacotherapy for stimulant abuse and dependence. *Addictive Behaviors, 29*, 1439–1464.

Grabowski, J., Rhoades, H., Stotts, A., Cowan, K., Kopecky, C., Dougherty, A., et al. (2004b). Agonist-like or antagonist-like treatment for cocaine dependence with methadone for heroin dependence: Two double-blind randomized clinical trials. *Neuropsychopharmacology, 29*(5), 969–981.

Grinspoon, L., & Bakalar, J. B. (1997). *Psychedelic drugs reconsidered.* New York, NY: The Lindesmith Center.

Grob, C. S., McKenna, D. J., Callaway, J. C., Brito, G. S., Neves, E. S., Oberlaender, G., et al. (1996). Human psychopharmacology of hoasca: A plant hallucinogen used in ritual context in Brazil. *The Journal of Nervous and Mental Disease, 184*(2), 86–94.

Grof, S. (2008). *LSD psychotherapy*. Santa Cruz, CA: Multidisciplinary Association for Psychedelic Studies.

Grof, S. (2009). *LSD: Doorway to the numinous*. Rochester, VT: Park Street.

Gual, A., & Lehert, P. (2001). Acamprosate during and after acute alcohol withdrawal: A double-blind placebo-controlled study in Spain. *Alcohol and Alcoholism, 36*(5), 413–418. doi:10.1093/alcalc/36.5.413.

Halpern, J. H., Sherwood, A. R., Passie, T., Blackwell, K. C., & Ruttenberer, A. J. (2008). Evidence of health and safety in American members of a religion who use a hallucinogenic sacrament. *Medical Science Monitor, 14*(8), 15–22.

Henningfield, J. E. (1995). Nicotine medications for smoking cessation. *New England Journal of Medicine, 333*: 1196–1203.

Higgins, G. A., & Fletcher, P. J. (2003). Serotonin and drug reward: Focus on 5-HT2C receptors. *European Journal of Pharmacology, 480*, 151–162.

Hoffer, A., & Osmond, H. (1967). *The hallucinogens.* New York, NY: Academic Press.

Hoffman, A. (2009). *LSD: My problem child.* Santa Cruz, CA: Multidisciplinary Association for Psychedelic Studies.

Hope, B. T., Nye, H. E., Kelz, M. B., Self, D. W., Iadarola, M. J., Nakabeppu, Y., et al. (1994). Induction of a long-lasting AP-1 complex composed of altered Fos-like proteins in brain by chronic cocaine and other chronic treatments. *Neuron, 13*, 1235–1244.

Hughes, J. C., & Cook, C. C. (2006). The efficacy of disulfiram: A review of outcome studies. *Addiction, 92*(4), 381–395.

Hyman, S. E., Malenka, R. C., & Nestler, E. J. (2006). Neural mechanisms of addiction: The role of reward-related learning and memory. *Annual Review of Neuroscience, 29*, 565–598.

Ichikawa, J., Ishii, H., Bonacorrso, S., Wiley, F. L., O'Laughlin, I. A., & Meltzer, H. Y. (2001). 5-HT2A and D2 receptor blockade increases cortical DA release via 5-HT1A receptor activation: A possible mechanism of atypical antipsychotic-induced cortical dopamine release. *Journal of Neurochemistry, 76*(5), 1521–1531.

Kalivas, P. W. (2004). Glutamate systems in cocaine addiction. *Current Opinion in Pharmacology, 4*(1), 23–29.

Kampman, K. M., Pettinati, H., Lynch, K. G., Sparkman, T., & O'Brien, C. P. (2003). A pilot trial of olanzapine for the treatment of cocaine dependence. *Drug and Alcohol Dependence, 70*(3), 265–273.

Keiser, M. J., Setola, V., Irwin, J. J., Laggner, C., Abbas, A. I., Hufeison, S. J., et al. (2009). Predicting new molecular targets for known drugs. *Nature: International Weekly Journal of Science, 462*, 175–181.

Kelley, A. E. (2004). Memory and addiction: Shared neural circuitry and molecular mechanisms. *Neuron, 44*, 161–179.

Kjellgren, A., Eriksson, A., & Norlander, T. (2009). Experiences of encounters with ayahuasca – "the vine of the soul". *Journal of Psychoactive Drugs, 42*(4), 309–315.

Koob, G. F., & Bloom, F. E. (1998). Neuroscience of addiction. *Neuron, 21*, 467–476.

Koob, G. F., & Le Moal, M. (1997). Drug abuse: Hedonic homeostatic dysregulation. *Science, 278*, 52–58.

Li, Y., Kolb, B., & Robinson, T. E. (2003). The location of persistent amphetamine-induced changes in the density of dendritic spines on medium spiny neurons in the nucleus accumbens and caudate-putamen. *Neuropsychopharmacology, 28*, 1082–1085.

Li, Z., Ichikawa, J., Dai, J., & Meltzer, H. Y. (2004). Aripiprazole, a novel antipsychotic drug, preferentially increases dopamine release in the prefrontal cortex and hippocampus in rat brain. *European Journal of Psychiatry, 493*(1–3), 75–83.

Li, Y., Sattler, R., Yang, E. J., Nunes, A., Ayukawa, Y., Aktar. S., et al. (2011). Harmine, a natural beta-carboline alkaloid, upregulates astroglial glutamate transporter expression. *Neuropharmacology, 60*(7–8), 1168–1175.

Lysis. (n. d.). In *Merriam-Webster's online dictionary.* Retrieved from http://www.merriam-webster.com/dictionary/lysis.

Mabit J. (2007). Ayahuasca in the treatment of addictions. In T. B. Robert & M. J. Winkelman (Eds.), *Psychedelic medicine (vol. 2): New evidence for hallucinogenic substances as treatments* (pp. 87-103). New York, NY: Praeger.

Marsch, L. A. (2002). The efficacy of methadone maintenance interventions in reducing illicit opiate use, HIV risk behavior, and criminality: A meta-analysis. *Addiction, 93*(4), 515–532. doi:10.1046/j.1360-0443.1998.9345157.x.

Matthews, A. M., Wilson, V. B., & Mitchell, S. H. (2011). The role of antipsychotics in smoking and smoking cessation. *CNS Drugs, 25*(4), 299–315.

McGregor, A., Lacosta, S., & Roberts, D. C. (1993). L-tryptophan decreases the breaking point under a progressive ratio schedule of intravenous cocaine reinforcement in the rat. *Pharmacology, Biochemistry and Behavior, 44*, 651–655.

McKenna, D. J., Towers, G. H. N., & Abbott, F. (1984). Monoamine oxidase inhibitors in South American hallucinogenic plants: Tryptamine and B-carboline constituents of ayahuasca. *Journal of Ethnopharmacology, 10*, 195–223.

Metzner, R. (1999). *Sacred vine of spirits: Ayahuasca*. Rochester, VT: Park Street Press.

Millan, M.J., Dekeyne, A., & Gobert, A. (1998). Serotonin (5-HT)2C receptors tonically inhibit dopamine (DA) and noradrenaline (NA), but not 5-HT, release in the frontal cortex in vivo. *Neuropharmacology, 37*(7), 935–955.

Molliver, M. E. (1987). Serotonergic neuronal systems: What their anatomic organization tells us about function. *Journal of Clinical Psychopharmacology, 7*(Suppl 6), 3S–23S.

Moore, R. Y., & Bloom, F. E. (1978). Central catecholamine neuron systems: Anatomy and physiology of the dopamine systems. *Annual Review of Neurosciences, 1*, 129–169.

Morton, W. A. (1999). Cocaine and psychiatric symptoms. *Primary Care Companion to the Journal of Clinical Psychiatry, 1*(4), 109–113.

Navarro, G., Moreno, E., Bonaventura, J., Brugarolas, M., Farré, D., Aguinaga, D., et al. (2013). Cocaine inhibits dopamine D_2 receptor signaling via sigma-1-D_2 receptor heteromers. *PLoS One, 8*(4), e61245.

Negus, S. S., & Mello, N. K. (2003a). Effects of chronic d-amphetamine treatment on cocaine and food-maintained responding under a second-order schedule in Rhesus monkeys. *Drug and Alcohol Dependence,* 70, 39–52.

Negus, S. S., & Mello, N. K. (2003b). Effects of chronic d-amphetamine treatment on cocaine and food-maintained responding under a progressive-ratio schedule in Rhesus monkeys. *Psychopharmacology, 167*, 324–332.

Osorio, F. L., Macedo, L. R., Sousa, J. P., Pinto, J. P., Quevedo, J., Crippa, J. A., et al. (2011). The therapeutic potential of harmine and ayahuasca in depression: Evidence from exploratory animal and human studies. In R. G. dos Santos (Ed.), *The ethnopharmacology of ayahuasca* (pp. 75–78). Kerala, India: Transworld Research Network. Retrieved June 21, 2013 from http://issuu.com/researchsignpost/docs/rafael.

Overman, G. P., Teter, C. J., & Guthrie, S. K. (2003). Acamprosate for the adjunctive treatment of alcohol dependence. *Annals of Pharmacotherapy, 37*(7), 1090–1099. doi:10.1345/aph.1C351.

Pahnke, W. N., Kurland, A. A., Unger, S., Savage, C., & Grof, S. (1970). The experimental use of psychedelic psychotherapy. *JAMA, 212*(11), 1856–1863.

Pierce, R. C., & Kumaresan, V. (2006). The mesolimbic dopamine system: The final common pathway for the reinforcing effect of DOA? *Neuroscience and Biobehavioral Reviews, 30*(2), 215–238.

Psyche. (n. d.). In *Merriam-Webster's online dictionary*. Retrieved from http://www.merriam-webster.com/dictionary/psyche.

Purves, D., Augustine, G. J., Fitzpatrick, D., & Hall, W. C. (Eds.). (2011). *Neuroscience*. Sunderland, CT: Sinauer.

Robinson, T. E., & Kolb, B. (1999). Alterations in the morphology of dendrites and dendritic spines in the nucleus accumbens and pre-frontal cortex following repeated treatment with amphetamine or cocaine. *European Journal of Neuroscience, 11*, 1598–1604.

Rollema, H., Chambers, L. K., Coe, J. W., Glowa, J. Hurst, R. S., Lebel, L. A., et al. (2007). Pharmacological profile of the alpha4beta2 nicotinic acetylcholine receptor partial agonist varenicline, an effective smoking cessation aid. *Neuropharmacology, 52*(3), 985–994.

Rothman, R. B., & Baumann, M. H. (2003). Monoamine transporters and psychostimulant drugs. *European Journal of Pharmacology, 479*, 23–40.

Rothman, R. B., & Baumann, M. H. (2006). Balance between dopamine and serotonin release modulates behavior effects of amphetamine-type drugs. *Annals of the New York Academy of Sciences, 1074*, 245–260.

Rothman, R. B., Blough, B. E., Woolverton, W. L., Anderson, K. G., Negus, S. S., Mello, N. K., et al. (2005). Development of a rationally designed, low abuse potential, biogenic amine releaser that suppresses cocaine self-administration. *Journal of Pharmacology and Experimental Therapeutics, 313*, 1361–1369.

Rothman, R. B., Blough, B. E., & Baumann, M. H. (2006). Dual dopamine/serotonin releasers as potential medications for stimulant and alcohol addictions. *AAPS Journal, 9*(1), E1–E10. doi:10.1208/aapsj0901001.

Rothman, R. B., Blough, B. E., & Baumann, M. H. (2008). Dual dopamine/serotonin releasers: Potential treatment agents for stimulant addiction. *Experimental and Clinical Psychopharmacology, 16*(6), 458–474.

Ruck, C. A., Bigwood, J., Staples, D., Ott, J., & Wasson, R. G. (1979). Entheogens. *Journal of Psychedelic Drugs, 11*, 145–146.

Substance Abuse Mental Health Services Administration. (2012). Results from the 2010 National Survey on Drug Use and Health: Summary of national findings. U.S. Department of Health and Human Services. Retrieved from http://www.samhsa.gov/data/NSDUH/2k10ResultsTables/NSDUHTables2010R/HTM/Sect1peTabs1to46.htm#Tab1.1A.

Schultes, R. E., Hofmann, A., & Ratsch, C. (1998). *Plants of the gods: Their sacred, healing, and hallucinogenic powers*. Rochester, VT: Healing Arts Press.

Shanon, B. Moments of insight, healing, and transformation: A cognitive phenomenological analysis. In this volume.

Shanon, B. (2002). *The antipodes of the mind: Charting the phenomenology of the ayahuasca experience*. Oxford: Oxford University Press.

Shulgin, Al, & Shulgin, An. (1997). *Tihkal: The continuation*. Berkeley, CA: Transform.

Smith, C. (1958). A new adjunct to the treatment of alcoholism: The hallucinogenic drugs. *Quarterly Journal for the Studies of Alcohol, 19*, 406–417.

Smith, F. L., Yu, D. S., Smith, D. G., Leccese, A. P., & Lyness, W. H. (1986). Dietary tryptophan supplements attenuate amphetamine self-administration in the rat. *Pharmacology, Biochemistry, and Behavior, 25*(4), 849–855.

Smith, R. L., Canton, H., Barrett, R. J., & Sanders-Bush, E. (1998). Agonist properties of N,N-dimethyltryptamine at serotonin 5-HT2A and 5-HT2C receptors. *Pharmacology, Biochemistry, and Behavior, 61*(3), 323–330.

Spanagel, R., Herz, A., & Shippenberg, T. S. (1992). Opposing tonically active endogenous opioid systems modulate the mesolimbic dopaminergic pathway. *Proceedings of the National Academy of Sciences, 89*, 2046–2050.

Stace, W. T. (1961). *Mysticism and philosophy*. London: Macmillan.

Stahl, S. M. (2008). *Stahl's essential psychopharmacology: Neuroscientific basis and practical applications*. New York, NY: Cambridge University Press.

Steinbusch, H. W. (1981). Distribution of serotonin-immunoreactivity in the central nervous system of the rat-cell bodies and terminals. *Neuroscience, 6*, 557–618.

Steiner, H., & Gerfen, C. R. (1996). Dynorphin regulates D1 dopamine receptor-mediated responses in the striatum: Relative contributions of pre- and postsynaptic mechanisms in dorsal and ventral striatum demonstrated by altered immediate-early gene induction. *Journal of Comparative Neurology, 376*, 530–541.

Strassman, R. J., Qualls, C. R., Uhlenhuth, E. H., & Robert, K. (1994). Dose response study of N,N-dimethyltryptamine in humans. II. Subjective effects and preliminary results of a new rating scale. *Archives of General Psychiatry, 51*(2), 98–108.

Strassman, R. (2001). *DMT: The spirit molecule*. Rochester, VT: Park Street.

Thomas, M. J., Kalivas, P. W., & Shaham, Y. (2009). Neuroplasticity in the mesolimbic dopamine system and cocaine addiction. *British Journal of Pharmacology, 154*(2), 327–342.

Trichter, S., Klimo, J., & Krippner, S. (2009). Changes in spirituality among ayahuasca ceremony novice participants. *Journal of Psychoactive Drugs, 41*(2), 121–134.

Ungerstedt, U. (1971). Stereotaxic mapping of the monoamine pathways in the rat brain. *Acta Physiologica Scandinavica Supplement, 367*, 1–48.

United Nations Office of Drugs and Crime. (2012). *World drug report*. New York, NY: United Nations. Retrieved June 21, 2013 from http://www.unodc.org/documents/data-and-analysis/WDR2012/WDR_2012_web_small.pdf.

W. W. (1994). The society of Alcoholics Anonymous (reprinted). *American Journal of Psychiatry, 151*(6), 259–262.

Wise, R. A. (1980). The dopamine synapse and the notion of "pleasure centers" in the brain. *Trends in Neurosciences, 3*, 91–95.

Wojnicki, F. H. E., Rothman, R. B., Rice, K. C., Glowa, J. R. (1999). Effects of phentermine on responding maintained under multiple fixed-ratio schedules of food and cocaine presentation in the Rhesus monkey. *Journal of Pharmacology and Experimental Therapeutics, 288*, 550–560.

Yokell, M. A., Zaller, N. D., Green, T. C., & Rich, J. D. (2011). Buprenorphine and buprenorphine/naloxone diversion, misuse, and illicit use: An international review. *Current Drug Abuse Reviews, 4*(1), 28–41.

Zhang, D., Zhang, L., Tang, Y., Zhang, Q., Lou, S., Sharp, F. R., et al. (2005). Repeated cocaine administration induces gene expression changes through the dopamine D1 receptors. *Neuropsychopharmacology, 30*, 1443–1454.

Zhihua, X., & Miller, G. M. (2007). Trace amine-associated receptor 1 is a modulator of the dopamine transporter. *The Journal of Pharmacology and Experimental Therapeutics, 321*, 128–136.

Zinberg, N. E. (1984). *Drug, set, and setting: The basis for controlled intoxicant use*. New Haven, CT: Yale University Press.

Chapter 8
Therapist and Patient Perspectives on Ayahuasca-Assisted Treatment for Substance Dependence

Anja Loizaga-Velder and Armando Loizaga Pazzi

Abstract This chapter is based on over 15 years of field observation by the authors and the findings of a theoretical and qualitative empirical study that included interviews with 15 therapists who used ayahuasca professionally in the treatment of addictions, as well as with 14 substance-dependent individuals who participated in ayahuasca-assisted treatment in varying contexts. The chapter will address the value of ayahuasca for substance-dependence treatment from a psychotherapeutic perspective, and the variables that may influence treatment outcome. Special attention is placed on the role of ritual and integration.

Introduction

This chapter explores the therapeutic value of ritual ayahuasca use for addiction treatment from a psychotherapeutic perspective and identifies variables that may influence treatment outcome. This article is derived from 15 years of field observation by the authors and the findings of a theoretical and qualitative empirical study conducted by Loizaga-Velder for her doctoral dissertation on therapeutic uses of ayahuasca in substance-dependence treatment (Presser-Velder 2013).

A. Loizaga-Velder (✉)
Institute for Medical Psychology, University of Heidelberg, Bergheimer Straße 20 69115 Heidelberg, Germany
e-mail: nierika@gmx.net
URL: http://www.nierika.info

A. Loizaga-Velder · A. L. Pazzi
Nierika Association, Chalmita, Mexico
e-mail: nierika52@gmail.com
URL: http://www.nierika.info

B. C. Labate and C. Cavnar (eds.), *The Therapeutic Use of Ayahuasca*,
DOI: 10.1007/978-3-642-40426-9_8, © Springer-Verlag Berlin Heidelberg 2014

Psychedelic plants have a long history of traditional use with spiritual, cultural, and therapeutic purposes among several indigenous peoples. The ritual use of such plants, particularly peyote and ayahuasca, is still alive in South and North America, and continues to provide effective culturally adapted treatment forms for different physical and psychological ailments, including substance dependence (Cabieses 1993; Calabrese 2013; Chiappe Costa 1979). As a consequence of the "cross-cultural transference of therapeutic approaches" (i.e., therapeutic practices developed in one cultural context are introduced to another), nonnative patients dissatisfied with conventional therapeutic offers also seek out healing rituals with psychoactive plants. Traditional ayahuasca interventions often times coexist with, or are complemented by, Western therapeutic strategies in different types of intercultural treatment projects. Furthermore, in the last decades, the use of ayahuasca in syncretic religious rituals has spread worldwide (Labate and Jungaberle 2011). Frequently, humanitarian and therapeutic support for substance-dependent individuals is also provided in these contexts (Labate et al. 2010).

Different modalities for substance-dependence treatment and management through ayahuasca rituals have been developed in both religious settings, which have an indirect focus on healing, and formal, structured therapeutic settings. Ayahuasca-assisted support for substance dependence is currently offered by indigenous healers, psychotherapists, and religious or shamanic ayahuasca circles in several countries of the American continent, including Peru, Brazil, Ecuador, Colombia, Argentina, Chile, Mexico, USA, and Canada. Such efforts are rooted in either indigenous Amazonian medicine traditions, the Brazilian ayahuasca religions, psychedelic-assisted psychotherapy, or consist of a hybrid combination of these. They include following modalities: (1) informal support, such as that offered by some religious groups in Brazil, who provide humanitarian services to substance-dependent individuals, including the option to participate in ayahuasca rituals; (2) outpatient programs that offer monthly ayahuasca sessions as complement to their therapeutic program, and (3) inpatient programs of various lengths that offer regular ayahuasca sessions as an integral part of the therapy. Structural aspects and professionalism vary considerably among existing programs.

Anecdotal reports by individuals who have overcome substance dependence by participating in religious or shamanic ayahuasca ceremonies indicate that there is a noteworthy therapeutic value to such practices. Results of preliminary outcome studies presented by two multidisciplinary treatment centers that provide ayahuasca-assisted treatment for substance dependence, Takiwasi in Peru, and IDEAA in Brazil (Fernández and Fábregas in this volume; Fernández et al. in this volume; Giove Nakazawa 2002; Mabit 2007), and outcomes of an observational study of ayahuasca-assisted treatment in a rural First Nations community in British Colombia, Canada (Thomas et al. 2013) are promising, considering the overall efficacy for addiction treatment in general. However, systematic clinical studies are required to confirm these findings.

Generating the Research

Using qualitative research methods based on a combination of personal field observation and problem-centered interviews (Witzel 2000), the qualitative study, described briefly here, aimed at gaining a better understanding of the therapeutic value of ayahuasca in addiction treatment from a psychotherapeutic perspective, and at identifying variables that may influence the outcome of ayahuasca-assisted treatment, based on both the subjective experiences of patients and on the perspective of experts in the field. In this context, the study focused primarily on therapeutic uses of ayahuasca that are rooted in traditional indigenous medicine and those derived from this. Other approaches were also included; however, they were not explored in the same depth.

Several field studies were conducted among a variety of existing therapeutic projects utilizing ayahuasca rituals to assist individuals to overcome substance dependence. The qualitative study included: (a) a review of the therapeutic conceptualization of seven therapeutic centers that apply ayahuasca in the treatment of addiction in diverse settings (traditional medicine-based, ayahuasca church-based, and hybrid projects, including psychotherapeutic support) and three therapists working in private practice, who complement psychotherapeutic substance-dependence treatment with ayahuasca rituals; (b) interviews with 15 professionals with expertise in both treatment of addictions and therapeutic ayahuasca use (4 traditional healers and 11 mental-health professionals with university degrees); and (c) interviews with 14 individuals who had undergone ayahuasca-assisted therapy for addiction in diverse settings[1]: traditional indigenous medicine (3 subjects), neoshamanic (1 subject) or a hybrid combination of traditional medicine and psychotherapy (10 subjects).

Research data for this study was evaluated and conceptually structured with qualitative data analysis according to Miles and Huberman (1994). A brief review and reflections on the most relevant findings will follow.

The Therapeutic Value of Ayahuasca from the Perspective of Therapists and Patients

The findings of this field study indicate that, for certain patients, and when used in appropriate contexts, ayahuasca can contribute to achieving abstinence from harmful drug use or to reducing drug-related harm in a significant way (i.e.,

[1] Interviewed patients were from diverse cultural backgrounds: Most were Latin American (Peruvian, Argentinean, Mexican, Colombian); 1 was from Spain, 1 from USA, 5 patients were from rural contexts, and 9 from urban contexts, with a wide spectrum of educational levels (incomplete elementary school to university degrees); ages ranged from 24 to 52 years old, with a mean average 41 years.

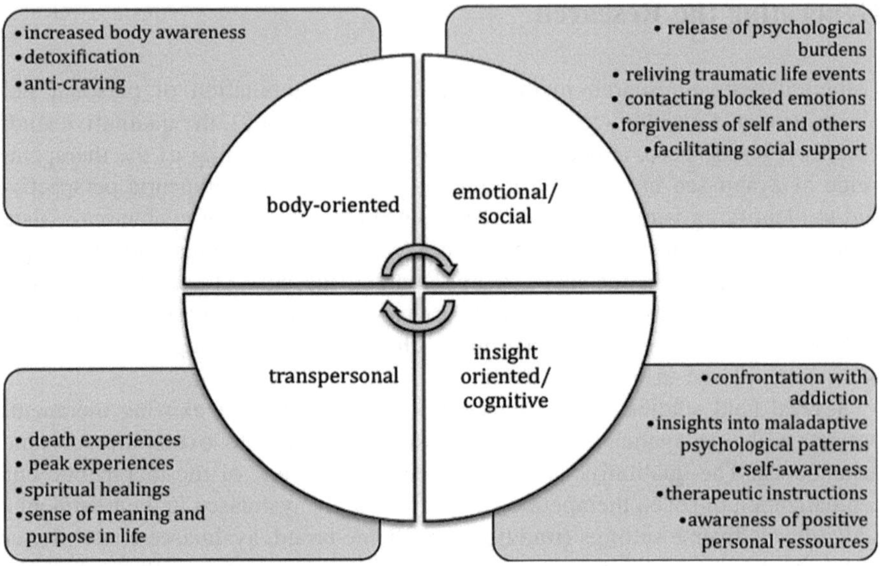

Fig. 8.1 Subjective ayahuasca experiences with therapeutic effects

consumption of less harmful substances and/or patterns of less frequent use). Ayahuasca-induced experiences can also promote deeper self-understanding, facilitate resolution of psychological issues underlying substance dependencies, and uncover positive psychological resources that the patient was unaware of, thereby increasing a sense of self-esteem and self-efficacy. All interviewed therapists referred to ayahuasca as a catalyst that can render therapeutic processes more effective and shorter, and sometimes allows for critical interventions when other strategies have failed.[2]

The following therapeutically relevant subjective experiences induced by ayahuasca rituals were observed in this study and synthesized in Fig. 8.1.

Patients reported a broad spectrum of ayahuasca-induced subjective experiences that they considered significant in relation to their recovery. These can be categorized in four interrelated, psychotherapeutically relevant aspects that include body-oriented, emotional/social, insight oriented/cognitive, and transpersonal. Most patients reported that the therapeutic effect of participating in ayahuasca rituals resulted from an integral synthesis of the above-mentioned types of experiences, their psychological processing, and their implementation into daily life.

From a Western psychotherapeutic point of view, the therapeutic value of ayahuasca seems to lie primarily in stimulating the following therapeutic processes: augmenting body awareness, reducing drug-craving, triggering different

---

[2] A less comprehensive version of some of these findings has been published in Loizaga-Velder, 2013.

types of emotional processes (catharsis, perception of previously suppressed emotions, generating inner resources for coping with emotions or urges to use), supporting introspection (self-analysis, eliciting consciousness of addiction and its adverse effects on oneself and others), and enhancing self-efficacy (becoming aware of positive aspects of oneself, thus improving self-esteem and confidence to stay sober). In the context of group treatment, ritual ayahuasca ingestion can also catalyze certain social processes that can contribute to recovery and recovery maintenance. All of the above-mentioned therapeutic processes are also found in the general treatment objectives and goals of various common psychotherapeutic approaches to the treatment of addictions. Some of these therapeutic aspects of ayahuasca in the treatment of substance dependence will be discussed below in detail.

Body-Oriented Aspects

One important therapeutic value identified in this study of ayahuasca for substance-dependence treatment is that ayahuasca-induced experiences can increase awareness of the body and facilitate a renewed relationship with the physical self. This can be valuable for the recovery process, as substance dependence involves not only psychological, but also physical factors. Body-oriented aspects can provide important resources for the relief of stress and emotional pain or trauma that is typically associated with substance dependence.

The majority of both therapists and patients interviewed attributed detoxifying and anti-craving qualities to ayahuasca and associated these effects primarily with the emetic effect of this plant preparation. This is a concept stemming from traditional Amazonian medicine, in which a number of other emetic plants are also employed for the purpose of detoxification (Giove Nakazawa 2002). Emetic plant preparations are also used in traditional healing contexts of other cultures for the treatment of addictions, such as at the Wat Tham Krabok monastery in Thailand (Schreiber 1999), where, as observed in this study, positive effects on withdrawal symptoms and attenuation of craving in opiate addicts have been also reported as a consequence of intense vomiting.

The majority of the patients interviewed pointed out that, in contrast to other previous recreational experiences with drugs, the experiences with ayahuasca were very difficult on the body and mind, and required significant effort. One patient describes it as such:

> Especially the first times [drinking ayahuasca] were very hard for me. It was very difficult to look inside myself… I was throwing up and throwing up, cleansing myself and then I went down to the bottom and was seeing all my things… The sensations were super strong for me, I was shivering like a dog in a cage crying and throwing up (Pedro[3]).

---

[3] All names are pseudonyms.

Another patient commented,

> The physical hardship I underwent during my ayahuasca session made me understand why ayahuasca is not addictive. I had never felt physically so bad (Omar).

In the reports of ritual participants, diverse types of emotions, memories, ideas, and visions that had meaning and relevance to their personal recovery process frequently accompanied the vomiting and diarrhea induced by ayahuasca. Several participants in this study described experiences of unloading psychological burdens, such as releasing guilt, psychological blockages, negative emotions, attitudes, and thoughts through the act of purging.

> In one session the spirit of the ayahuasca came into my mouth in the form of a serpent. I just let it happen. She went deep into me and made me throw up. I vomited bitter and acid stuff, rage, and many emotions. After vomiting, I felt very liberated and renewed, as if I was again 15 years old (Presser-Velder 2000, p. 158).

Far from being regarded as an undesirable side effect, vomiting was conceived of as a component of the ayahuasca experience with important therapeutic value, providing patients with a sense of relief and of a "new beginning," accompanied by a lasting sensation of "mental clarity" as exemplified in the following statements: "For a long time I didn't vomit with ayahuasca, but when I finally did, I felt much more peaceful… vomiting was very helpful, it unties your knots… It was what helped me the most" (Tomas); "When I take ayahuasca, I purge everything… afterwards I come down again and I start to think clearer" (Jaime).

In some patients, the motivation to stay clean or sober was facilitated by the sensation of detoxification and purification experienced after purging. Furthermore, several patients reported that drug craving diminished significantly or ceased completely after meaningful ayahuasca experiences:

> Since then [an ayahuasca session three years ago], I don't feel any desire to smoke. I even feel disgusted and it's no effort for me to be clean. It's unbelievable for me and for people who know me, because I couldn't picture myself without smoking before that session. I had tried to quit by so many means and nothing had helped (Ernesto).

Such anti-craving effects were reported by some as being permanent and by others as temporary and gradually fading after varying amounts of time (several days to weeks or months). All patients interviewed associated this anti-craving effect to the psychological and spiritual processes triggered by the ayahuasca experience, as in the following case:

> After the first ayahuasca session I was not drinking any alcohol for two weeks. It was not even on my mind…not drinking came naturally…there was no void that needed to be filled anymore… I found that life had a meaning (Steve).

The subjective experiences of attenuation of withdrawal symptoms, diminished craving, and increased physical well being as a result of vomiting during the ayahuasca experience can be regarded also as a form of "symbolic healing." Moermann (1979) has proposed that metaphors or symbols can alter cognitive, emotional, and behavioral structures and that they can also influence biochemical processes in the body through a psycho-physiological interconnection. Symbolic healing, as such, is a therapeutic factor present in most indigenous medicinal traditions that also plays a role in modern biomedical healing processes.

In addition to the above-mentioned psychological factors, pharmacological factors may also play a role in the observed therapeutic effects of ayahuasca. The ayahuasca compound acts temporarily on several neurological pathways associated with craving and other aspects of substance abuse (Brierley and Davidson 2012; Liester and Prickett 2012, in this volume). These pharmacological aspects may come into play, particularly among individuals who regularly partake in ayahuasca rituals, such as members of ayahuasca churches and participants in structured therapeutic programs that include regular ayahuasca ingestion. The neurobiology of ayahuasca-assisted treatment is, however, not yet fully understood. Further research on the anti-craving properties of ayahuasca is especially relevant to substance-dependence treatment, because craving and relapse are strongly related.

Emotional and Psychosocial Aspects

The modified state of consciousness induced by ayahuasca can act as a catalyst for diverse emotional processes, which may range from deep sadness, terrorizing fears, and rage to profound calmness, well being, and bliss. Ayahuasca lowers the threshold for conscious control, allowing subconscious material to arise and become conscious, and may also trigger catharsis of blocked emotions. In contrast to the perceived need to escape from painful or negative emotions through substance use, during the ayahuasca-modified state of consciousness, patients tend to focus on the continued exploration of emotional issues.

> I felt the most exhausting and intense emotions, which I had kept locked inside myself for decades. And, even though it was the hardest thing to experience, I always felt grateful and full of love… Because of that, I did not resist and fully trusted the experience (Ernesto).

Approximately two-thirds of the patients interviewed reported experiences of biographical recapitulation. Painful and traumatic life events represent predominant psychotherapeutic issues among substance-dependent patients. During the state of consciousness induced by ayahuasca, memories of such events are brought into awareness and, in many cases, can be experientially re-lived, while at the same time associated painful emotions and anxiety can be liberated and transformed. Some patients reported that these experiences helped them release resentments and guilt by promoting feelings of forgiveness of self and others:

> I had to learn to love myself and forgive myself and more than anything, forgive my family. This was needed for getting well… I realized things I had done in my life to myself and to others, and I asked myself, "How could I have done that?" At that moment, I expelled everything while I vomited or cried and then these things vanished… I carried a giant bag of guilt, but there I got rid of the guilt and I felt better (Pedro).

Many of the patients reported that ayahuasca helped them to reflect on relationship dynamics with significant others. These reflections were often accompanied by increased empathy and a motivation to overcome interpersonal issues. One example follows:

> I started to think a lot about my family and friends and the things that I had done to [them]. With this plant [ayahuasca] I could feel situations through their feelings. Like how my mom felt when she discovered my bag of marijuana. I could see this without judging and without being me (Daniel).

The ayahuasca-generated insights and psycho-emotional processes associated with the ayahuasca experience seemed to have improved the quality of interpersonal relationships in some patients, which in turn fostered positive emotional feedback that could help counteract the typical isolation of addiction. The shared modified state of consciousness of an ayahuasca ceremony can also enhance the patient–therapist relationship, as reported by both patients and therapists in this study, especially when the therapist is facilitating or co-facilitating the ayahuasca ceremony, facilitating a type of nonverbal bonding that is typically experienced in ayahuasca ceremonies by participants. The strength of the therapeutic alliance has been identified as one of the universal factors that contribute significantly to positive treatment outcomes (Lambert 2004).

The notion of fellowship is the therapeutic backbone of many approaches to substance-dependence treatment, such as varied types of therapeutic communities and self-help recovery groups like Alcoholics Anonymous (AA) or Narcotics Anonymous (NA). Social support for recovering patients, or in C. G. Jung's words, "the protective wall of human community" (Alcoholics Anonymous World Services 1984), is an important factor for achieving and maintaining recovery. The collective participation in ayahuasca rituals can facilitate group therapeutic processes that are significant in addiction treatment. Social support and social norms regarding substance use seem to play an essential role in the observed therapeutic effects on substance-dependence issues reported by participants in ceremonies of the ayahuasca churches. Sharing the experience of a nonordinary state of consciousness and collectively managing the "ayahuasca ordeal" often catalyzes social processes that are relevant to recovery by generating group cohesiveness. An interviewed therapist related this in the following way: "In the ayahuasca session you become a community… it [the session] creates a sense of belonging to a family or a group…. it is an experience that is lived through together" (Medical Doctor Fernando).

This sense of belonging can lead to increased participation in activities with a peer group that holds positive, health-oriented values. This can also be strongly motivational and may significantly support the integration of insights into lasting behavioral changes. Ayahuasca communities seem to provide support for the handling of psychosocial stress, which can have a psycho-hygienic function by preventing relapse and providing a social safety net as that found in other type of self-help groups. The participation in ayahuasca ceremonies seems to be particularly effective in curbing the abuse of substances that are not accepted in the peer group (e.g., tobacco use in certain ayahuasca church communities such as UDV).

Insight-Oriented and Cognitive Aspects

The findings of this study also indicate that ayahuasca-induced states of consciousness allow for a shift in perspective, which can foster a renewed perception of self and may trigger insights into one's own psychodynamics and the capabilities of finding creative solutions to one's psychological problems.

Many interviewed patients reported experiences of enhanced cognitive functioning, referred to as "mental clarity" or "exceptional lucidity." Patients described elaborate inner dialogs, shifts in perspective, and therapeutically relevant insights that came to them through the ayahuasca experience. All of the patients stated that ayahuasca facilitated self-reflection. It also provided insights and helped them transform maladaptive psychological patterns and addiction pathways by revealing different perspectives on their problems. The fact that the insights were self-generated led patients to feel empowered to assume a more proactive role in their recovery, a factor also highlighted and valued by most therapists interviewed.

Patients and therapists alike emphasized that ayahuasca can function as an "inner mirror" that allows one to readily accept previously denied aspects of the psyche that are usually difficult to address in therapeutic contexts. This is especially important in addiction therapy, where confronting denial mechanisms usually plays an essential role in treatment. Trying to break through denial mechanisms can be problematic, as this effort is likely to create further resistance. However, it seems that confrontation stemming from within or from a perceived spiritual source, such as "Mother Ayahuasca," "Mother Earth" or "God," can be better received, integrated, and contained by patients, as reported here:

> Ayahuasca showed me that I did not know myself…. I saw myself as through a camera or a mirror, and I was looking at myself…as if being in the presence of somebody who knows exactly who I am and how I felt, and knew what I was doing with my life (Carlos).

Nearly all patients reported that the ayahuasca experience confronted them directly with their addiction. Some testimonies follow: "I felt the presence of a spiritual guide. This guide let me know that I did have a problem with alcoholism; before this, I was denying it. I got a strong feeling that I wanted to change" (Steve); "The awareness of my addiction became ever so real and the acceptance and strength as the only way to handle this aspect of myself" (Alonso);

> The plant showed me that I was trapped in my alcoholism, that I was a slave to alcohol…. The downward path on which I was going [alcoholism] and the other path which I could choose to go was revealed to me….[I realized that] hand in hand with my alcoholism was my idleness, rage, superficialities, egoism, etc. I could say that each ayahuasca intake was

> touching my insides and showing me what I was doing wrong…the way in which these things were revealed to me was fundamental, almost shocking, very precise, and so wise, that it left no room for doubting my need for change and recovery (Omar).

In addition to being directly confronted with their addiction, most patients also reported becoming aware of other dysfunctional aspects of themselves that had previously remained unconscious. Becoming aware of one's dysfunctional patterns is a fundamental first step towards overcoming them; an idea shared by various psychological schools. Ayahuasca seems to be effective in eliciting or enhancing this process in patients undergoing substance abuse treatment, as exemplified by the following interview excerpt:

> The plants…don't just attack your addiction. In reality, the problem is not the addiction itself, the addiction is a consequence of many problems in your life… Using plants is an introspection inside yourself…. They open things inside of you…to arrive at a point where you have developed a trauma or a complex…what has blocked you and diverted your path toward alcohol or drugs (Sergio).

All patients interviewed noted that they received some sort of therapeutic instruction during their ayahuasca experience that, when implemented, became relevant for their recovery and general personal growth. These instructions were perceived to come from some direct and literal or metaphorical messages.

Patients and therapists alike reported that ayahuasca could bring into consciousness not only negative aspects, but also positive personal resources that they were not aware of or had previously neglected. This contributed to a more objective and complete self-image, enhancing a sense of self-efficacy and positive self-regard. Both cognitive and emotional aspects of this more positive outlook on the self seem to complement each other and contribute to better emotional functioning; an important factor for recovery from addictions. These processes are illustrated in the next two examples: "Ayahuasca helps you to have trust in yourself, to feel good about what you are doing" (Sebastian); "My approach to life is much more optimistic. I am generally happier and tend not to doubt myself because I have much more self-confidence" (Steve).

Transpersonal Aspects

The therapeutic effect of spiritual experiences on addictions has been recognized throughout the various psychological orientations to addiction treatment. The acknowledgment of the limitations of the human being and the search for healing through that which transcends the individual is the basis for the 12-step fellowships such as AA and NA that have influenced dependence treatment worldwide. Among the different approaches to understanding this disorder, substance dependence has been conceptualized as a type of self-medication for an existential void and for a sense of meaninglessness that may be best addressed and fulfilled through spiritual means (Miller 1999; White and Laudet 2006). Spiritual concerns are also addressed in substance-dependence treatment programs through practices such as transcendental meditation, based on Eastern spirituality, and Native American spiritual practices, such as sweat lodges, talking circles, and Native American Church peyote ceremonies in culturally specific programs serving native populations. Research has provided evidence that spiritual factors, such as authentic spiritual experiences and spiritual orientation to recovery, can contribute positively to addiction treatment outcome (Project MATCH Research Group 1997; White and Laudet 2006).

Throughout this study, spiritual aspects of the ayahuasca experience were reported to have been pivotal for the recovery process by both therapists and patients. A majority of the patients interviewed stated that by participating in ayahuasca ceremonies, they had been able to establish a vivid spiritual connection with a divine or spiritual power (God, nature, the Virgin Mary, Jesus, Buddha, the cosmos, etc.). This had a deep positive impact on their substance dependence and life in general. One example follows:

> It was the most profound spiritual awakening to come face to face with the divine self within all of us. The notions of God, life, and love became direct experience of my inner self and for the first time I could dialog with this spiritual force. This was tremendously empowering and reassuring to my spiritual self. A sense of wonder and perfection overcame me and well being seemed the natural way to be (Alonso).

Spiritual peak experiences were often accompanied by a sense of bliss and profound peace and/or a sense of relief from confusion, promoting lasting feelings of wholeness and inner balance. Patients also reported vivid inner experiences related to existential values such as humility, gratitude, compassion, love, joy, and an appreciation for life. Some patients experienced "spiritual cleansings and healings" or received support from spiritual allies or helpers, which, in some cases, helped to counteract the hopelessness that they felt with regard to previous unsuccessful attempts at quitting drug abuse. Patients also reported that they gained a new sense of meaning and purpose in life through these experiences that invigorated their motivation to stay sober. For many, spiritual experiences had reportedly transformed their consciousness in a way that allowed them to overcome craving for drugs without effort.

> What really helped me was the spiritual connection I got from the ayahuasca ceremonies…. They gave me a sense of a spiritual nature in life, which made me realize that I did not want to binge-drink anymore, because life is much more important than that…. They [ayahuasca ceremonies] made me feel that there was a presence of someone who loved me unconditionally and who gave me the strength to stop myself from drinking or drinking too much…. The experience gave me a spiritual basis for my life and made me realize that life had a purpose and meaning…. I began to reevaluate my life…. The fact that there is something more to life than just the material world. Before ayahuasca, I had felt lost, alone, and a bit hopeless in life; but…since I participated in my first ayahuasca ritual, I have a spiritual link to call upon. I can look back on my experience and that feeling of being in touch with God and realize that life isn't empty, and then I no longer feel the strong desire to drink (Steve).

Death experiences, such as feeling that one was dying or seeing oneself as dead, were another type of transpersonal experience given therapeutic relevance by half of the patients interviewed. Patients stated that death experiences reminded them of the value of life and confronted them with the necessity to make profound change in their lifestyle. As reported by one patient:

> The encounter with the medicine was the most powerful experience I have ever lived. I have always lived on the edge and I am used to strong emotions, but never something similar to this. One of my intentions was to quit smoking cigarettes and, during my healing process, the spirit of ayahuasca showed me visions of the future if I continued smoking. I saw my daughters' faces in my funeral. I could see their pain and feel their suffering. I felt a huge irresponsibility, because even when you know you might die from smoking, only when you experience your own death, you can understand. I faced my darkest fears and I had to deal with them. But every time I passed through one of my fears, a revelation came to me as a reward (Ernesto).

This concludes the portion of this chapter that describes an overview of the therapeutic effects of ayahuasca-assisted therapy identified in the cited study. Consistency in observations by other research groups (see Giove Nakazawa 2002; Pfitzner 2008; Fernández et al. in this volume) on the above-described therapeutic effects of ayahuasca suggest that ayahuasca use in ceremonial contexts has identifiable therapeutic qualities that can be valuable in the treatment of addictive disorders.

Variables that may Influence Treatment Outcome

It is important to point out that ayahuasca is not a panacea for substance dependence, but is rather a therapeutic tool with an outcome depending on how it is used and to whom and by whom it is administered. Ayahuasca-assisted treatment is useful only for certain individuals and under certain circumstances. The experience, and hence the psychotherapeutic effects, can be influenced by what has been identified in the context of substance-assisted therapy and drug use in general as the drug, set, and setting triad. Treatment outcome can be furthermore influenced by complementary therapeutic strategies that include aftercare. Social support and the degree to which the experiences are integrated and the lessons implemented in the everyday life of the patients are other variables that influence treatment outcome. The following figure illustrates factors identified in this study (Fig. 8.2).

Ayahuasca-related. The quality of the ayahuasca preparation, its composition, and an appropriate proportion of MAO-Inhibiting and DMT-containing plants can influence the experience significantly. Both an adequate initial dose and, if necessary, subsequent doses, should be individually adapted to each ritual participant's constitution, sensitivity, and therapeutic process.

Patient-related. Patient-related factors that are known to influence substance abuse treatment in general can also be relevant in determining outcomes in ayahuasca-assisted treatment. These include the severity of addiction, motivation,

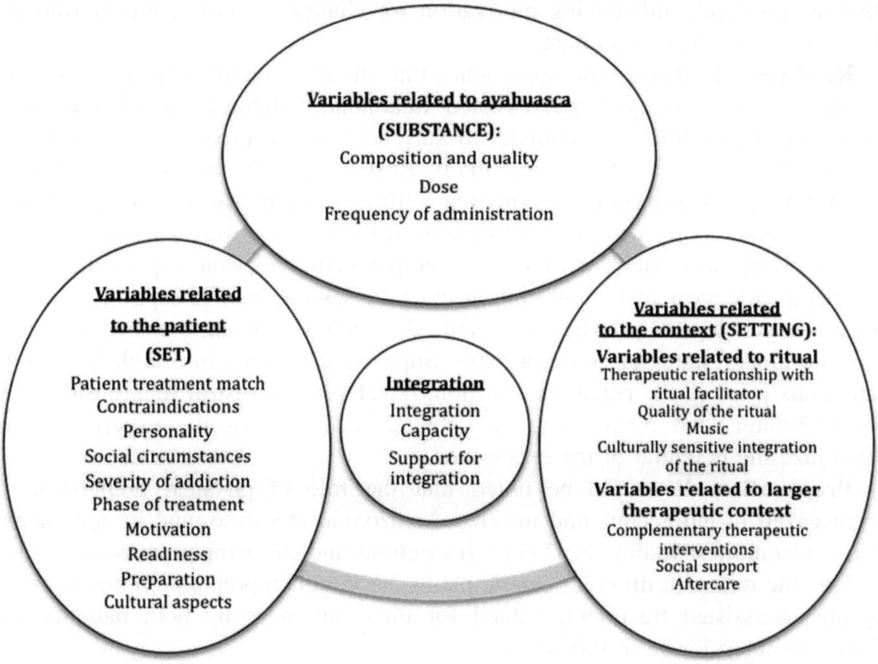

Fig. 8.2 Variables that influence treatment outcome

active engagement in the treatment process, and psychological readiness for change. Social support networks, premorbid life structures, and patient-treatment matching are also relevant in determining successful outcomes. Furthermore, factors specific to treatments that involve nonordinary states of consciousness, such as voluntary participation, readiness and preparation for the experiences, capacity for integration, and cultural factors, may play a role as well. Some of these patient-related variables will be described below in more detail.

Patient-treatment match. Ayahuasca is not necessarily the best treatment option for all patients with substance dependence. Treatment programs and patients both benefit from careful screening for patients who are unlikely to respond well to the treatment and to the characteristics of the specific therapeutic environment the treatment is embedded in. Special attention must be paid to patients for whom ayahuasca use may be counter-indicated, which include patients with certain physical conditions, psychotic patients, those with severe personality disorders, and patients using certain prescription drugs.

Motivation. Initial motivation is an important factor in the successful outcome of ayahuasca-assisted treatment. Generally speaking, patients with a high intrinsic motivation to overcome their substance dependence are more likely to benefit from ayahuasca-assisted treatment. Nevertheless, it is in the best interest of the patient to consider that confrontational ayahuasca experiences may induce psychological distress, positively influencing motivation for change in some patients who are otherwise resistant to treatment.

Readiness. In therapeutic approaches that involve nonordinary states of consciousness, such as ayahuasca-assisted treatment, voluntary participation is a necessary precondition for patients to surrender to the process, without which effective therapeutic work is very unlikely. Resistance to the ayahuasca experience can be therapeutically counterproductive. Willingness and psychological readiness of the patients to go within, and to confront themselves, were also factors considered to be necessary for inducing therapeutically relevant experiences. Psychotherapeutic work and counseling prior to the sessions can be supportive in this regard. Psychological preparation should also include education about the nature of nonordinary states of consciousness. Supporting patients in establishing clear intentions prior to the ritual intervention, developing a trustful relationship with the facilitator, and maintaining an open attitude towards the experience can maximize the potential of the experience.

Preparation. It should be noted that the role of physical preparation is emphasized in indigenous and mestizo Amazonian medicine, and in approaches derived from these traditions. Dietary restrictions and cleansing processes that may include the intake of different emetic plants are common preparation practices for ayahuasca-assisted treatment, valued for their outcomes by both patients and therapists interviewed in this study.

Cultural aspects. It was the experience of all therapists interviewed that traditional ayahuasca ceremonies were as therapeutically effective for individuals from Western cultural backgrounds as for mestizo or indigenous participants. It is, however, important to consider that interactions between the cultural predispositions of the participants can influence the focus and content of the experience and its interpretation. Some Western participants may not have the necessary cultural references to understand and deal with some complex, abstract, and symbolic contents of the ayahuasca experience. Therapeutic support for the preparation for, and integration of, their experience can be particularly relevant in these cases. Cultural and subcultural norms regarding the use of specific psychoactive substances may also play a role in final outcome.

Context-related. Treatment outcomes were also attributed to the ayahuasca rituals and the broader therapeutic context they were embedded in, the adequacy and quality of which can influence treatment outcomes significantly.

Ritual. Within the holistic point of view of indigenous medicine, ayahuasca is not conceptualized as an isolated pharmacological treatment, but rather as a ritual intervention supported by a psychedelic plant compound and complementary therapeutic strategies. The therapeutic potential of ayahuasca is conceived as embedded in its ritual use, and as unfolding better in this interrelation.

Ritual can be defined as a formalized symbolic procedure with subjective and cultural meaning, and the purpose of transcendence. As long as rituals are alive and have not become stereotyped, they serve the following purposes: They establish sacred spaces and times, they provide a framework and an outlet for strong emotional reactions, they connect individuals with a group, and they maintain or re-establish health and natural order.

Ayahuasca rituals rooted in indigenous medicine have been developed based on experience of the effects of ayahuasca, and can, in the view of several therapists interviewed, provide the ideal setting for the containment and the therapeutic guidance of ayahuasca-induced nonordinary states of consciousness. A few of the therapists interviewed preferred working in contexts adapted to Western culture; yet, they all maintain certain elemental aspects of the traditional ritual.

The quality of the context in which ayahuasca is ingested can be an important influence on treatment outcomes. Adequate ayahuasca rituals serve the purpose of containing and guiding intense modified states of consciousness and of providing a sense of safety, protection, and containment for the experience. Only when feeling safe can patients surrender to the experience and engage in their inner journey. The role of ritual was described by one of the patients interviewed in the following words:

> I feel that the fact that we all come together and bless the place and bless ayahuasca and pray, I think all that makes it a place where you feel healthier…. It doesn't matter how many things you can see as long as you are in a place where you can say, "Okay, this is where it has to happen," and this feeling of security makes it so that you can transcend and calm yourself and take your time…in a circle where all the energy is contained, and you can't escape…the ritual setting gives you a space where you can go further (Daniel).

Rituals provide a focus for the experience that may be primarily therapeutic or spiritual. Promoting a clear intention in participants at the beginning of the session and sharing a common purpose and treatment goals can improve therapeutic outcomes. The facilitators' skills and sensitivity during the session, as well as his or her ability to build rapport, and the adequacy of therapeutic strategies and interventions, may strongly influence the experience.

Music. Music was considered by all participants interviewed to be of critical importance. Music modulates the intensity of the experience and can suggest specific states of consciousness and emotional responses. Simple instrumental music or medicine songs called *icaros* constitute the essence of traditional healing ayahuasca practices. Icaros are usually sung with specific therapeutic intentions according to the patients' processes during the ceremony (Bustos 2008; Giove Nakazawa 1993). One traditional healer compared the function of icaros in an ayahuasca ceremony to the function of the oars of a canoe, without which the canoe would be at the mercy of the currents of the river (Presser-Velder 2000). Icaros and other types of music, such as religious hymns or world music, live or recorded, are meant to deepen or steer the ayahuasca trance, inducing and modulating visions and emotions and stimulating subconscious material on different levels.

Adequate frequency and spacing of the ayahuasca-assisted interventions. It is worth noting that, although in a few testimonies the first ayahuasca sessions led to a therapeutic breakthrough, in many of the cases reviewed, a single ayahuasca session was not sufficient to induce sustained therapeutic results. Instead, therapeutic outcomes resulted from participation in several ayahuasca rituals. Findings indicate that the best outcomes can be obtained when the number of ayahuasca sessions and intervals can be adapted to individual needs and processes, and is not predetermined by treatment protocols.

Interestingly, some patients perceived a therapeutic continuity between sessions, exemplified by following statements: "I could not name one most important experience, all of them were as one more step in a greater process, that provided physical, psychological, and spiritual support [for recovery]" (Pablo).

Aftercare. Aftercare is especially relevant in treatments that involve modified states of consciousness such as ayahuasca-supported treatment. Integration of not only the ayahuasca experiences, but also of the treatment experience as a whole, can be challenging and may require ongoing therapeutic support by therapists familiar with ayahuasca. Aftercare aims to prevent relapse by keeping the patient away from high-risk environments and helping the patient to establish supportive social contexts, achieve occupational stability and confront everyday challenges. Outside therapeutic settings, social support networks, as in the case of ayahuasca churches or shamanic ayahuasca circles, can cover some functions of therapeutic aftercare in a way similar to AA and other sobriety based self-help strategies. In addition to conventional therapeutic support as part of their aftercare plan, some treatment participants reported that the availability of ayahuasca ceremonies as part of their recovery-maintenance strategy helped in relapse prevention and in coping with drug urges and situations of personal distress.

Integration. All therapists, traditional healers, and modern-trained therapists alike who were interviewed agreed on the observation that qualified assistance in processing the ayahuasca experience and implementing insights into participants' daily life was a critical factor in achieving sustained treatment results and minimizing undesired effects such as ego inflation. As illustrated by one therapist and one patient, respectively:

> [If there is no integration] whatever insights, whatever understandings people may reach will be lost, because the nature of the mind is such. The ordinary, everyday mind floods in very quickly after the experience, so the experience can soon become just a memory. You have to have some integration, you have to have some program, you have to have a daily practice [in order to archive sustained therapeutic outcomes] (Medical Doctor, T10).

> Integration of the experiences is not easy. It is way easier to watch the ayahuasca visions like a movie on TV and keep going the next day the same way as before. But if you want to integrate the ayahuasca visions, you need to jump over your shadow and work hard.... I cannot integrate all immediately, sometimes it needs time.... For some of the visions, I will need my whole life to make them become real (Presser-Velder 2000, p. 165).

The term "integration" is oftentimes used to refer to different aspects of a process that includes making sense out of the experience, filtering the content, assimilating and accommodating the experience psychologically, and implementing insights into lasting changes. All patients who participated in programs that offered complementary psychotherapy for the purpose of processing and analyzing the content of the ayahuasca experiences considered that such sessions were very important in helping them to fully understand and deepen the meaning of the ayahuasca experience. This was perceived to be especially so in regards to complex visions and metaphorical messages received during the session.

> Ayahuasca is not magic. I had to face my psychologist with all my baggage of shame and misery that the plant would show me and then we would work through everything.... The process with my therapist was fundamental. I believe that if one takes plants without therapeutic support, it is like finding a treasure, but not the key to open it. Psychotherapy was good in helping me interpret, completely accept, and implement what the plant was teaching me (Omar).

Group sharing has a very important function because it provides an opportunity to witness other participants' processes, facilitating identification with them and reinforcement of the commitment to implement positive changes in one's life.

> The group also helps when they tell you that they, too, were able to let go of terrible habits and feel much better. That helps a lot, talking with people who drank alcohol and managed to get out of their inner hell, that helps one to not relapse (Omar).

According to patient reports, journaling about the experience can also be very beneficial, and some patients reported that re-reading the notes of the experience years later continues to shed light on different levels of understanding.

It should also be noted that some of the interviewed ritual participants did not attend structured therapeutic programs and did not receive any psychotherapeutic support in addition to their ayahuasca experience. Yet, they apparently had sufficient inner resources for integration or augmented these through their social contexts and reached certain levels of integration through informal conversations after the ayahuasca session about the content and insights with other ritual participants.

Final Thoughts

In well-structured settings, ayahuasca experiences can contribute to the process of recovery from substance dependence by triggering interrelated physical, psychological, and spiritual processes that are valued in the various existing therapeutic approaches to addiction treatment. Reviews of the therapeutic effects of psychedelics in addiction treatment indicate that psychedelics are valuable therapeutic tools if used appropriately (Grof 1980; Halpern 2007; Hämmig 2008; Krebs and Johansen 2012). In this regard, the findings of this study are consistent with previous research in the field.

Ayahuasca typically induces nonordinary states of consciousness that involve changes in perception, emotion, cognition, and behavior. These changes can lead to increased awareness of the body and can stimulate psychological processes that provide resources for the relief of stress, emotional pain, or trauma that are typically associated with substance dependence. Ayahuasca experiences can also trigger therapeutically relevant insights, contribute to improvement of interpersonal relationships, promote personal growth and awareness of positive psychological resources, and enhance a sense of self-efficacy in patients. Furthermore, anti-craving effects were consistently reported, which seem to originate in both psychological and neurophysiologic mechanisms. The findings of this study can be also related to studies which suggest that participation in ayahuasca rituals can have positive effects on depression and anxiety (Dobkin de Rios et al. 2005; Halpern et al. 2008; Osório et al. 2011; Palladino 2009; Santos et al. 2007; Palhano-Fontes et al., in this volume); psychological conditions that are often related to the development of substance dependence and relapse.

However, in the substance-dependence treatment field, no pharmacological treatment has shown lasting success in the treatment of addictions without accompanying psychosocial interventions. This is also true for ayahuasca. For the purpose of substance-dependence treatment, ayahuasca rituals should ideally be embedded in individualized treatment programs that include psychosocial strategies. Moreover, in the opinion of the authors, ayahuasca-assisted treatment should not be reduced to a type of self-administered pharmacological intervention, but rather should be preserved as a plant-supported ritual intervention with foundations in traditional medicine that benefits from complementary psychotherapy.

Ayahuasca is best understood as a therapeutic tool and, as with any potent tool, there are risks associated with its use. This is especially true when contraindications are not respected or when ayahuasca is used by individuals who are unable to handle its effects, or if it is used in inadequate and unprofessional contexts. However, when these considerations are taken into account, it seems that ayahuasca can be an effective and reasonably safe therapeutic tool for treating substance dependence.

These results, however, are preliminary and need to be verified through studies that involve systematic data collection with standardized outcome measures. Stigma related to psychedelics as therapeutic agents should not preclude the objective evaluation of treatment outcomes; rather, these should be considered from an ethical and scientific perspective, as the search continues for novel treatment strategies that could be effective in relieving the suffering of substance-dependent individuals.

References

Alcoholics Anonymous World Services (Ed.). (1984). *Pass it on: The story of Bill Wilson and how the A.A. message reached the world.* New York, NY: Author.

Brierley, D., & Davidson, C. (2012). Developments in harmine pharmacology- implications for ayahuasca use and drug-dependence treatment. *Progress in Neuropsychopharmacology & Biological Psychiatry*. doi:10.1016/j.pnpbp.2012.06.001.

Bustos, S. (2008). *The healing power of the Icaros: A phenomenological study of ayahuasca experiences*. Doctoral Dissertation, The California Institute of Integral Studies, San Francisco, CA.

Cabieses, F. (1993). *Apuntes de medicina tradicional: La racionalización de lo irracional*. Lima, Peru: Consejo Nacional de Ciencia y Tecnología.

Calabrese, J. D. (2013). *A different medicine: Postcolonial healing in the Native American Church*. New York: Oxford University Press.

Chiappe Costa, M. (1979). El empleo de alucinógenos en la psiquiatría folklórica. In C. A. Seguin (Ed.), *Psiquiatría folklórica: Shamanes y curanderos* (pp. 176–186). Lima, Peru: Edición Centro de Proyección Cristiana.

Dobkin de Rios, M., Grob, C. S., Lopez, E., da Silviera, D. X., Alonso, L. K., & Doering-Silveira, E. (2005). Ayahuasca in adolescence: Qualitative results. *Journal of Psychoactive Drugs, 37*(2), 135–139.

Fernández, X., & Fábregas, J. M. Experience of treatment with ayahuasca for drug addiction in the Brazilian Amazon. In this volume.

Fernández, X., dos Santos, R. G., Fábregas, J. M., Cutchet, M., Fondevila, S. González, D., Bouso, J. C. Psychotherapeutic assessment of the effects of ritual ayahuasca use on drug dependency: A pilot study. In this volume.

Giove Nakazawa, R. A. (1993). Acerca del Ícaro o canto chamánico. *Revista Takiwasi, 2*, 7–29.

Giove Nakazawa, R. A. (2002). *La liana de los muertos al rescate de la vida: Medicina tradicional Amazónica en el tratamiento de toxicomanías*. Tarapoto, Peru: Revista Takiwasi.

Grof, S. (1980). *LSD psychotherapy*. Pomona, CA: Hunter House.

Halpern, J. H. (2007). Hallucinogens in the treatment of alcoholism and other addictions. In M. J. Winkelman & T. B. Roberts (Eds.), *Psychedelic medicine: New evidence for hallucinogenic substances as treatments* (Vol. 2, pp. 1–14). Westport, CT: Praeger.

Halpern, J. H., Sherwood, A. R., Passie, T., Blackwell, K. C., & Ruttenber, A. J. (2008). Evidence of health and safety in American members of a religion who use a hallucinogenic sacrament. *Medical Science Monitor, 14*(8), 15–22.

Hämmig, R. (2008). Psychedlika-unterstützte Suchttherapien. In H. Jungaberle, P. Gasser, J. Weinhold, & R. Verres (Eds.), *Therapie mit psychoaktiven Substanzen* (pp. 223–236). Bern, Switzerland: Huber.

Krebs, T. S., & Johansen, P. O. (2012). Lysergic acid dietthylamide (LSD) for alcoholism: Meta-analysis of randomized controlled trials. *Psychopharmacology (Berl), 26*(7), 994–1002. doi:10.1177/0269881112439253.

Labate, B. C., & Jungaberle, H. (Eds.). (2011). *The internationalization of ayahuasca*. Zurich, Switzerland: LIT Verlag.

Labate, B. C., Santos, R. G., Anderson, B. T., Mercante, M., & Barbosa, P. C. R. (2010). The treatment and handling of substance dependency with ayahuasca: Reflections on current and future research. In B. C. Labate & E. MacRae (Eds.), *Ayahuasca, ritual, and religion in Brazil* (pp. 205–227). London, England: Equinox.

Lambert, M. J. (2004). *Bergin and Garfield's handbook of psychotherapy and behavior change* (5th ed.). New York, NY: Wiley.

Liester, M. B., & Prickett, J. (2012). Hypotheses regarding the mechanisms of ayahuasca in the treatment of addictions. *Journal of Psychoactive Drugs, 44*(3), 200–208.

Liester, M. B., & Prickett, J. Four hypotheses regarding ayahuasca's mechanisms of action in the treatment of addictions. In this volume.

Loizaga-Velder, A. (2013). A psychotherapeutic view on therapeutic effects of ritual ayahuasca use in the treatment of addiction. *MAPS Bulletin, 23*(1), 36–40.

Mabit, J. (2007). Ayahuasca in the treatment of addictions. In M. J. Winkelman & T. B. Roberts (Eds.), *Psychedelic medicine: New evidence for hallucinogenic substances as treatments* (Vol. 2, pp. 87–106). Westport, CT: Praeger.

Miles, M. B., & Huberman, A. M. (1994). *Qualitative data analysis: An expanded sourcebook* (2nd ed.). Thousand Oaks, CA: Sage.

Miller, W. R. (1999). *Integrating spirituality into treatment*. Washington, DC: American Psychological Association.

Moermann, D. E. (1979). Anthropology of symbolic healing. *Current Anthropology, 20*(1), 59–80.

Osório, F., Horta de Macedo, L., Machado de Sousa, J. P., Porfirio Pinto, J., Quevedo, J., de Souza Crippa, J. A., et al. (2011). The therapeutic potential of harmine and ayahuasca in depression: Evidence from exploratory human and animal studies. In R. Guimarães dos Santos (Ed.), *The ethnopharmacology of ayahuasca* (pp. 75–85). Trivandrum, India: Transworld Research Network.

Palhano-Fontes, F. P., Alchieri, J. C., Oliveira, J. P. M., Lobao Soares, B., Hallak, J. E. C., Galvao-Coelho, N., & de Araujo, D. B. The therapeutic potentials of ayahuasca in the treatment of depression. In this volume.

Palladino, L. (2009). *Vine of the soul: A phenomenological study of ayahuasca and its effect on depression*. Doctoral Dissertation, Pacifica Graduate Institute Santa Barbara, CA.

Pfitzner, F. (2008). *Amazonische Heilkunde in der Behandlung der Drogensucht—Eine explorative Studie*. Saarbrücken, Germany: Verlag Dr. Müller.

Presser-Velder, A. (2000). *Das therapeutische Potential der rituellen Verwendung sakraler Heilpflanzen*. Diplomarbeit (degree thesis), University of Koblenz-Landau, Landau, Germany.

Presser-Velder, A. (2013). *Treating substance dependencies with psychoactives. A theoretical and qualitative empirical study on therapeutic uses of ayahuasca*. Doctoral Dissertation, Ruprecht-Karls-Universität Heidelberg, Heidelberg, Germany.

Project MATCH Research Group. (1997). Matching alcoholism treatments to client heterogeneity: Project MATCH three-year drinking outcomes. *Alcoholism, Clinical and Experimental Research, 22*(6), 1300–1311.

Santos, R. G., Landeira-Fernandez, J., Strassman, R. J., Motta, V., & Cruz, A. P. (2007). Effects of ayahuasca on psychometric measures of anxiety, paniclike and hopelessness in Santo Daime members. *Journal of Ethnopharmacology, 112*(3), 507–513.

Schreiber, T. (1999). *Eine psychologische Studie über Suchttherapie mit Nicht-Asiaten im buddhistischem Kloster Wat Tham Krabok in Thailand*. Diplomarbeit (degree thesis), University of Koblenz-Landau, Landau.

Thomas, G., Lucas, P., Capler, R., Tupper, K., & Martin, G. (2013). Ayahuasca-assisted therapy for addictions: Results from a preliminary observational study in Canada. *Current Drug Abuse Reviews, 6*(1), 30–42.

White, W., & Laudet, A. (2006). Spirituality, science and addiction. *Counselor Magazine, 7*(1), 56–59.

Witzel, A. (2000). The problem centered interview. *Forum qualitative social research, 1*(1), Art 22. Retrieved from http://www.qualitativeresearch.net/index.php/fqs/article/viewArticle/1132/2521[20.11.2010,10:30].

Chapter 9
Effect of Santo Daime Membership on Substance Dependence

Beatriz Caiuby Labate, Rafael Guimarães dos Santos, Rick Strassman, Brian T. Anderson and Suely Mizumoto

Abstract Previous clinical research on hallucinogen-assisted psychotherapy reported efficacy in treating substance abuse disorders, similar to what has been reported in naturalistic studies of peyote use among Native American Church members. Urban use of the Amazonian hallucinogenic brew, ayahuasca, is

---

This paper is a translation from the original Spanish published in 2013 as, "Efectos de la pertenencia al Santo Daime sobre la dependencia a sustancias psicoativas," in B. C. Labate and J. C. Bouso, (Eds.), *Ayahuasca y Salud* (pp. 302–310). Barcelona: Los Libros de La Liebre de Marzo.

B. C. Labate (✉)
Centro de Investigación y Docencia Económicas–CIDE Región Centro, Circuito Tecnopolo Norte s/n, Col. Hacienda Nueva 20313 Aguascalientes, Ags, México
e-mail: blabate@bialabate.net
URL: http://www.bialabate.net; http://www.neip.info

B. C. Labate
Institute of Medical Psychology, University of Heidelberg, Heidelberg, Germany

R. G. dos Santos
International Center for Ethnobotanical Education, Research and Service (ICEERS), Halsteren, The Netherlands
e-mail: banisteria@gmail.com
URL: http://banisteria.blogspot.com

R. Strassman
Department of Psychiatry, University of New Mexico School of Medicine, Albuquerque, New Mexico, USA
e-mail: rickstrassman@earthlink.net
URL: http://www.rickstrassman.com; http://www.cottonwoodresearch.org

R. Strassman
Cottonwood Research Foundation, Gallup, New Mexico, USA

B. T. Anderson
School of Medicine, Stanford University, Stanford, USA
e-mail: bta5ht@gmail.com

B. T. Anderson
Núcleo de Estudos Interdisciplinares sobre Psicoativos (NEIP), São Paulo, Brazil

B. C. Labate and C. Cavnar (eds.), *The Therapeutic Use of Ayahuasca*,
DOI: 10.1007/978-3-642-40426-9_9,

increasingly common in syncretic Brazilian ayahuasca religions, and anecdotal reports suggest recovery from substance dependence among those who participate in their rituals. We sought to assess more quantitatively the effects of Brazilian ayahuasca-using church membership on substance dependence. We employed a modified questionnaire using DSM-IV criteria to determine the presence of substance dependence within a sample of members of a branch of the Santo Daime Brazilian ayahuasca religion. Nearly half of these church members reported substance dependence before joining the religious organization; of these, 90 % reported cessation of use of at least one substance upon which, before church membership, they reported dependency. While these preliminary data require confirmation using more rigorous criteria, they suggest a potential role for ayahuasca, within a particular context, in the treatment of substance dependence.

Introduction

The adjunctive use of hallucinogens in the treatment of substance abuse was an active research area in the 1960s and early 1970s (Bogenschutz and Pommy 2012). With the resumption of clinical hallucinogen research in the US and Europe (Strassman 1995), hallucinogens' potential utility in treating these disorders may again be considered.

Ayahuasca is an Amazonian brew usually composed of two plants, one of which contains the hallucinogen N,N-dimethyltryptamine (DMT), while the other contains reversible monoamine oxidase-A inhibiting harmala alkaloid beta-carbolines, allowing oral activity of DMT (McKenna et al. 1984). A relatively recent phenomenon is the development of mostly urban, Brazilian ayahuasca religions; syncretic churches that incorporate ayahuasca as their religious sacrament (Labate and Araújo 2004). Preliminary data from one of these ayahuasca-using churches, the União do Vegetal (Grob et al. 1996), suggest a beneficial effect of church membership on substance abuse disorders. In this article we describe our initial, more formal, inquiry into the relationship between substance dependence and membership in a Brazilian ayahuasca religion.

S. Mizumoto
Department of Psychiatry, Federal Univeristy of São Paulo (UNIFESP), São Paulo, Brazil
e-mail: suely_mizumoto@yahoo.com.br

S. Mizumoto
The Research Group on Mental Health, State University of Santa Cruz of Bahia (UESC-BA), Ilhéus, Brazil

Methods

Participants. We studied the *Centro Eclético da Fluente Luz Universal Raimundo Irineu Serra* (CEFLURIS), a denomination of the Santo Daime Brazilian ayahuasca religion where several of the authors already had personal contacts receptive to the project. The study team presented the research protocol to the national directorship of CEFLURIS, who subsequently authorized the study and provided logistical support. Because of proximity to the research team, we chose to interview congregants of several member churches of the São Paulo and Minas Gerais regions. Participants were informed of the nature and objectives of the study, and all gave voluntary informed consent. Members of CEFLURIS consume ayahuasca in religious ceremonies that take place usually biweekly. According to our field observations, the group's official teachings promote abstention from maladaptive use of psychoactive substances.

Eighty-three individuals (41 men and 42 women) between the ages of 18 and 40 years participated in the survey. Thirty-six (44 %) had been church members for at least 3 years.

Instrument. The survey distributed to CEFLURIS members was a self-administered instrument based upon the *Diagnostic and Statistical Manual of Mental Disorders* (DSM-IV) (American Psychiatric Association, 2000) that we modified and translated into Portuguese (available upon request). At first, we included marijuana in the list of potentially abused substances, but before beginning the survey, excluded it out of concern that CEFLURIS' placement of it into their category of "sacred" plants (MacRae 1998) would reduce participants' forthrightness regarding other substances.

Participants were asked to indicate which of the following substances they currently use or formerly used: (a) alcohol, (b) tobacco, (c) sedatives/tranquilizers, (d) heroin/morphine, (e) cocaine (via nasal insufflation), (f) crack cocaine (via smoking), (g) amphetamines, (h) MDMA (Ecstasy) or LSD, (i) solvents, (j) others. Due to the very small numbers of individuals reporting use of MDMA, solvents, LSD, and heroin, we placed all subjects' responses regarding these substances into "others."

Seven subsequent questions assessed present and past patterns of use. In cases where respondents answered five questions affirmatively regarding DSM-IV criteria for dependence, we considered them dependent upon that particular substance. Recovery was determined by a negative response to the question: "Are you currently using this drug?"

Data collection. We recruited participants in Santo Daime churches before the start of their religious ceremonies, or at social gatherings of the community. We did not indicate the survey's specific content in order to avoid selection bias. The study was carried out in 1998. Participants anonymously deposited completed surveys in receptacles used especially for this purpose.

Results. Thirty-eight individuals (46 %) did not meet our criteria for a history of substance dependence. Seven (9 %) had never used any of the listed substances, and 31 (37 %) had used one or more substances, but did not meet criteria for dependence.

Forty-one individuals (49 %) met our criteria for a history of substance dependence. The remaining 5 % included 3 individuals (4 %) who did not answer questions regarding patterns of use, and 1 (1 %) who responded only that he/she was using ayahuasca to treat his/her AIDS. Note that someone who had been dependent on, for example, 2 substances, and stopped using only 1 of them, was considered as having "recovered," whether or not he/she continued dependence upon other substance(s): This explains the discrepancies in percentages reported below.

Of the 41 individuals who had a history of substance dependence, 37 (90 % of this subset) self-reported recovery from 1 or more substances, and 4 (10 %) reported continued dependence. Nineteen percent of the 41 individuals reported recovery from tobacco dependence, 27 % from alcohol, 24 % from cocaine, 8 % from crack cocaine, 5 % from "other" substances (MDMA, solvents, LSD, and heroin).

Discussion

We found a high rate of self-reported recovery from substance dependence, 90 %, among members of the CEFLURIS Brazilian ayahuasca religion. While this report can be considered only preliminary for a number of reasons discussed below, it does suggest that consumption of ayahuasca in a ritual setting has beneficial effects upon substance dependence disorders.

This study is limited by several factors. It is retrospective, rather than prospective, and is subject to selective recollection and reporting of substance use patterns. We had no collateral informants to confirm or refute self-reported patterns of use; neither did we have urine or blood toxicology data to support assertions by participants that use had ceased. Length of recovery from substance dependence also was not determined. We did not assess whether some individuals' use continued, but no longer in a dependent manner.

There were no control groups, either matched individuals outside of CEFLURIS, or perhaps more salient, individuals who joined CEFLURIS but later dropped out. In addition, all Santo Daime members use ayahuasca; thus, it was not possible to find a non-ayahuasca-using control group within the religion in order to determine the role of church membership alone on substance use relative to ayahuasca use within the church.

We also were unable to assess the patterns of use of marijuana within this cohort because of the dynamic and ambivalent nature of CEFLURIS' relationship to it. The CEFLURIS community had previously used marijuana in rituals as a religious sacrament, especially within the Amazon rainforest where their central headquarters are located. This use of marijuana drew criticism from other Brazilian ayahuasca religious communities (Goulart 2004), particularly during negotiations with the Brazilian government when the latter was deciding whether to grant permission for ayahuasca use to these organizations. As a result, the national directorship of CEFLURIS prohibited marijuana use in religious ceremonies (MacRae 1998). Marijuana use became irregular, external to the ritual context, and less openly discussed. Our decision not to poll respondents' use of marijuana has relevance to our primary findings because of the suggestion that marijuana may be effectively substituted for other drugs of abuse, arguably with less morbidity (Labigalini et al. 1999; Sifaneck and Kaplan 1995).

The efficacy of ayahuasca as a treatment for substance use disorders in religious or secular contexts has previously been suggested by Mabit (2002) and Grob et al. (1996). In the report of Grob et al. comparing 15 members of the UDV Brazilian ayahuasca religion with 15 carefully matched controls, 73 % of UDV members had a past history of "significant" alcohol-related problems, one-third had a formal diagnosis of alcohol abuse, 27 % had abused stimulants, and 53 % were tobacco dependent. He reported that all the subjects who regularly attend UDV ceremonies no longer abused these substances (Grob et al. 1996, 1999).

Preliminary data from Takiwasi, a residential treatment center in Peru that uses ayahuasca in a setting that combines indigenous shamanism and Western psychotherapy to treat substance abuse, particularly coca paste dependence and alcoholism, reveal that 31 % of over 200 patients who had at least one ayahuasca session experienced resolution of their substance abuse problems. Twenty-three percent continued using, but less severely; 23 % were unchanged or worse; 23 % were lost to follow-up (Mabit 2002).

There are several possible explanations as to how participation in ayahuasca-using rituals may help reduce substance abuse. Neurobiologically, ayahuasca increases platelet serotonin uptake/transporter sites (Callaway et al. 1994), low levels of which are found in brains of alcoholic subjects. In addition, serotonin transporter sites affect responses to cocaine (Sora et al. 2001) and adaptation to stress and fear (Wellman et al. 2007) in non-human species. Ayahuasca may thus modify relevant CNS 5-HT systems in a salutatory manner in substance abusing/dependent individuals.

Psychodynamic models have been employed to interpret beneficial results found in treatment studies using other classical hallucinogens, such as LSD, in substance use disorders involving alcohol and heroin (Pahnke et al. 1970; Savage and McCabe 1973). It is important to note that in these studies, hallucinogens were used as adjuncts to the psychotherapeutic process, rather than as primarily psychopharmacological interventions used in, sometimes, unsupportive clinical settings (Smart et al. 1966).

Religious conversion often results in reduced patterns of harmful use of various substances (Paloutzian et al. 1999). To the extent that such effects are obtained by the use of ayahuasca, either in religious or secular settings, they may be involved in the beneficial effects noted by others and us. Our findings may thus be analogous to those suggesting a reduced incidence of alcohol abuse in members of the Native American Church. In this case, the hallucinogenic mescaline-containing peyote cactus is used in a religious context (Albaugh and Anderson 1974).

Ayahuasca contains both the powerful classical hallucinogen N,N-DMT (Strassman et al. 1994), as well as the beta-carboline monoamine oxidase-A inhibitors, harmine, harmaline, and tetrahydroharmine (McKenna et al. 1984). While it is most likely that DMT plays the predominant role relevant to psychological and behavioral changes, little is known of the human psychopharmacology of the harmala alkaloids contained in ayahuasca (Naranjo 1969), nor of their synergism with DMT.

Our data suggest a high rate (90 %) of resolution of substance dependence disorders in members of a Brazilian ayahuasca religion. While provocative, they require validation using better-controlled methodologies. Future studies should examine the interplay between the set and setting of the religious use of ayahuasca and responses to the brew that contribute to recovery. By so doing, it may be possible to develop models that optimize the use of ayahuasca in the treatment of substance use disorders by combining Western medical approaches with those found to be useful in indigenous and religiously-oriented settings.

References

Albaugh, B. J., & Anderson, P. O. (1974). Peyote in the treatment of alcoholism among American Indians. *American Journal of Psychiatry, 131*, 1247–1251.

American Psychiatric Association (2000). *Diagnostic and statistical manual of mental disorders*. (4th ed., text rev.). Washington, DC: American Psychiatric Association.

Bogenschutz, M. P. & Pommy, J. M. (2012). Therapeutic mechanisms of classic hallucinogens in the treatment of addictions: From indirect evidence to testable hypotheses. *Drug Test Analysis, 4*, 543–555.

Callaway, J. C., Airaksinen, M. M., McKenna, D. J., Brito, G. S., & Grob, C. S. (1994). Platelet serotonin uptake sites increased in drinkers of ayahuasca. *Psychopharmacology, 116*(3), 385–387.

Goulart, S. L. (2004). *Contrastes e continuidades em uma tradição amazônica: as religiões da ayahuasca*. (Unpublished doctoral thesis). State University of Campinas, Brazil.

Grob, C. S., McKenna, D. J., Callaway, J. C., Brito, G. S., Neves, E. S., Oberlaender, G., et al. (1996). Human psychopharmacology of hoasca, a plant hallucinogen used in ritual context in Brazil. *Journal of Nervous and Mental Disorders, 184*, 86–94.

Grob, C. S. (1999). The psychology of ayahuasca. In R. Metzner (Ed.), *Ayahuasca: Human consciousness and the spirits of nature* (pp. 214–249). New York, NY: Thunder's Mouth Press.

Labate, B. C., & Araújo, W. S. (Eds.). (2004). *O uso ritual da ayahuasca* (2nd ed.). Campinas, Brazil: Mercado de Letras.

Labigalini, E., Rodrigues, L. R., & Silveira, D. X. (1999). Therapeutic use of cannabis by crack addicts in Brazil. *Journal of Psychoactive Drugs, 31*(4), 451–455.

Mabit, J. (2002). Blending traditions: Using indigenous medicinal knowledge to treat drug addiction. *Newsletter of the Multidisciplinary Association of Psychedelic Studies, 12*(2), 25–32.

MacRae, E. (1998). Santo Daime and Santa Maria: The licit ritual use of ayahuasca and the illicit use of cannabis in a Brazilian Amazonian religion. *International Journal of Drug Policy, 9*, 325–338.

McKenna, D. J., Towers, G. H. N., & Abbott, F. (1984). Monoamine oxidase inhibitors in South American hallucinogenic plants: Tryptamine and β-carboline constituents of ayahuasca. *Journal of Ethnopharmacology, 10*(2), 195–223.

Naranjo, C. (1969). Psychotherapeutic possibilities of new fantasy-enhancing drugs. *Clinical Toxicology, 2*(2), 209–224.

Pahnke, W. N., Kurland, A. A., Unger, S., Savage, C., & Grof, S. (1970). The experimental use of psychedelic (LSD) psychotherapy. *Journal of the American Medical Association, 212*(11), 1856–1863.

Paloutzian, R. F., Richardson, J. T., & Rambo, L. R. (1999). Religious conversion and personality change. *Journal of Personality, 67*, 1047–1079.

Savage, C., & McCabe, O. L. (1973). Residential psychedelic (LSD) therapy for the narcotic addict: A controlled study. *Archives of General Psychiatry, 28*(6), 808–814.

Sifaneck, S. J., & Kaplan, C. D. (1995). Keeping off, stepping on, and stepping off: The stepping stone theory reevaluated in the context of the Dutch cannabis experience. *Contemporary Drug Problems, 22*, 483–512.

Smart, R. G., Storm, T., Baker, E. F. W., & Solursh, L. (1966). A controlled study of lysergide in the treatment of alcoholism: I. The effects on drinking behavior. *Quarterly Journal for the Study of Alcohol, 27*(3), 469–482.

Sora, I., Hall, F. S., Andrews, A. M., Itokawa, M., Li, X. F., Wei, H., et al. (2001). Molecular mechanisms of cocaine reward: Combined dopamine and serotonin transporter knockouts eliminate cocaine place preference. *Proceedings of the National Academy of Science USA, 98*(9), 5300–5305.

Strassman, R. J., Qualls, C. R., Uhlenhuth, E. H., & Kellner, R. (1994). Dose-response study of N, N-dimethyltryptamine in humans II: Subjective effects and preliminary results of a new rating scale. *Archives of General Psychiatry, 51*, 98–108.

Strassman, R. J. (1995). Hallucinogenic drugs in psychiatric research and treatment perspectives and prospects. *Journal of Nervous and Mental Disease, 183*(3), 127–138.

Wellman, C. L., Izquierdo, A., Garrett, J. E., Martin, K. P., Carroll, J., Millstein, R., et al. (2007). Impaired stress-coping and fear extinction and abnormal corticolimbic morphology in serotonin transporter knock-out mice. *Journal of Neuroscience, 27*(3), 684–691.

Chapter 10
Experience of Treatment with Ayahuasca for Drug Addiction in the Brazilian Amazon

Xavier Fernández and Josep María Fábregas

Abstract This article presents the experience of the Institute of Applied Amazonian Ethnopsychology (IDEAA), which was created by a group of Spaniards in the Brazilian Amazon in order to study and implement the use of ayahuasca in processes of personal growth and addiction treatment. It begins with a brief description of their basic assumptions, as well as the sources of knowledge underlying the practice, such as transpersonal psychology, Santo Daime, shamanism, and Eastern disciplines. The following section shows the relationship of activities carried out in the rituals, then goes more deeply into the healing process, through a therapeutic model based on minimal accompanying intervention. Through an analysis of the content, we are introduced to the fundamental themes of ayahuasca sessions with addicts, which are discussed and related to the dynamics of transformation. The text concludes with clinical field observations that have emerged after years of practice.

Translated by Gayle Highpine and revised by Clancy Cavnar.
This chapter is a translation from the original Spanish published in 2013 as, "Experiencia de un tratamiento con ayahuasca para las drogodependencias en la Amazonia brasileña," in B. C. Labate and J. C. Bouso (Eds.), *Ayahuasca y Salud* (pp. 392–423). Barcelona: Los Libros de La Liebre de Marzo.
X. Fernández—Deceased

X. Fernández
Instituto de Etnopsicología Amazónica Aplicada (IDEAA), Amazonas, Brazil

J. M. Fábregas (✉)
Instituto de Etnopsicología Amazónica Aplicada (IDEAA) and Centro de Investigación y Tratamiento de las Adicciones (CITA), CITA Clínica, Mas Mia s/n 08319 Dosrius Barcelona, Spain
e-mail: miafabregas@gmail.com

B. C. Labate and C. Cavnar (eds.), *The Therapeutic Use of Ayahuasca*,
DOI: 10.1007/978-3-642-40426-9_10, © Springer-Verlag Berlin Heidelberg 2014

Introduction

In the year 2000, the IDEAA Institute was created by Barcelona psychiatrist Josep María Fábregas in order to study and implement the structured use of ayahuasca in the development of processes of self-knowledge and personal development, as well as in the treatment of various disorders, mainly addiction and its associated problems.

The first stage took place in Belo Horizonte, Minas Gerais, Brazil. That served as a pilot project for IDEAA prior to its final location in the interior of the Amazon jungle. In 2002, it moved to Prato Satin, which takes its name from the stream on whose banks it stands. That stream joins the Mapiá River, the same river that, several kilometers downstream, leads to the Vila Céu do Mapiá; the Mapiá River is, in turn, a tributary of the Purus River. All this land is within the protected space of La Floresta Pauni, in the state of Amazonas.

IDEAA is defined as a place where traditional or ancestral knowledge lives together with advances in contemporary psychology, using a pluralistic approach that allows the convergence of different methods. In the words of director J. M. Fábregas:

> IDEAA is a journey of personal improvement, expansion of consciousness, of knowledge; a learning path…a place suitable for this process of looking inside; introspection. We intend that experience with visionary substances be comfortable and safe, as well as fruitful and deep.

One aspect that characterizes the IDEAA concept is the work of integration of what one has learned with the visionary plants. This is understood in two ways: firstly as psychological integration, through work done after the experience with ayahuasca to develop the introspective material using meetings, writing, drawing, etc.; and, secondly, through designing tasks where the knowledge may be applied, such as activities that serve to channel the experience in daily life: community work, yoga, meditation, and other activities. This integration work gives importance to the individual process. It is taken into account that each case is different; personal differences are respected, without diminishing the group work and community integration. The process intended is introspective meditation, with the collective purpose of inner knowledge.

Conception

The sources of knowledge that have inspired the development of the Institute fall within three great frames of reference: the shamanism of the native tradition, the syncretic doctrines of the Daime,[1] and modern contributions from psychology.

[1] Santo Daime: a syncretic religious doctrine that uses ayahuasca in its rituals. For a broad view of the subject, see Labate and Araújo (2004) and MacRae (1992).

The more traditional side, with the teachings of shamanism, has left its mark in the inclination toward nature. In some rituals carried out in the jungle, the heritage of the native vision of taking ayahuasca, in which contact with nature is immediate, can be recognized. It should be recalled that at the beginning, the Institute was visited by trained shamans of the Shipibo, Asháninka, Shuar, and Navajo ethnic groups. In addition, the relevance of the moments of silence in the session can also be seen as a legacy of the austere shamanic rituals.

The roots in the Amazon tradition can also be seen through the importance of the diet, and the notion of purging as a natural process of detoxification. Although not strictly imposed, the diet is taken into account in the preparation of the work, and it is recommended to avoid certain foods such as meat and eggs, excess sugar, salt, fat, and coffee. Sometimes, too much heavy food causes hard physical cleaning in the form of vomiting and diarrhea. Abuse of food is closely linked with the compulsion to drug dependency; however, the will of the users is respected in choice of food. In this sense, the therapeutic work is closer to reflection than to repression.

Within the influence of the indigenous tradition, we find the use of *kambô,*[2] as well as anecdotally reported use of other plants such as peyote (*Lophophora williamsii*) and cebil (*Anadenanthera colubrina*). These have yet to become part of the repertoire of practices employed by the Institute, but are specific opportunities to expand knowledge of modified states of consciousness.

The second great influence—and certainly more noticeable—is that represented by the Santo Daime community of the town of Céu do Mapiá. Their geographical proximity, an hour by road, establishes a close neighborly relationship that has resulted in certain modes of collaboration and participation. Within the program of the Institute, there exists the possibility to experience some works of the Daimista community, with the aim of completing the process of seeking and healing. The official works of *hinarios,*[3] *concentrações,*[4] and *curas*[5] are the main ceremonies, while sessions of the spiritist[6] or Umbanda[7] line are oriented toward the final stages of the process, when users have reached a more elaborate knowledge of the complex Daimista cosmology.

The teachings transmitted by the community contain a notable body of knowledge about the drink, from its preparation and conservation to the tempos of

---

[2] *Kambô,* also called "frog vaccine," consists of an inoculation of the venom of the frog *Phyllomedusa bicolor*, based on a belief that in controlled doses it can reinforce the defenses of the organism.

[3] The *hinário* (hymnal) work is a session in which a determined collection of hymns is danced and sung.

[4] The *concentração* (concentration) work alternates periods of singing with periods of silent meditation, called concentrations.

[5] The *cura* (healing) works are intended to seek health at all human levels, including the spiritual.

[6] Referring to spiritist practices, based on the teachings of Allen Kardec, among others.

[7] Umbanda is a doctrine that fuses Candomblé, Christianity, and Kardecist Spiritism.

the rituals, comprising an apprenticeship in the proper use of the plants. However, the most outstanding aspect of the community of Mapiá may perhaps be their spiritual teachings. As some users have noted, contact with the people and their work has allowed them to come to terms with feelings and values that had long seemed empty after their drug abuse. In the words of Josep Cunyat, a veteran ex-user, "Tired and exhausted words like love, forgiveness, etc., are taking on meaning for people who have been very confused and very lost in life, and who suddenly begin to feel those words." In this way, the Santo Daime doctrine provides certain elements that allow the integration of the content of experiences that prove difficult to understand and that occasionally may require outside support to frame such ineffable realities. Feelings and experiences of union, membership, equality, and brotherhood, where the collective sense can compensate for the usual excess of self-centeredness, have also been identified in Daimista sessions.

The people of Céu do Mapiá transmit a wide knowledge of modified states of consciousness and transcendental realities, from their position as curators of the personal experience of their members. The cosmology of the Santo Daime incorporates an understanding of the numinous areas, such as the notion of an immaterial or astral plane, a natural conception of healing, and references to Christian, Amazonian, and African entities. It also emphasizes the transmission of universal values: love, justice, truth, harmony, etc., in addition to the conditions for fruitful transpersonal work, such as the value of intention, firmness, the group, and respect for certain policy prescriptions in diet and abstinence.

The third influx comes from the Western world, both from science and from the knowledge of modified states of consciousness from therapeutic currents such as humanist psychology, gestalt therapy, and especially transpersonal psychology, which proposes a synthesis of the human being through transcendent states experienced beyond the personal sphere. It incorporates the perennial knowledge of traditions of Eastern knowledge and explores peak experiences. Some formulations, such as the recent integral view of psychology, propose balancing the different facets of the human being. No doubt the practice of the Institute moves into this approach because it includes disciplines such as yoga, meditation, and tai chi.

One of the premises in the transpersonal approach is the idea of giving the individual the conditions for creating his or her own healing, thus favoring active processes of self-regeneration. There is an alternative to the approach of using external actions, often drugs, to be received by a patient in a passive way to eradicate a symptom. The help is intended not simply to delete the external expression of a problem, but to fashion his or her healing from within; in this case, through the self-knowledge generated by ayahuasca, where inconvenience and difficulties are seen as stops on the way to self-realization, knowledge, and health. Reference to deep or transpersonal realities allows the compression of the experiences of those who are immersed in processes of great difficulty. The person who passes through those states may be surprised or overwhelmed at the extent of the experience, so a referential framework is shown as an aid that can reassure and channel the experience toward integration.

In addition to psychology, the science around ayahuasca and psychonautic[8] and entheogenic[9] currents has influenced the activities of the Institute. Currently, several research projects are being carried out to evaluate different aspects of the effects of ayahuasca and the results of its consumption by humans. These three main areas have contributed to the development of the project in a dynamic way, although we have also witnessed problems of interference between the different ways of understanding drug addiction, healing, or the process involved in treatment. The strong emphasis on the diet on the part of the shamans was not entirely incorporated, perhaps due to the fact that intensive retreats were not practiced, but rather regular weekly ceremonies, which made it impossible to maintain the constant cleansing diet.

Another discrepancy between frames of knowledge has been in the way disease is understood. While therapeutic ideas stress the responsibility of the individual in his or her own healing, the spiritist conception, widespread in the area, states the importance of certain "suffering spirits" who are capable of deviating the impulses of the individual toward drug abuse. These notions, seemingly incompatible, produced friction and debates, creating the possibility of extending cognitive horizons in a creative coexistence of cultural synergies, wherein respect for other ways of understanding life could be practiced.

In summary, and in synthesis, we can say that the practice of the Institute focuses on processes of knowledge, self-examination, and healing, opening spaces for complementary integration of secular work with visionary plants, in a practice that is of integral character and respectful of personal processes. As an institute of ethnopsychology, it assumes the ecological attitudes and natural practices of the environment that surrounds it, with special attention to the study of ayahuasca.

Program

At the *Bom Dia* (Good Morning) meeting, held every morning except Sunday, the day's activities are organized with a review of the health and the feelings of each person. In case of difficulties, solutions to practical problems are encouraged, from the care of wounds to the organization of community tasks to the preparation of the rituals, among other concerns. It is a very open meeting, where each person may express himself freely, the guide being simply a moderator who gathers the initiatives of the group.

---

[8] Jünger was the first to use the term "psychonaut," meaning "navigator of consciousness." It is used at present to refer to researchers and artists who use psychoactive substances as means of introspective self-exploration.

[9] This is related to the neologism "entheogen," proposed by, among others, Wasson and Ott, in 1979, to designate visionary or shamanic substances or those substances capable of producing a similar modified state of consciousness. It means, "generating the divine within" and was born of the intent to clarify that visionary substances are not strictly hallucinogenic.

On Monday afternoons, the weekly appraisal meeting is organized. In it, the Institute's users[10] frame their purposes and compare their actions throughout the week with goals set forth the previous week. The most common is the intention to reduce or quit tobacco—putting their compulsion to the test—or to adjust the diet, eliminating sugar, bread, etc. These initiatives demonstrate advances in the capacity to make choices.

The yoga classes, which begin at dawn, are sessions of the hatha form, a specialty that especially focuses on postural techniques and work on the physical dimension. Blockages and restrictions left by years of drug addiction are quickly revealed; every day it is an effort for users to face this class and confront problems such as the habit of not rising early or personal complexes of resistance. Yoga enables integration of the ayahuasca experience with the corporal body, materializing the grasp of metaphysical nature into more tangible realities. This idea is implicit in the very name of the discipline, which etymologically means union.

Zen meditation allows a few moments of total cessation of thought, creating the possibility of listening to the mind in its natural state. It is worth noting that this discipline is very difficult for people with problems of addiction, especially cocaine, because they are confronted with exaggerated mental agitation. This practice serves as a complement to the session with ayahuasca, providing training in posture, attention, and breathing.

The morning is dedicated to community works and daily chores. Since the life of the addict is motivated, to a large extent, by self-gratification, group and community actions are understood as counterweight to a life of extreme individualism. These tasks include household chores such as gathering fruit, raking roads, taking care of the garden, etc. Those who have a skill or profession can offer their services to the group. In the therapeutic scheme, the presence of professionals who have collaborated with the Institute has contributed more than a structured set of activities: They have had close coexistence with users. The techniques employed by IDEAA include individual psychotherapy; workshops on emotions, breathing techniques, psychodrama, and bibliotherapy; and family constellation therapy. To that are added other practices such as massage, colonic irrigation, shiatsu, and naturopathy.

Around noon, the intensity of activity lessens, and after lunch, users normally return to their cabins.[11] This tone is maintained throughout the afternoon, interrupted only by Portuguese classes, recycling workshops, tai chi classes, or meditation. Retreating to individual cabins for introspection is one of the fundamental slogans of IDEAA. There, each user has an opportunity to create a space for reflection. Reading, and, above all, writing, are highly recommended, because

[10] The term "user" alludes to those who "use" IDEAA, both people with definite problems like addictions or other psychological complications and people without specific disorders who seek a process of personal growth.

[11] The cabins are constructed of wood with thatched roof in the traditional Amazonian style. They are 15 sq m, and in IDEAA they are the home of each user, creating an individual space for collecting oneself and introspection.

experience has shown that one of the best ways to integrate, develop, and fix the material in the mind is the creation of a personal diary. The Institute provides a model: a "blog notebook," which looks at the vital moments of the person, developing the story of his life in sections, and giving rise to a kind of autobiography. Also recommended is a diary of experiences, which gathers what the user has been learning during the sessions. The goal is to experience condensation, remembrance, and to understand the relationship of elements, creating the opportunity to transfer information from a non-ordinary state of consciousness to more earthly levels, making possible the practical application of the knowledge learned.

One task that, no doubt, deserves special attention is the preparation and execution of the session with ayahuasca. Every Saturday, a *chapéu*[12] work is conducted, in a hat-shaped circular construction under which the inhabitants of IDEAA gather once a week. The day is dedicated to the communal preparations for the session, and each person assumes a task, from the preparing of the fire to the creation of a floral center.

The session is the axis of IDEAA activities, and in its practice lies the essence of its purpose. It is a ritual that incorporates diverse elements, but it is not saturated with ornamentation, because the collective purpose is self-examination, which is brought about by meditation and concentration. In this space, the participants sit in a circle where, together but individually, they attempt to look inside themselves. Preferably, this is done with eyes closed, and the only rule is not to disturb the others, because the subtlety of the journey requires great respect for the privacy of each member. The intention is a confrontation with one's self, away from the evasions that so abound in everyday life and in addictive habits. For this reason, experience shows, the richest and most profound experiences occur most frequently in those who remain inside the circle without being disturbed by desires, distractions, lectures or other forms of escape from the encounter with one's self. The work consists of three occasions of drinking. It is possible to lie down in the hammock or sit by the fire, but the seated position is recommended to maintain a conscious attitude. The group usually consists of a guide, a caregiver, and about a dozen members. Evocative music is alternated with silences that favor internal confrontation. It closes with an effusive interchange of emotions, among hugs and congratulations, after the rigors of the internal battle.

The next day, usually Sunday, is a day of rest and integration. The evening is divided between evaluations of the research projects into the effects of the sessions, and the phase of integration, with a time for reflecting on the experience. But most important is the integration meeting, in which each person has the opportunity to narrate his or her experience and the results and conclusions they have drawn from it. Attendance is compulsory, but participation is voluntary, and everyone is free to express what he or she considers necessary. It is a space to exercise listening; inviting sincerity, openness, and sharing without value

[12] *Chapéu* is Portuguese for "hat."

judgments. The guide acts discreetly, and on occasion can give feedback that summarizes a scattered discourse, or that pulls out an important element to display an external vision that may help serve as a reflection, without interfering in a solely personal process. In addition to the main work of *chapeu,* there are other modalities that include: the cabin work, the *mata* work, the morning work, and the *roçado* work.

The cabin work is an individual session where the user receives ayahuasca in his or her cabin to develop an internal search through meditation, while the guide remains vigilant against any eventuality. It has few ritual elements—almost limited to the opening and a closing of the session—creating an opportunity conducive to interior contact. Since it usually happens with several people at one time, the group union is maintained from a distance. The relationship between the guide[13] and the user in this session has a special character, giving rise to an unusual complicity.

The *mata*[14] work uses the jungle as context. It is usually planned as a hike up to some *roçado,* or special enclave, where a simple meditation takes place, or a hammock is put up to lie down in, with musicians possibly incorporated into the sparse ritual. Most often done during the day, works in the forest have the vitality of synchrony with the natural environment.

In 2005, an extension of IDEAA was created in a rural house near Barcelona, as a base for preparing participants prior to the trip, and as a place to welcome them back after the Amazon experience. This initiative arose from observing the difficulties that users have had in adapting themselves back to the city. In this place, contact with nature, yoga practice, and community living help to retain the way of life and integrate it into everyday reality.

Here can be found the services of therapists, evaluations of research projects, and, especially at the beginning, the interviews that make up the process of preparation, information, and assessment. Future participants are evaluated with the help of psychometric instruments to learn in-depth about their motivations, their inclinations, and their capacities to properly fit into the project. Candidates have been excluded for not showing firm motivation, or for some severe psychopathology such as psychosis or severe personality disorders. People with psychiatric medication would be told to spend a period of phasing out their medication prior to travel, due to possible incompatibilities with ayahuasca; not just pharmacological incompatibility, but incompatibility in therapeutic conceptualization.

---

[13] Both in the ayahuasca sessions and in the integration meetings, the word "guide" is used to describe the figure who leads and accompanies the work of the users. The knowledge of the guides comes both from experiences with Daimista and shamanic traditions and Western training, such as that developed in the Society for Ethnopsychiatry and Cognitive Studies (Sociedad de Etnopsicología y Estudios Cognitivos, or SdEA), directed by Josep María Fericgla, which has brought together the majority of the guides and therapists who work in IDEAA.

[14] *Mata* means "forest" in Portuguese.

Because of their great diversity, there is no typical profile of users. However, most participants have been men, of Spanish origin, with an average age of over 30 years, asking for help for a cocaine problem. Very often, there are cases of dual psychopathology, i.e., a psychological problems associated with the drug dependency.

After the evaluation period, a few weeks pass until the trip, which takes about 3 days from Spain. When a new group arrives, a space is created for their adaptation, which normally takes from 1 to 3 weeks. Tropical conditions, the jungle, language, life in community, and, for many, the first contact with ayahuasca, combine to make a situation that is new and unfamiliar, so a careful period of adjustment is necessary. The moments of initial adaptation are usually conditioned by the predisposition of the user, and if that is negative, it can result in a long series of clashes. These first 3 or 4 weeks tend to be a time of optimism, except for those who find it difficult to adapt to the forest for various reasons; phobias, resistances, or other discomforts.

The first drinks of ayahuasca usually do not meet all expectations. Due to resistances, defenses, difficulty in recognizing the effect or in learning how to experience it, several sessions are often necessary for the full effects of the drink to be felt. After about a month, the individual is immersed in his personal process, when all his problems, with many associated difficulties emerge; before the realizations that the experience with ayahuasca can generate comes the polar opposite, "acting out,"[15] which, in the case of addicts, is especially charged. Users may feel the desire to leave the boundaries of the Institute, or present behaviors aimed at distracting themselves, ranging from staying up late to eating and smoking too much.

In this process of continuous catharsis, difficulties of acceptance, resistances to change, and development of conflict within each user, the boundaries of personal living spaces may be violated, because people live very closely in this village of fifteen people. Difficulties emerge among companions who are finding themselves immersed in the same coexistence; boundaries become too diffuse to establish conventional forms of therapeutic management. Therefore, the process ends up settling into a dynamic mode, with companions, guides or references engaged in closely participating attention.

An analysis has been completed of the content from users' accounts in the integration meetings described to explore the themes in the experiences of ayahuasca users with addictions. While this analysis might require its own paragraph, it has been included in the section on "process" for expository reasons.

A corpus has been used containing transcripts of the testimonies of 20 people, four women and sixteen men, who participated in the integration meetings between September 2003 and January 2004, with a total of 218 works or individual sessions analyzed. The technique used was that of thematic categorical analysis (Bardin 1977), which operates by grouping texts based on analogous content.

---

[15] "Acting out" [English in original] is used in therapeutic language to refer to the unconscious tendency to exteriorize internal conflicts with excessive willfulness and without reflection.

A qualitative approach has been chosen for several reasons. First of all: the need to capture the semantic richness of the experiences, especially taking into account the total subjectivity of these experiences, as well as the presence of socio-cultural variables. In addition, since it is a relatively little studied area, a qualitative approach is useful as an exploratory approach to the phenomenon. The investigator assumed a constructivist perspective of meaning and the phenomenological nature of the experiences of the user. A justification for the qualitative studies in research on psychoactive substances can be found in MacRae (2004), "The continuous appreciation of the analysis of this type of material depends on contextualization and assessing the conditions in which data were collected, thus reintroducing an inevitable human and 'subjective' element" (p. 5).

Despite the enormous range of experiences found, six fundamental thematic blocks have been identified that can be sorted by degree of relevance in the following way: review of the past, psychological insights,[16] experiences of emotional character, death experiences, experiences with nature, and transcendental experiences.

A large space is devoted to the emergence of past events, ranging from childhood experiences to the circumstances of the user's life with drugs:

> What I saw is the brutal disorder that I have had in my life. My life passed before me like a portrait. It can be summed up in one word: chaos. I have had to think about it and I analyzed it. From high school it was already a disaster: three expulsions, I was jailed. My youth was another disaster. I have passed my life drugging myself. Ayahuasca is scaring me, it is making me see very heavy things from my past, that would need to be forgiven.... One of the most violent situations I experienced was when I disappeared from home for more than one month and a half, (I was squatting with some colleagues), and when I came back my parents had given me for dead. My mother had a heart attack from the pressure she suffered all the time I was gone, and I had to go to the hospital and her crying and hugging me as she told me "you're alive, you're alive." Today I would like to hear her voice. I have come to get rid of all the shit (H. E.).

As subsections of the biographical review, the constant reference to family figures stands out, most of these stories referring to the damage caused by years of abuse. Revisiting traumatic episodes is another repeated subtheme:

> I was taken to the situation when my parents separated. I was three years old and I woke up one night and I was alone and I began to look for my mother in the cabinets and even in the trash. This is a flashback I had tonight, as if I really were in the situation anew, looking for my mother. I had feelings of rage because thirty years later, I have this pain and it made me want to scream. I have anger towards this pain that I do not know how to get out of me. I realize that it is pain from the lack of love from my mother (B. E.).

In spite of how hard it is to revisit those memories, the most people value these experiences and feel the need to go through them on their way to healing. The most common way of understanding them is as a phase of cleaning:

---

[16] "Insight" [English in original] signifies a sudden idea of intense clarity or penetration that may be associated with intuition.

> The feeling I dragged up from that era was a strange feeling, especially toward my father, who was a very hard man. I was calling him and an idea came to me very clearly: I did the best I could… The conclusion I draw is that one chooses how to take things… It was a work of cleansing. Forgotten images of the past, of childhood, of the schoolyard came to me, too (S. J.).

Another significant theme refers to experiences that clarify conflicts or personal qualities and give conscious insights into patterns of psychological functioning. Although this content is closely linked with the previous theme, it is considered relevant enough to stand alone as a theme, because sometimes it does not relate directly to the review of the past. "I see that I need the recognition of others. I've always felt alone, even in relationships with girls. First I have to think about recognizing myself before seeking recognition from others" (J. R.); "I saw myself as a cocoon, a true idiot, a self-centered, very isolated, very alone, sad, the sadness I dragged around. Then I said, 'damn, how is it that I have not seen before, how was I so blind?'" (S. J.).

Insights about patterns of abuse and dependence can be distinguished within this category: "I discovered that I drugged myself out of laziness, and as a reward after working. I was rewarding myself in the worst way" (M. A.); "My purpose was the compulsions, and this is my way to seek affection. I filled that void with food, lines of cocaine, etc." (A. J.); "I've done a lot of damage with drugs and now ayahuasca is helping me to return to my identity, which the drugs moved me away from" (B.E.); "I am useless. I am not capable of anything. I am very discouraged. I didn't use to be that way. I am now facing myself without drugs. I am realizing how I am in reality" (S. E.).

A distinct theme is the experiences of death, which often were felt in a literal way, at least at first. Usually they contained images of one's own death:

> It was a very hard work. I found myself in a tremendous situation. I lived my burial. I was in a coffin and my whole family, including the family that I have not seen for years, they wept for my death (H. E.).

"I thought that I would never return to my place on Earth. And it is confusing, as I went from one subject to another, I saw myself dead and tasted blood in my mouth" (B. E.).

Occasionally, these images were accompanied by pleasant feelings or lack of fear: "I had a vision in which I saw myself as a chrysalis. I felt dead and I saw myself dead, tossed on the grass, and I had eyes all over the body. Nothing scary, I felt good" (B. A.).

> I had a vision of myself, I was in a coffin, my death—this is the second time this has happened to me—and I saw a light. It did not give me any fear. I saw myself floating in the depths of silence. I opened eyes to cut this short, and it was impossible, something was sucking me outward (B. E.).

Elements relating to a later stage of liberation and rebirth appear associated with bright visions:

> I became a skeleton, a very unpleasant feeling. I had to touch it and everything. I felt it and I felt down to the pure bone…my death, so real, so filthy, so inhumane. I died drowning me in vomit…and I saw inside the coffin and tried to see my face, my hair, and all I saw was a skeleton. I looked at the nameplate and saw my name G. S. R. Very afraid. I tried to leave, because I had already seen enough, and enter a fantasy instead…. Watching you (referring to the group), you gave me the good role that I was entering; I saw an image of myself dressed in white, very pure. I touched my flesh and I found myself in a place enveloped in light, returning to be born (G. S. R.).

Reference to emotions and recovery is constant during the healing process, constituting another important thematic grouping: "Felt grief, sadness, rage, my habitual loneliness, and I felt very ashamed" S.; "I went to the fire and I felt the ability to be able to love. It cost me great effort to feel that" (M. A.).

> There are repeated allusions to persons significant in the context of emotional recovery: I remembered my people, my family and friends, others I have had to leave. I remembered much of my mother… I felt joy, sadness and love. I felt much. J. came to give me a hug and I felt super-full… All the feelings that I had, I want to gather them and write them down. Very well. I am very happy (M. A.).

Within this broad human emotional spectrum are frequent statements of appreciation: "I had blamed my father for my pain, but yesterday I had gratitude" (J. R.);

> Yesterday I felt gratitude toward my mother, in a memory of mine, and I felt that I should return the gratitude to her. And this morning I have done it, an offering in the river. I am grateful to G., who has been by my side and remains there and is a friend forever. And my sister who helped me to be here and was grateful that I was permitted to continue. I feel satisfied with what I've got. I am thankful to myself, it is the first thing that I have done well in many years (B. M.).

> The emphasis on the capacity to forgive and be forgiven is remarkable:

> For the first time I forgave several things. I forgave a girlfriend I had. For the police who hit me, I relived the hostilities, and the ability I had to do things that would make them beat me so much. I relived the story from the point of view of the cop and forgave him (B. A.).

In certain cases, especially toward the end of the process, explicit references are made to the feeling of love:

> Memories came to me of when I was small, my parents, my sisters, how it was before, it was very affectionate, such a kind of love, affection, well, exploded inside, totally burned, I opened and this was very decisive to follow" (M. A.).

> It was a work of many feelings. I worked much with the love, the love that I have towards everything and everyone, I have it, although it seems that I sometimes hate. I realized that if I hate it is because of love. I fought with people whom I love, if I didn't have regard for them I wouldn't fight with them (G. O.).

The nature experiences constitute a clearly significant thematic block, where we find an interesting variety of experiences, many of which relate to the jungle: feelings of intimacy with it, of connection, of fear, of being one with it or part of it, of the absence of anguish in the jungle, of its beauty, its forces, etc. Other types of experience with nature are also found: of everything being alive, of reconciliation with nature, of nature as a live being, of projection or transposition of human qualities into animals or plants, of awareness of our place in the world, of being one more animal, etc.: "Everything is alive; the jungle was tiny… I saw how the Earth breathed and I turned to see the trees and their leaves living and moving" (D. J.).

> I have done a work of connecting with nature. The wind and rain presented themselves to me. I saw how a frog came out of the ground and sank into the water. I saw how the roots were sucking. I saw how the trees danced (O. J.).

Comments praising the color green were often heard: "Green. The range of greens. People of the color green. All very soft, very simple and very pretty. I rolled in the grass. A pleasure to caress it, touch it. I grounded myself in the earth" (G. O.); "I believe that within the forest there is a very special force, very wild. As I think about it, I go there and enjoy it. Green is so important (C. P.).

It should be noted that the experiences of nature were very frequent in the *mata* works, set in the jungle. As for images or experiences of animals, we find a variety; from hazardous or gruesome animals to mythical images or power animals such as unicorns, lions, and eagles as well as constant references to snakes.

Feelings of union, connection, fullness, serenity, and transcendent, oceanic, transpersonal or spiritual experiences manifest themselves at a second level of relevance, but it is also difficult to express such ineffable experiences. Some people are reserved about sharing these experiences, although it is also possible that these states are not often reached because of the long biographical review necessary. However, it is clear that they form part of the experience of the work:

> I was connected to a higher force that filled me with a peace that had not experienced. I was not tangled up in interior dialogs; I saw everything clear and simple. The tendency I have of complicating things that seen from another point of view can be simple. I have filled out a lot (S. J.).

In some stories, experiences can contain some transpersonal element, even if they are not specific:

> I had a purge. I felt very sick to my stomach, and the poop, and the food, I saw it all as a life cycle. I saw a dead cockroach. The cockroach dies, and nothing happens. I saw a great chain of eating, shitting, and dying and nothing happens; and if the planet explodes in the cosmos nothing happens to it, then I realized that nature has no pain, that pain is invented by us, that poor children in Africa don't matter and I don't either, nor my own pain, of course. An acceptance of pain and of the cycle of life, very positive, that nothing happens (F. A.).

This section encompasses a wide variety of experiences. Especially noteworthy are the experiences of emptiness[17]: "I had a strange moment, as in nothing, in a

[17] This emptiness, different from what we mentioned as a result of the abuse of drugs, refers to an experience described and valued by the Zen Buddhist tradition as a state of profound perception of the nature of reality. It can manifest in a paradoxical form as empty and full at the same time, since this emptiness makes the phenomenal world possible.

vacuum, but full at the same time. There was no thought, or sensations or emotions, and I liked it, enjoyed it. It was a very positive work" (T. O.).

The main themes have been described here. It is likely, however, that certain contents were not easily verbalized or have been omitted, which could be the case, for example, with regard to entities, spirits, and other non-consensus realities. We recognize this limitation, especially taking into account the fact that those experiences are usual with ayahuasca, but have low relative frequency in our analysis.

A clearly secondary theme is references to difficulties at the sessions, especially in the first ones:

> Too much tension in the fetal position. I was also very aware of all. And it bothered me that I felt bad, and I was afraid of being afraid. I had a hard time, but I prefer this to not learning anything (W. P.).

Allusions to the body and its care appear occasionally: "It has shown me where I am screwed really… It is marking me where it hurts me now. My conclusion is that I have to take care of myself" (H.E.); "The physical body we have is a gift and should take care of it. I think that I'm waking up and beginning to appreciate it" (B. E.).

There are also experiences of one's personal potential: "I have started to break down barriers within myself, and I saw that I could do things that were unthinkable within myself. I have had to quit taking on the role of sick person."

References to ayahuasca itself present with moderate frequency, with nuanced expressions regarding the way it manifests its abilities. In some cases, it takes the form of a person: a woman, an Indian, etc. As a note, experiences of reliving one's own birth—also called "perinatal experiences" and studied in depth by Grof (1994)—have been collected in passing, but didn't become a theme of widespread influence.

From the results of the analysis, a number of considerations have emerged that will be described in the discussion section. Although we understand that the process of self-examination does not end, after 3–6 months, users return to their places of origin to start another process of adaptation and further integration. The difficulties at this stage are multiple; after the Amazon experience, a sense of satisfaction at having resolved various psychological problems is common, but this development still needs opportunities to evolve and become a reality.

The reencounter with everyday life is hard. Besides the change in continents, there is a change from a natural environment to urban spaces, and from rural society to a consumer society. Difficulties in adapting to the world of family and work can make users tumble into a desire to revert to old patterns of drug use. For this reason, the project offers a support network group, as well as the possibility of spending time in IDEAA-Barcelona, which serves as a bridge between the jungle and the city.

The research project developed by the Institute has a final phase of follow-up after 1 year that includes, among other evaluations, a semi-structured interview through which the user can assess his or her experience and the impact of the various elements of his or her process. In this case, a preliminary analysis has been made based on interviews with six people who completed the process successfully.[18] Given the small sample, the value of this analysis is purely exploratory and illustrative.

To the question about the impact of ayahuasca in their process and how they defined it, answers revolve around the idea of confronting or facing oneself, or learning more about oneself: "The ayahuasca, for the possibility that it has to make you see yourself as in a mirror" (O. E.); "For ayahuasca, the word for me is, 'a marvel.' To see your own self, to take on and confront yourself and deal with what comes to you, and to try to change" (H. E.);

> It gave me the opportunity to find myself within myself, and to confront myself and take on the negative aspects of my personality and to work with this. I got very messy; I think I had total chaos in my head, not knowing where to begin and deepen. I knew that I needed a total mental restructuring, but wasn't sure what was going wrong inside me, if was at the emotional level, if it was rage, sadness, grief, hate… (Referring to the important part of the process) taking on my "I," taking on my own self, taking on my fears and confronting myself and wanting to move forward, after this explosion of nature, which I believe is the fundamental substance in ayahuasca, yes (E. G.).

> I could see; I could see myself as though from outside myself, I could really see what I wanted to be. I reached what I want to be and what I was at that moment. It helped me to change (S. A.).

In general, evolution is shown in the way life is understood, from a change of values to a turnaround in the existential sense: "Before, I only believed in myself. Now, I realize there are many things to believe in and which can help you continue forward" (H. E.); "It influenced (the process in my life) by making me realize that there are things in life that are worth it; then you come here and you become aware of things" (M. A.).

> I was a person who didn't believe in anything, it was very hard to move forward in life if all that existed was what I saw with the eyes, I had nothing to grab onto. The fact of beginning to believe in something more, in a force greater than what I had at the time (O. E.).

Reconstruction and restructuring is another constant; primarily, keeping in mind that some of them had practically destroyed their lives:

> Having this opportunity I personally think has saved my life. It has saved me, above all, from falling back into drugs; it has helped me to know very well what they are, the path of drugs, and it has saved me. I was a person completely void in recent years, sick, empty, dependent, with zero quality of life, and with terrible judicial problems. Having to reconstruct myself at a clinic, in a community, was not enough, it wouldn't have lasted two days had I not met this substance (ayahuasca) in this privileged place and had the opportunity to restructure myself from within and from there to rebuild my life little by little" (E. G.).

[18] Referring to cases where abstinence from the principal drug of abuse was maintained for at least 1 year.

"Ayahuasca has allowed me to be a person and to go back and remake everything again, like a child who has to learn everything beginning with eating and walking" (S. J.).

Summarizing his own experience, Órfila talks about impermanence and temporality as some of the keys in the process of learning with ayahuasca. This fragment, by way of illustration, synthesizes the work that many have made relocating in life:

> Everything is present, but this present will be charged with the past and future. You cannot live the present without having resolved the past and without knowing how to project the illusion without expectations in the future.

Discussion of the Analysis

With regard to the themes of the process, the enormous work of biographical review necessary for users who undergo treatment for drug dependence and abuse has been demonstrated. For some, the life stories were filled with conflicting events, while for others substances of abuse had managed to suppress the impact and sometimes even the memory of those events. In the evolution of these stories, therefore, it seems obligatory to travel back to the past that has been opened in order to be resolved after a phase of cleansing. The unfolding of past events gives perspective and allows insight, revealing patterns of operation through the wealth of memory that emerges into consciousness. Shanon (2002) provides precise details about the cognitive dynamics of this process:

> In each case, the ayahuasquero saw images, each of which representing a certain point of his biography. The flashes did not emerge in chronological order, but juxtaposed thematically. This juxtaposition revealed some patterns of personality and behavior of the ayahuasquero of which he was not previously aware (p. 114).

In individuals who arrive at later stages of resolution it can be observed that a compression of old conflicts, realized through the personal history, gives an elevated perspective on the drug-addicted past that offers a sense of freedom from blame. By this time, the importance of recognition and acceptance as premises for handling conflicts has been made clear, with moments of high therapeutic value.

The experiences of death, on their part, point to a tortuous path of healing and regeneration. Difficult biographies at times need a "final" cleansing from where rebuilding can begin. Grof (2005) has explored both themes in the general context of modified states of consciousness. This author describes in depth the high therapeutic value of these experiences:

> The experience of psychological death tends in great measure to eliminate suicidal tendencies and ideation. Intense aggressive and self-destructive impulses are consumed in many dramatic experiential sequences in the process of death and rebirth… After the experiences of the death of the ego and of cosmic unity, abuse of alcohol and narcotics as well as suicidal tendencies are seen as tragic errors caused by a spiritual yearning for transcendence that previously had not been recognized and had been misunderstood (p. 297).

In the process with ayahuasca, the theme of death has been referred to by Shanon (2002) and also by Villaescusa (2006), in his study of the effects of short-term intake of ayahuasca; both used samples from subjects without clinical problems. It should be added that many of the experiences in the biographical review, such as the experiences of death, have a wide presence in this analysis with the dependent population, perhaps more than in people without defined problems, as in the samples used by these authors. The preponderance of issues about nature or natural elements has also been clearly found by Shanon (2002).

Throughout the process of acceptance and change, the emotions seem to be heavily involved. In the intense review of the past, repressed feelings or feelings not fully felt often emerge. Everything that had been lived without feeling penetrates consciousness, asking for an opportunity to actualize itself and stop being a pending account. This psychological recycling serves to rebalance the psyche of the person, through the release of conflicting emotions that were avoided during the years of emotional anesthesia with substances of abuse, which prevented the natural flow of emotions in life. Once the past has been purged and the ability to feel has been recovered, the individual is free to live in the present with a greater range of feelings. In this sense, an emotional actualization process seems to be produced. Riba (2004) has found a physiological correlate in the relationship between memory and emotions during his clinical studies on the effects of ayahuasca using the LORETA[19] technique. Activity changes were registered in brain waves on certain areas, such as the paralimbic system, involved in processes of attention, emotion, and memory. Villaescusa (2006) found an increase of awareness of emotions in urban Westerners, while Fericgla (1997) has highlighted the role of emotions in the effects of ayahuasca, describing it as an emotional self-education. Thus, ayahuasca may be indicated for emotional problems such as blocks or trauma.

Moments of acceptance and recognition appear to be key elements in resolving conflicts. Later in the treatment, the discovery of the ability to forgive both oneself and others is shown as a valuable therapeutic experience. This, coupled with other changes in the emotional sphere, leads to an evolution in the processes of users. The first months are dominated by intense biographical review within a phase of cleansing, while for those who have passed 3, 6, and 9 months, experiences of reconciliation, of serenity, etc., are found with more frequency. However, this progression is not linear, and one or another element may alternate, so after sessions of great fullness, one is likely to relive the past and continue the cleansing process.

Experiences of high therapeutic value noted among drug addicts include biographical review, insights, and experiences of emotions or of death. Compared to data from subjects without addictions, other types of experiences are relatively less frequent, such as those related to human culture, mythology, religion, philosophy,

[19] A technique for registering brain waves, LORETA is an acronym for Low Resolution Brain Electromagnetic Tomography.

metaphysics, and metamorphosis (such as those, for example, found by Shanon 2002). It is possible, therefore, that users with dependency need to delve into their therapeutic processes prior to evolving into other subjects.

Experiences of high therapeutic value noted among drug addicts include biographical review, insights, and experiences of emotions or of death. Compared to data from subjects without addictions, other types of experiences are relatively less frequent, such as those related to human culture, mythology, religion, philosophy, metaphysics, and metamorphosis (such as those, for example, found by Shanon 2002). It is possible, therefore, that users with dependency need to delve into their therapeutic processes prior to evolving into other subjects.

Final Thoughts

We started by describing IDEAA as a pluralistic place, where different ways of conceiving healing and knowledge of visionary plants have been combined together. This pluralistic quality can be seen as its character and its weakness at once, because, although it has been a place of meeting among different frameworks, people, and cultures, it is also a challenge to undertake a process of intense difficulty without the constant support of a consistent framework. However, this organization has allowed freedom and has shown an ability to adapt to circumstances. It has also made it possible for each user to be the creator of their own process—only accompanied and assisted—with the result of meeting with their self, and ultimately deeper self-knowledge.

Although external aid in the process is recognized as essential, some forms of conventional psychotherapy have been inadequate; even the description of treatment can lead to confusion. The figure of the guide, facilitator or caregiver is conceived simply as a companion to the personal discovery process. In everyday life, their role is to give whatever support is necessary, with flexible limits, or to adopt a role that encourages the reflection of conflicts like a mirror, helping the process with ayahuasca to crystallize in everyday life. Interventions are restricted to the unavoidable, because the experience with ayahuasca allows reflection of conflicts and encounter with an interior orientation from which limits can be set. Only on certain occasions, as in the performance of rituals, is the position of guide adopted, whose presence is without a doubt essential. Fabregas reflects on these figures:

> They are companions, they are references, they are guides in this respect; more than guides for reference. A guide would be a marked path, while a reference may be something that is out there, even behind, allowing you to locate yourself and to orientate yourself, putting your personal experience and knowledge at your disposition.

At the same time, this figure is necessary, recognizing that at the forefront of a session there is always a guide:

> In any experience with visionary substances he is an indispensable presence... The honesty and the ability of that guide determine the success of the experience; creates security or gives accurate direction; or, on the other hand, a manipulative or dishonest guide can achieve much in the short term but quickly finds a limit. I think that experiences have to be accompanied; not guided, directed or conducted, but accompanied... I would not recommend unaccompanied individual experiences.

In a way, we are dealing with a process so intimate, so profound, so ineffable, that it does not require frames or rigid figures who may interfere with the very personal space where the knowledge is generated. The result of this approach is a flexible therapeutic support, with little hierarchy, minimal management, horizontal in nature, where the "therapist" is a facilitator, a companion in the human processes, or a reference guide.

However, facing certain stormy experiences, references or evocative ideas are necessary to allow us to understand the complexity of those states. Certain notions of the perennial philosophy, Daimista cosmology or transpersonal psychology are displayed as an aid to understanding, for example, the numerous experiences of death that are integrated to be seen as the symbolic process of death and rebirth. The same can be said of experiences of emptiness, torment, dissolution of self, etc.; that, upon being mentioned by the companion, help the person in search of meaning, which he can usually find himself. But the territory of consciousness is perhaps too vast to be classified, and some experiences within little-explored regions naturally only lead to silence.

Concerning frameworks of knowledge, IDEAA has a framework currently and constantly in construction. Included with regard to this dynamism, within the Brazilian scene, is the recent analysis of Araujo (1999), which studies the Daimista group Barquinha as a "cosmology in construction," whereas Labate (2004) describes reinvention of uses or new ways of conceiving the work with ayahuasca that are built through creating spaces of intersection among different cultural, therapeutic, and religious references.

Regarding the role of the various elements involved in the process; obviously, ayahuasca is not the only help that the person receives. Yoga, the activities of the Institute, and the presence of the Amazon jungle, with its people, undoubtedly influence the recovery process. However, both IDEAA and the area in general are structured around the ritual ingestion of this beverage, a practice of high social relevance and assiduity.

Users stress the role of the ayahuasca—always assuming its structured, focused, and ritualized use—at the same time valuing their own responsibility in their evolution, without underestimating the value of the entire structure of the Institute. Recalling that they often recognize the value of ayahuasca as an aid in confronting themselves, we can say that the process takes place as a game of mirrors: The individual recognizes the value of the substance, and the ayahuasca reflects and reunites the human being, without forgetting the essential conditions.

With regard to these, it has been shown that, in addition to accompanying persons, a structure or setting is necessary so that the process is conducted in the best conditions of security. It would be very time-consuming to specify all the factors involved, which, in any case, are well known, but it is worthwhile to stress the importance of spaces of integration, in which lessons take meaning and reach the possibility of becoming realities. Meetings, writing, reading, drawing, yoga, and meditation are some of the ways that been validated. Absence of such conditions may increase the dangers inherent in working with modified states of consciousness: inflation of the ego, narcissism, a tendency to act out, etc. Fericgla (2003) made a deeper analysis of these difficulties, claiming that integration will prevent these states. With regard to the need for a context in structured use of a visionary substance, Fabregas explains:

> Sometimes people have difficulties with the acceptance of the ritual of the setting, because they experience it as a limit, as an imposition. But when they have a little more perspective, it changes from compression to an understanding that those limits are what give the security to then let go, knowing that one won't be able to fall, and in contrast, when there are no limits, one is afraid of oneself, and that fear is what prevents the crossing. Therefore, I think that setting is essential in the use of visionary substances. I believe in a ritual use of the substance, a paradoxical process may occur, in which structure becomes destructuring.

To summarize: One can say that it is indispensable to employ structure and guidance with ayahuasca, which includes the presence of experienced figures, a purpose that orients the search, and an appropriate environment that allows the safe development of the session. For the individual, many conditions influence his evolution, but without doubt, motivation stands out. Experience has shown that people who financed their own process make greater use than those who are borne by families. Also, it can be said that there is evidence of a better outcome in people close to their forties than in young users. The explanation may be that that many older individuals seem to have "bottomed out" in terms of their troubled lives, while those in their twenties often were far from true renunciation. In addition, younger people have less psychological structure, something very valuable when dealing with the difficulties of the process. We should add that, for Westerners, leaving the Amazon environment is unavoidable, and the barriers to keep the lines of knowledge acquired are as difficult to overcome as they are rewarding to surpass.

Based on the above, it seems that people with disputes in the emotional sphere, such as unresolved personal stories and traumatic events, could benefit from the use of ayahuasca. Related to this, Fábregas reveals interesting clinical observations out of his extensive experience:

> Ayahuasca has indications, doubtful cases, and contraindications, and among the indications, beyond any doubt, are emotional blockages and traumatic biographical experiences. In a case of rape for example, among all the treatments that I know, all the tools of psychology, a visionary substance would be indicated because it offers the possibility of reliving the emotions of the situation,...of allowing the experience to be relocated in a different way, and of replacing that memory in a different way.... As a contraindication, I personally abstain from giving ayahuasca to the psychotic.

It even deepens the issue by testing other possible therapeutic approaches. He continues,

> (A visionary substance) is a very valuable tool, with psychotherapy when the painful nucleus is entered, rejection and avoidance occur, and medication makes no sense because only the symptom is corrected, not the situation, which is covers but does not cease to act. In contrast, the possibility of making that catharsis, that emotional discharge, and above all the deep experience of the situation from a different perspective is a therapeutic luxury without equal.

If the process developed using ayahuasca has shown a clear validity, it is in the search for existential meaning. Both people hovering around 40 and addicts who questioned their way of living have found through the Amazon brew messages about the meaning of life, help in finding their place in the world, and help adapting and restructuring their lives. This aspect is strongly related to the transpersonal experiences and contact with nature, because both have the effect of reformulating the vision of the world, resulting in perceptible changes in values and attitudes. Here it can be said that the IDEAA concept seems to have functioned successfully with people seeking to recover spaces of meaning, fulfillment, and satisfaction in their lives after a long period following the abandonment of drugs.

Although not much can be said about the profiles indicated or contraindicated, it seems a shared premise that seriously psychotic people and those with severe character disorders lack the structure or minimal psychological stability required to work with ayahuasca. On the other hand, it is difficult and perhaps inappropriate to try to predict the effect of drinking ayahuasca based on diagnostic profiles, because some problems of the psychotic type have been traversed and resolved successfully. Among the arrivals, it is undeniably necessary to distinguish between real pathologies and the known spiritual emergency.[20]

To mention difficulties encountered in the practice of the Institute, two especially complex cases cannot be forgotten. Although they were seen at different times, both shared a dual diagnosis and a relatively early age, around age twenty. Despite the fact that neither of them has been blocked in their process, during their stay at the Institute they complicated cases considerably, especially in terms of the day-to-day operation. This leads us to reflect on the psychological structure indispensable in the intense Amazonian process, which includes a series of situations of high innovation, but also taking into account that their difficulties in these cases could not be attributed to ayahuasca. One of them carried a strong habit of anxiolytic psychiatric medication that he could not stop easily, leading him to suffer a prolonged withdrawal syndrome. The second case was surprising, involving consumption of substances not permitted within the Institute, especially cannabis; illustrating the relationship between this consumption and his state of stupor and disconnection.

In addition to the users presenting a problem with drugs, a considerable proportion of the demands of IDEAA comes from people seeking help for other disorders or a path of human evolution. Individuals with other dependencies, such

[20] Grof has described spiritual emergencies as evolutionary crises of growth: sharp, sudden, and erupting to change everyday habits and relationships in an uncomfortable and painful way.

as sex, pathological consumption, or eating disorders, have been helped, although cases of the latter have been particularly resistant.

Although the results of these introspective processes are difficult to measure objectively, conclusions may be expected from future studies. Field observations on the consequences of the process require more experimental verification, which may derive from the studies currently being made on IDEAA participants through quantitative measures in various areas of psychology. Research is the key to assess the true nature and effects of the human processes generated through the visionary beverage. Discoveries are expected that are capable of overcoming our current limitations, weaving together knowledge that has been transmitted through the efforts of many rising generations.

References

Araújo, W. S. (1999). *Navegando sobre as ondas do Daime: História, cosmologia e ritual da Barquinha*. Campinas, Brazil: Editora da Unicamp.

Bardin, L. (1977). *El análisis de contenido*. Madrid: Akal.

Fericgla, J. M. (Ed.). (1997). *Al trasluz de la ayahuasca*. Barcelona: Los libros de la Liebre de Marzo.

Fericgla, J. M. (Ed.). (2003). *Epopteia: Avanzar sin olvidar*. Barcelona: Los libros de la Liebre de Marzo.

Grof, S. (1994). *La Mente Holotrópica. Los niveles de la conciencia humana*. Barcelona: Kairós.

Grof, S. (2005). *Psicoterapia con LSD. El potencial curativo de la medicina psiquedélica*. Barcelona: La Liebre de Marzo.

Labate, B. C. (2004). *A reinvenção do uso da Ayahuasca nos centros urbanos*. Campinas, Brazil: Mercado de Letras.

Labate, B. C., & Araújo, W. S. (Eds.). (2004). *O uso ritual da ayahuasca* (2ª ed.). Campinas, Brazil: Mercado de Letras.

MacRae, E. (1992). *Guiado pela lua: Xamanismo e uso ritual da ayahuasca no culto do Santo Daime*. São Paulo: Brasiliense.

MacRae, E. (2004). Abordagens qualitativas na compreensão do uso de psicoativos. In L. A. Tavares, A. R. Almeida, A. N. Filho, E. MacRae, & O. S. Ferreira (Eds.), *Drogas, tempos, lugares e olhares sobre seu consume* (pp. 27–48). Salvador: Edufba.

Riba, J. (2004). Effects of the South American psychoactive beverage ayahuasca on regional brain electrical activity in humans: A functional study using low-resolution electromagnetic tomography (LORETA). *Neuropsychobiology, 50*(1), 89–101.

Shanon, B. (2002). *The Antipodes of mind: Charting the phenomenology of ayahuasca experience*. NY: Oxford University Press.

Villaescusa, M. (2006). Efectos subjetivos a corto plazo de tomas de ayahuasca en contexto occiental urbano. *Enteogenia: Revista libre cultura y estudios psiconáuticos, 1*(May/June), 13–26.

Chapter 11
Assessment of the Psychotherapeutic Effects of Ritual Ayahuasca Use on Drug Dependency: A Pilot Study

Xavier Fernández, Rafael Guimarães dos Santos, Marta Cutchet, Sabela Fondevila, Débora González, Miguel Ángel Alcázar, Jordi Riba, José Carlos Bouso and Josep María Fábregas

Abstract Using personality, psychopathology, and neuropsychological assessment instruments, our team assessed the therapeutic effects of an ayahuasca ritual treatment. Data was collected at the Institute of Applied Amazonian Ethnopsychology (IDEAA), in the Brazilian Amazon Basin. Psychological assessments were obtained both before and at the end of the treatment. The ayahuasca treatment lasted between 3 and 9 months and included biweekly ayahuasca consumption. The sample consisted of 13 patients (8 men, 5 women) with a mean age

---

X. Fernández—Deceased

X. Fernández · M. Cutchet
Instituto de Etnopsicología Amazónica Aplicada (IDEAA), Amazonas, Brazil
e-mail: mcutchet@gmail.com

R. G. dos Santos
International Center for Ethnobotanical Education, Research & Service (ICEERS), Halsteren, The Netherlands
e-mail: banisteria@gmail.com
URL: http://banisteria.blogspot.com

M. Cutchet
Centro de Investigación y Tratamiento de las Adicciones (CITA), Barcelona, Spain

S. Fondevila
Universidad Complutense de Madrid, Madrid, Spain
e-mail: sabellissima@gmail.com

D. González
Institut Hospital del Mar d'Investigaciones Mèdiques, IMIM, Barcelona, Spain
e-mail: debora.gonzalez@gmail.com

M. Á. Alcázar
Universidad Autónoma de Madrid, Madrid, Spain
e-mail: miguelangel.alcazar@uam.es

J. Riba
Neuropsicología Humana Experimental, IIB-Sant Pau, Barcelona, Spain
e-mail: jriba@santpau.cat

B. C. Labate and C. Cavnar (eds.), *The Therapeutic Use of Ayahuasca*,
DOI: 10.1007/978-3-642-40426-9_11,

of 35 years. Nine had a diagnosis of drug abuse and/or dependence; one of borderline personality disorder, and 3 were at IDEAA for personal growth. Results showed that the "Impulsiveness," "Disorderliness," "Anticipatory Worry," and "Shyness with Strangers" subscales of the *Temperament and Character Inventory* presented statistically significant reductions after treatment, while the "Self-Directedness," "Responsibility," "Purposefulness," and "Congruent Second Nature" subscales presented significant increases. The psychopathology subscales "Positive Symptoms," "Obsessive–Compulsive," and "Anxiety" of the *Symptom Check-List-90-Revised*, were significantly diminished after treatment, as well as all subscales of the *Frontal Systems Behavior Scale:* "Total," "Apathy," "Disinhibition," and "Executive Dysfunction." In addition, the "Resistance to Interference" measure of the *Stroop Color and Word Test*, the *Purpose in Life Test*, and the "Transcendent Dimension," "Meaning and Purpose in Life," "Mission in Life," and "Material Values" subscales of the *Spiritual Orientation Inventory* presented statistically significant increases after treatment. Despite important limitations, such as the small sample size and the lack of a control group, the present pilot study provides preliminary evidence suggesting psychotherapeutic effects of ritual ayahuasca treatment in drug-related disorders.

Keywords Ayahuasca · Hallucinogens · Ritual · Spirituality · Drug dependence · Personality · Psychopathology · Cognition · Psychosocial well being · Psychotherapy · Therapeutic assessment

Introduction

Anecdotal evidence suggests that the ritual use of ayahuasca, either in the traditional indigenous and *mestizo* contexts, in the syncretic Brazilian religions, or in diverse neo-shamanic practices, and in clinics like the Takiwasi Center in Peru, may help the treatment of drug-related disorders (see Bouso and Riba, in this

J. C. Bouso
International Center for Ethnobotanical Education, Research & Service (ICEERS), Halsteren, The Netherlands
e-mail: jcbouso@gmail.com
URL: http://iceers.org

J. C. Bouso
Institut Hospital del Mar d'Investigaciones Mèdiques (IMIM), Barcelona, Spain

J. María Fábregas (✉)
Instituto de Etnopsicología Amazónica Aplicada (IDEAA), Centro de Investigación y Tratamiento de las Adicciones (CITA), CITA Clínica, Mas Mia s/n 08319 Dosrius Barcelona, Spain
e-mail: miafabregas@gmail.com

volume). Nevertheless, to the best of our knowledge, there is neither any efficacy study, nor a longitudinal research devoted to assess, within the same study, personality, psychopathology, executive functions and neuropsychological status, life attitudes, and spirituality, in drug-dependent individuals after a ritual treatment program with ayahuasca.

This chapter presents preliminary data obtained at the Institute of Applied Amazonian Ethnopsychology Instituto de Etnopsicología Amazónica Aplicada(IDEAA). The Institute was created by one of the authors, Fábregas. It is placed at the Brazilian Amazon basin, near the Mapiá River, a tributary of the Purús River in the municipality of Pauiní, in the Amazon State (Fernández and Fábregas, in this volume). The aim of this text is to describe an observational study on the variations on personality, psychopathology, and neuropsychological measures in individuals treated with ayahuasca in the IDEAA setting.

Methods

Volunteers. Thirteen Spanish volunteers over 18 years of age (eight men and five women) with a mean age of 35 years participated in the study. The sample included nine patients with drug abuse and/or dependence disorder (D) mainly related with the consumption of heroin and cocaine derivatives (hydrochloride salt, cocaine paste, and crack cocaine); one with borderline personality disorder (BPD), and three individuals who were at IDEAA for personal growth(PG). The sample included people with a medium–high socioeconomic status, i.e., all volunteers had higher-than-average income and all were high school graduates. Most participants had no previous experience with ayahuasca. All subjects with dependence disorders were very problematic drug users with long and prolific delictive careers, who were considered hopeless by their families and their social environment, and that had previously failed in other treatments for their drug-related problems.

All volunteers signed a written informed consent allowing their clinical data to be used for scientific purposes, as long as their anonymity was preserved. Data was collected in Spain before and after the volunteer's travel to IDEAA. Data collection was performed from October 2004 to November 2008.

Study Design and Variables. Patients stayed in IDEAA for at least 3 months (mean: 4½ months; range: 3–9 months). During this time, patients consumed ayahuasca at IDEAA between 1 and 2 times per week, and also in a Santo Daime community near the institute (mean: 2–3 times per month; range: 1–15 times per month). Study evaluations were performed before and after the ayahuasca treatment. As this is not a clinical study, but an observational one, questionnaires were not equally administered to all volunteers. The criteria for choosing which questionnaires should be applied were based on the clinical expertise of the IDEAA team (see below).

In this study, personality was assessed using the *Temperament and Character Inventory-Revised* (*TCI-R*) ($N = 10$; 9D + 1BPD). The psychopathological status of the volunteers was evaluated with the *Symptom Check-List-90-Revised* (*SCL-90-R*) (*N* = 9; 9D), and their neuropsychological performance and behavior was assessed with the *Stroop Color and Word Test* (*N* = 13; all sample), the *Letter-Number Sequencing* (*LNS*) from the *WAIS-III* (*N* = 12; 9D + 1 BPD + 2PG), and the *Frontal Systems Behavior Scale* (*FrSBe*) (*N* = 11; 9D + 1BPD + 1PG). Life attitudes and spirituality were assessed with the *Purpose in Life Test* (*PLT*) (*N* = 9; 9D) and the *Spiritual Orientation Inventory* (*SOI*) (*N* = 9; 9D). Our group used these scales and questionnaires in previous research (Bouso et al. 2011, 2012). The questionnaires used are briefly described below:

Personality traits. *Temperament and Character Inventory* (*TCI-Revised*). The *TCI-R* is based on the psychobiological model of personality developed by Cloninger, Svrakic, and Przybeck (1993). The temperament dimensions are assumed to be independently inheritable and to manifest in early development, while the character dimensions are assumed to be influenced more by sociocultural learning and maturation. The *TCI-R* has 240 Likert-type items with five response options, assessing seven dimensions of personality and 29 sub-dimensions. The four primary dimensions of temperament and their facets are: (1) Harm Avoidance (HA): HA1-Anticipatory Worry versus Uninhibited Optimism; HA2-Fear of Uncertainty versus Confidence; HA3-Shyness with Strangers versus Gregariousness; HA4-Fatigability and Asthenia versus Vigor; (2) Novelty Seeking (NS): NS1-Exploratory Excitability versus Stoic Rigidity; NS2-Impulsiveness versus Reflection; NS3-Extravagance versus Reserve; NS4-Disorderliness versus Regimentation; (3) Reward Dependence (RD): RD1-Sentimentality versus Insensitivity; RD3-Attachment versus Detachment; RD4-Dependence versus Independence; and (4) Persistence (P).

The three dimensions of character are: (1) Self-Directedness (SD): SD1-Responsibility versus Blaming; SD2-Purposefulness versus Lack of Goal-Direction; SD3-Resourcefulness; SD4-Self-Acceptance versus Self-Striving; SD5-Congrugent Second Nature; (2) Cooperativeness (C): C1-Social Acceptance versus Social Intolerance; C2-Empathy versus Social Disinterest; C3-Helpfulness versus Unhelpfulness; C4-Compassion versus Revengefulness; C5-Integrated Conscience; and (3) Self-Transcendence (ST): ST1-Self-Forgetfulness versus Self-Conscious Experience; ST2-Transpersonal Identification versus Self-Isolation; ST3-Spiritual Acceptance versus Rational Materialism.

Psychopathological status. *The Symptom Check-List-90-Revised* (*SCL-90-R*). The *SCL-90-R* (Derogatis 1994) is a self-report questionnaire that assesses nine psychopathological symptomatic dimensions, including 90 Likert-type items that are scored from 0 to 4: Somatization (SOM), Obsessive–Compulsive (O–C), Interpersonal Sensitivity (I–S), Depression (DEP), Anxiety (ANX), Hostility (HOS), Phobic Anxiety (PHOB), Paranoid Ideation (PAR), and Psychoticism (PSY). The scale also provides three additional psychopathological indices: General Severity Index (GSI), Positive Symptoms Distress Index (PSDI), and Positive Symptoms Total (PST). For all the scales, higher scores imply worse symptomatology.

Neuropsychological performance and behavior. *The Stroop Color and Word Test.* The *Stroop* test (Golden 1994) assesses conflict monitoring and resolution (resistance to interference), cognitive abilities involving the anterior cingulate-dorsolateral prefrontal system and the rostroventral prefrontal cortex (Melcher et al. 2008). In this test, subjects must first read a list of color names ("red," "green," "blue") written in black ink. When this is completed, a list of X's, each printed in red, green, or blue, is presented and the subject must indicate the color of the X. Finally, a third list is presented to the participant containing a list of the same color names, but printed this time in an incongruent ink color. As with the second list, the participant is asked to indicate the color in which each element is printed. The subject is given 45 s, and the numbers of correctly read items from the first list and correctly reported items from lists two and three are recorded. Dependent variables are the total number of words read (W), the total number of correctly identified colors in the second list (C) and the total number of color incongruent words read (IW). Finally, a "Resistance to Interference" measure (RI) is calculated according to the following formula: $RI = IW - (C \times W/C + W)$. Better performance is reflected as higher scores on IW and RI.

The Letter-Number Sequencing (LNS) from the WAIS-III. The *LNS* (Wechsler 1997) is a measure of working memory, a task involving dorsolateral, ventrolateral, and orbitofrontal prefrontal cortices (Barbey et al. 2011). Subjects are verbally presented with a random series of numbers and letters that they have to report back in a specified order, i.e., numbers in ascending order and letters in alphabetical order. Series of increasing length are presented to the subject until an error is committed. The score is the maximum number of elements in the series correctly reported by the participant. Higher scores indicate better performance.

The Frontal Systems Behavior Scale (FrSBe). The *FrSBe* (Grace and Malloy 2001) is a rating scale designed to measure behaviors associated with damage to the frontal lobes and systems of the brain. This questionnaire was used to assess hypothetical frontal lobe alterations that could potentially go undetected with classical neuropsychological tests, but that could have an impact on everyday life. Both self- and relative-administered versions exist. In the present study, the self-administered version was used. The questionnaire comprises 46 Likert-type items with five response options. The items are distributed into three subscales: Apathy/Akinesia (14 items), Disinhibition/Emotional Dysregulation (15 items), and Executive Dysfunction (17 items). Higher scores reflect worse frontal function. A global score is computed by adding up the scores of the individual scales.

Life Attitudes and Psychosocial Well Being. *Purpose in Life Test (PLT).* The *PLT* (Crumbaugh and Maholick 1976) is a measure of a subject's perceived "meaning of life" versus "existential vacuum" and is based on Victor Frankl's Logotherapy. It consists of 20 items; each rated on a 7-point scale ranging from 1 (low purpose) to 7 (high purpose). The total score can range from 20 (low purpose) to 140 (high purpose).

Spiritual Orientation Inventory (SOI). The *SOI* (Elkins et al. 1988) is a measure of spirituality based on the humanistic model and is designed to assess the spirituality of those affiliated with traditional religion. It is an 85 Likert-type item self-report questionnaire. Items are distributed into nine major components: Transcendent Dimension, Meaning and Purpose in Life, Mission in Life, Sacredness of Life, Material Values, Altruism, Idealism, Awareness of the Tragic, and Fruits of Spirituality. Each item has seven response options.

All volunteers gave their written informed consent to participate.

Statistical analysis. Because different questionnaires were administered to varying numbers of volunteers, statistical results are presented accordingly. Scores of the assorted questionnaires and scales were analyzed using paired Student's *t* tests of repeated measures comparing the scores obtained by each subject before and after the treatment. In all tests performed, differences were considered statistically significant for *p* values lower than 0.05.

Results

Personality traits. The "Impulsiveness" ($p = 0.042$), "Disorderliness" ($p = 0.022$), "Anticipatory Worry" ($p = 0.029$), and "Shyness with Strangers" ($p = 0.011$) subscales of the *TCI-R* presented statistically significant reductions after the ayahuasca treatment ($N = 10$; 9D + 1BPD) (Table 11.1).

On the other hand, the subscales "Self-Directedness" ($p = 0.007$), "Responsibility" ($p = 0.021$), "Purposefulness" ($p = 0.030$), and "Congruent Second Nature" ($p = 0.015$) presented increases after the ayahuasca treatment ($N = 10$; 9D + 1BPD) (Table 11.1). There were no statistically significant differences on the other subscales.

Psychopathological Status. On the *SCL-90-R* ($N = 9$; 9D), the subscales "Positive Symptoms Total" ($p = 0.029$), "Obsessive–Compulsive" ($p = 0.006$), and "Anxiety" ($p = 0.045$) presented statistically significant reductions after the ayahuasca treatment (Table 11.2). There were no statistically significant differences on the other subscales.

Neuropsychological Performance and Behavior. The "Resistance to Interference" ($p = 0.026$) subscale of the *Stroop* test ($N = 13$; all sample) presented a

Table 11.1 TCI-R scales means with significant statistical results ($N = 10$)

TCI-R scales	Before treatment	After treatment	Student t test
Impulsiveness	27.20	23.00	*
Disorderliness	21.00	19.50	*
Anticipatory worry	29.80	26.80	*
Shyness with strangers	21.00	17.10	*
Self-directedness	131.10	147.50	**
Responsibility	30.50	33.10	*
Purposefulness	21.40	24.70	*
Congrugent second nature	31.80	38.50	*

* $p < 0.05$; ** $p < 0.01$

Table 11.2 SCL-90-R subscales means and statistical results ($N = 9$)

SCL-90-R subscales	Before treatment	After treatment	Student t test
GSI	0.61	0.35	ns
PSDI	1.46	1.37	ns
PST	32.22	18.37	*
SOM	0.65	0.55	ns
O-C	0.75	0.33	**
I-S	0.53	0.36	ns
DEP	0.67	0.37	ns
ANX	0.63	0.26	*
HOS	0.44	0.14	ns
PHOB	0.47	0.19	ns
PAR	0.59	0.29	ns
PSY	0.43	0.22	ns

GSI: General Severity Index; PSDI: Positive Symptoms Distress Index; PST: Positive Symptoms Total; SOM: Somatization; O-C: Obsessive-Compulsive; I–S: Interpersonal-Sensitivity; DEP: Depression, ANX: Anxiety; HOS: Hostility; PHOB: Phobic Anxiety; PAR: Paranoid Ideation; PSY: Psychoticism; ns: non-significant; * $p < 0.05$; ** $p < 0.01$

statistically significant increase after the ayahuasca treatment. There were no statistically significant differences on the other *Stroop* subscales.

LNS measures ($N = 12$; 9D + 1BPD + 2PG) did not show statistically significant differences before and after the ayahuasca treatment.

All subscales of the *FrSBe*—"Total" ($p = 0.001$), "Executive Dysfunction" ($p = 0.000$), "Apathy" ($p = 0.001$) and "Disinhibition" ($p = 0.019$)—indicated statistically significant reductions after the ayahuasca treatment ($N = 11$; 9D + 1BPD + 1PG) (Table 11.3).

Life Attitudes and Spirituality. There was a statistically significant increase in the *PLT* scores after the ayahuasca treatment ($N = 9$; 9D; $p = 0.001$) (Table 11.4).

The subscales "Transcendent Dimension" ($p = 0.004$), "Meaning and Purpose in Life" ($p = 0.006$), "Mission in Life" ($p = 0.008$), "Sacredness of Life" ($p = 0.031$) and "Fruits of Spirituality" ($p = 0.004$) of the *SOI* ($N = 9$; 9D) showed statistically significant increases after the ayahuasca treatment (Table 11.4). There were no statistically significant differences on the other *SOI* subscales.

Table 11.3 FrSBe subscales means and statistical results ($N = 11$)

FrSBe subscales	Before treatment	After treatment	Student t test
Total	111.09	88.54	**
Executive Dysfunction	45.91	35.54	**
Apathy	35.55	27.90	**
Disinhibition	32.91	27.27	*

* $p < 0.05$; ** $p < 0.01$

Table 11.4 PLT and SOI subscales means and statistical results ($N = 9$)

	Before treatment	After treatment	Student t test
PLT	96.44	114.44	**
SOI subscales			
Transcendent dimension	3.57	5.29	**
Meaning/purpose in life	4.84	5.58	**
Mission in life	4.04	5.19	**
Sacredness of life	5.03	5.56	*
Material values	4.57	4.72	ns
Altruism	4.94	4.96	ns
Idealism	4.40	4.61	ns
Awareness of the tragic	5.04	5.37	ns
Fruits of spirituality	3.78	5.26	**

ns: non-significant; * $p < 0.05$; **$p < 0.01$

Discussion

The overall results of this study suggest that the ritual treatment with ayahuasca as was performed at IDEAA led to some therapeutic benefits that included amelioration of several psychological dimensions related to drug dependence as measured by validated questionnaires and scales.

Personality Traits

In the personality assessment using the *TCI-R*, differences were found in some of the temperament sub-dimensions, which are believed to be genetically determined. Scores in the "Impulsiveness" subscale were significantly reduced after the ayahuasca treatment. Since high scores in "Impulsiveness" have been associated extensively with drug use (Pedrero-Pérez and Mota 2008; Verdejo-García et al. 2008), the reductions showed in the "Impulsiveness" subscale, together with significant reductions in the sub-dimensions "Disorderliness," "Anticipatory Worry," and "Shyness with Strangers," may reflect less risk-taking behavior, more ordered pattern of behaviors, and less anxiety and shyness after ritual treatment with ayahuasca.

Regarding the character dimensions, participants scored significantly higher in the dimension "Self-Directedness," and in the subscales of "Responsibility," "Purposefulness," and "Congruent Second Nature" after the ayahuasca treatment. These findings may also reflect positive and therapeutic behavior modifications directed to more self-regulation, responsibility, orientation, congruency, and motivation to change. In fact, perhaps the most interesting personality result, from a clinical point of view, may be the higher scores achieved by subjects in the dimension "Self-Directedness" after the ayahuasca treatment, since this change may predict long-term beneficial outcomes. "Self-Directedness" is consistently found to be low in drug abusers (Pedrero-Pérez and Mota 2008), so its increase after the ayahuasca treatment may be reflecting the efficacy of the treatment. Higher scores in "Self-Directedness" may also reflect that the treatment enhanced the inner potentialities of the patients. It would be interesting to develop long-term efficacy studies in order to see if this change in personality is permanent.

One eventual radical consequence of permanent change in the "Self-Directedness" trait may be related to a major change not only in terms of treatment outcome, but also in terms of a more difficult kind of change; that is, in the kind of psychiatric diseases that have no or little cure, known as the "personality disorders." Patients suffering from personality disorders commonly have low scores in "Self-Directedness," and it is common to find a combination of low scores in "Self-Directedness" and high scores in "Self-Transcendence" in many types of personality disorders (Gutiérrez et al. 2008). Notably, more than half of the patients with drug-related disorders have some kind of personality disorder (Herrero et al. 2008), and it is also very common that this patient group has low scores in "Self-Directedness" and high scores in "Self-Transcendence" independent of the drug abused (Pedrero-Pérez and Mota 2008).

Our subjects did not significantly change their scores in the "Self-Transcendence" dimension after the ayahuasca treatment, besides being involved in several ayahuasca ceremonies. Since patients with drug-related disorders often present high "Self-Transcendence" scores and ayahuasca consumption frequently induces extreme spiritual experiences, the reason we did not see changes in the "Self-Transcendence" dimension after the ayahuasca treatment may be that our subjects already had high scores in that dimension. In fact, the scores obtained for our subjects both at the beginning and at the end of the treatment are considered as high "Self-Transcendence" scores for the normative data of the general Spanish population (Gutiérrez-Zotes et al. 2004), and also higher than the ones found in other studies where this personality trait has been assessed in Spanish addicts.

It is interesting to note that higher scores obtained in "Self-Directedness" by our subjects after the treatment were indicators of good treatment outcomes. In our previous long-term ayahuasca study, this variable was lower in the ayahuasca-using groups compared with control groups (Bouso et al. 2012), even while they used less drugs than controls (Fábregas et al. 2010). Perhaps we are attending to two different approaches here to treat drug abuse: one, the religious use of ayahuasca (Grob et al. 1996; Halpern et al. 2008), and the other, the psychotherapeutic approach (for an overview, see Loizaga-Velder and Loizaga Pazzi, in this volume).

Although the religious and the psychotherapeutic approaches are not mutually exclusive, especially in the context of the ritual use of ayahuasca (Labate et al. 2009; Goulart 2011), we separate the two contexts here for practical reasons: the religious context, more associated with a doctrine and a group of individuals that give encouragement and support for personal changes; and the psychotherapeutic context, more associated with the individual's own strength to overcome difficulties. In this perspective, in the religious approach, the "Self-Directedness" dimension would be lower because it is the doctrine of the group that drives the subject's behaviors, and, while following a doctrine, subjects would be protected from temptations to abuse drugs. On the other hand, in a psychotherapeutic approach, it is the subject that would take control of his or her personal situation and, accordingly, psychotherapeutic techniques are focused on subjects gaining self-control over their situations.

In summary, the increments in the "Self-Directedness" scores and the absence of significant changes in the "Self-Transcendence" scores may indicate a benefit in terms not only of treatment outcome, but also in terms of benefits of patients with personality disorders. Future prospective studies are needed in order to eventually confirm or to refute this interesting finding.

Psychopathological Status

Regarding the psychopathological status of the volunteers as measured by the *SCL-90-R*, it can be observed in Table 11.2 that the subscales "Positive Symptoms Total," "Obsessive–Compulsive," and "Anxiety" were significantly reduced after the ayahuasca treatment, suggesting a reduction of some psychopathological symptoms as measured by the *SCL-90-R* after the ayahuasca treatment.

Previous studies with healthy long-term users of ayahuasca, including adolescents and adults, suggest that these individuals present low levels of psychopathology, and may even present better metal health status compared to the control groups used in the studies (*Studies with adults*: Grob et al. 1996; Barbosa et al. 2005; Halpern et al. 2008; Barbosa et al. 2009; Bouso et al. 2012; *Study with adolescents*: da Silveira et al. 2005; for a review of adult and adolescent studies see Labate et al. 2009; Barbosa et al. 2012). The psychopathological data are supported by increasing preclinical and clinical evidence demonstrating anxiolytic and antidepressive potentials for ayahuasca or some of its isolated alkaloids (dos Santos et al. 2007; Osório et al. 2011; Palhano-Fontes et al. in this volume).

Neuropsychological Performance and Behavior

Scores in the "Resistance to Interference" subscale of the *Stroop* test were significantly higher after the ayahuasca treatment. This subscale is associated with visuoperceptive functions involved in discriminating interference. Specifically, this part of the *Stroop* test consists of rapidly naming the color of a word that is written in another color, exemplifying the capacity to inhibit reading, a highly automated process. In a broader sense, the significant increase in the "Resistance to Interference" subscale after the ayahuasca treatment could indicate an improvement in some aspects of the executive functions.

In line with the *Stroop* data, all subscales of the *FrSBe* showed statistically significant reductions after treatment. Since the *FrSBe* is a behavioral questionnaire, these data suggest that patients increased their planning and execution abilities; while, at the same time, they reduced their apathy in the behavioral level.

Deficits in executive functions related to attention, cognitive flexibility, memory, and processing speed, are commonly reported among drug-dependent individuals. The data presented in our pilot study suggests that the ayahuasca treatment improved, or at least normalized, the cognitive and executive functions among our patient group.

On the other hand, there was neither difference on the other *Stroop* subscales nor in the *LNS* measures before and after the ayahuasca treatment. The absence of significant differences in the neuropsychological tests may indicate the overall safety profile of ayahuasca for cognition. These data are in line with the subject's interviews, and with studies with healthy long-term consumers of ayahuasca (Grob et al. 1996; Barbosa et al. 2005; da Silveira et al. 2005; Halpern et al. 2008; Barbosa et al. 2009; Bouso et al. 2012; for a review of adult and adolescent studies see Labate et al. 2009; Barbosa et al. 2012).

Life Attitudes and Spirituality

There was a statistically significant increase in the *PLT* scores after the ayahuasca treatment. Moreover, the subscales "Transcendent Dimension," "Meaning and Purpose in Life," "Mission in Life," and "Material Values" of the *SOI* also showed statistically significant increases after the ayahuasca treatment.

These data might indicate that patients increased their motivation for pursuing new and less harmful goals in life, associated with an increase in the transcendent aspects of life. Increases in mystical-type and religious experiences, similar to those described by our group of volunteers, are comparable to the ones that had been described in human research with hallucinogenic compounds like LSD and psilocybin. These experiences have been related to improvements in several mental health measures (Grof 2001; Griffiths et al. 2006, 2008, 2011; MacLean et al. 2011).

Limitations

Despite the promising results suggesting that a ritual treatment involving ayahuasca might present psychotherapeutic value for people with drug-related disorders, the present study has several limitations.

First, the small sample size may have decreased statistical power and increased the probability of false positive results. Second, there was no comparison group, and third, data from some volunteers was lost because of the difficulties of the fieldwork conditions in the middle of the Amazon. Nevertheless, independent of the statistical differences, what seems most interesting is the observation of the clinical changes that the patients experienced after the ayahuasca treatment: objective clinical changes measured with personality, psychopathological, and neuropsychological rating scales.

The observed changes might not be entirely related to the ayahuasca treatment, but could also be explained by the fact that the subjects had stayed several months in a relatively isolated environment where there were few possibilities of obtaining drugs, and the observed changes could just be the consequence of the passage of time. Nevertheless, the observed changes in personality measures, above all in impulsivity and in self-directedness, suggest that those changes were more a consequence of the therapeutic program than the mere passage of time. In any case, the positive changes observed at the end of the treatment in personality, psychopathological, and neuropsychological assessments indicate that the global experience was positive and beneficial for the subjects, as also shown by their subjective narratives (Fernández and Fábregas, in this volume).

Today, according to our fieldwork observation some years after the experience, all 13 subjects are completely integrated in society. Moreover, two of them are ayahuasca leaders in their local communities. Future studies should try to replicate the present findings using a control group and also including follow-up assessments.

Conclusions

Despite its limitations, and recognizing the exploratory nature of this observational pilot study, our results suggest that the ritual use of ayahuasca in a therapeutic context may have beneficial psychotherapeutic effects in several mental health dimensions. This statement is further illustrated by the fact that clinical changes suggesting therapeutic effects were observed in several psychological areas, including personality, psychopathology, cognition, life attitudes, and spirituality. These preliminary results give support for continuous investigations on the possible therapeutic use of ayahuasca.

References

Barbey, A. K., Koenigs, M., & Grafman, J. (2011). Orbitofrontal contributions to human working memory. *Cerebral Cortex, 21*(4), 789–795.

Barbosa, P. C., Giglio, J. S., & Dalgalarrondo, P. (2005). Altered states of consciousness and short-term psychological after-effects induced by the first time ritual use of ayahuasca in an urban context in Brazil. *Journal of Psychoactive Drugs, 37*(2), 193–201.

Barbosa, P. C., Cazorla, I. M., Giglio, J. S., & Strassman, R. (2009). A six-month prospective evaluation of personality traits, psychiatric symptoms and quality of life in ayahuasca-naïve subjects. *Journal of Psychoactive Drugs, 41*(3), 205–212.

Barbosa, P. C., Mizumoto, S., Bogenschutz, M. P., & Strassman, R. J. (2012). Health status of ayahuasca users. *Drug Testing and Analysis, 4*(7–8), 601–609.
Bouso, J. C., & Riba, J. Ayahuasca and the treatment of drug addiction. In this volume.
Bouso, J. C., González, D., Fondevila, S., Cutchet, M., Fernández, X., Barbosa, P. C. R., Riba, J. (2012). Personality, psychopathology, life attitudes and neuropsychological performance among ritual users of ayahuasca: A longitudinal study. *PLoS ONE, 7*(8), e42421.
Bouso, J. C., Fábregas, J. M., González, D., Fondevila, S., Fernández, X., Cutchet, M., et al. (2011). Long-term effects of ritual use of ayahuasca on mental health. In B. C. Labate & H. Jungaberle (Eds.), *The internationalization of ayahuasca* (pp. 167–184). Zurich: LIT Verlag.
Cloninger, C. R., Svrakic, D. M., & Przybeck, T. R. (1993). A psychobiological model of temperament and character. *Archives of General Psychiatry, 50*(12), 975–990.
Crumbaugh, J. C., & Maholick, L. T. (1976). *The purpose in life test*. Murfreesboro, TN: Psychometric Affiliates.
da Silveira, D. X., Grob, C. S., Dobkin de Rios, M., Lopez, E., Alonso, L. K., Tacla, C., et al. (2005). Ayahuasca in adolescence: A preliminary psychiatric assessment. *Journal of Psychoactive Drugs, 37*(2), 129–133.
Derogatis, L. R. (1994). *Symptom Checklist-90-R: Administration, scoring and procedures manual*. Minneapolis: National Computer System.
dos Santos, R. G., Landeira-Fernandez, J., Strassman, R. J., Motta, V., & Cruz, A. P. (2007). Effects of ayahuasca on psychometric measures of anxiety, panic-like and hopelessness in Santo Daime members. *Journal of Ethnopharmacology, 112*(3), 507–513.
Elkins, D. N., Hedstrom, L. J., Hughes, L. L., Leaf, J. A., & Saunders, C. (1988). Toward phenomenological spirituality: Definition, description, and measurement. *Journal of Humanistic Psychology, 28*(4), 5–18.
Fábregas, J. M., González, D., Fondevila, S., Cutchet, M., Fernández, X., Barbosa, P. C., Bouso, J. C. (2010). Assessment of addiction severity among ritual users of ayahuasca. *Drug and Alcohol Dependence, 111*(3), 257-261.
Fernández, X., & Fábregas, J. M. "Experience of treatment with ayahuasca for drug addiction in the Brazilian Amazon." In this volume.
Golden, C. J. (1994). *Stroop: Test de colores y palabras*. Madrid: TEA.
Goulart, S. L. (2011). The notion of cure in the Brazilian ayahuasca religions. In R. G. dos Santos (Ed.), *The ethnopharmacology of ayahuasca* (pp. 23-53). Trivandrum, India: Transworld Research Network. Retrieved June 9, 2013 from http://www.trnres.com/ebook/uploads/rafael/T_12998350262%20Rafael.pdf.
Grace, J., & Malloy, P. F. (2001). *Frontal Systems Behavior Scale: Professional Manual*. Lutz, FL: Psychological Assessment Resources, Inc.
Griffiths, R. R., Richards, W. A., McCann, U., & Jesse, R. (2006). Psilocybin can occasion mystical-type experiences having substantial and sustained personal meaning and spiritual significance. *Psychopharmacology (Berl), 187*(3), 268–283.
Griffiths, R. R., Richards, W. A., Johnson, M. W., McCann, U., & Jesse, R. (2008). Mystical-type experiences occasioned by psilocybin mediate the attribution of personal meaning and spiritual significance 14 months later. *Journal of Psychopharmacology, 22*(6), 621–632.
Griffiths, R. R., Johnson, M. W., Richards, W. A., Richards, B. D., McCann, U., & Jesse, R. (2011). Psilocybin occasioned mystical-type experiences: Immediate and persisting dose-related effects. *Psychopharmacology (Berl), 218*(4), 649–665.
Grob, C. S., McKenna, D. J., Callaway, J. C., Brito, G. S., Neves, E. S., Oberlaender, G., Boone, K. B. (1996). Human psychopharmacology of hoasca, a plant hallucinogen used in ritual context in Brazil. *Journal of Nervous and Mental Disease, 184*(2), 86-94.
Grof, S. (2001). *LSD psychotherapy*. Santa Cruz, CA: Multidisciplinary Association for Psychedelic Studies.
Gutiérrez, F., Navinés, R., Navarro, P., García-Esteve, L., Subirá, S., Torrens, M., et al. (2008). What do all personality disorders have in common? Ineffectiveness and uncooperativeness. *Comprehensive Psychiatry, 49*(6), 570–578.

Gutiérrez-Zotes, J. A., Bayón, C., Montserrat, C., Valero, J., Labad, A., Cloninger, C. R., & Fernández-Aranda, F. (2004). Inventario del Temperamento y el Carácter-Revisado (TCI-R). Baremación y datos normativos en una muestra de población general. *Actas Españolas de Psiquiatría, 32*(1), 8-15.

Halpern, J. H., Sherwood, A. R., Passie, T., Blackwell, K. C., & Ruttenber, A. J. (2008). Evidence of health and safety in American members of a religion who use a hallucinogenic sacrament. *Medical Science Monitor, 14*(8), SR15-22.

Herrero, M. J., Domingo-Salvany, A., Torrens, M., Brugal, M. T., Gutiérrez, F., ITINERE Investigators. (2008). Personality profile in young current regular users of cocaine. *Substance Use and Misuse, 43*(10), 1378-94.

Labate, B. C., Rose, I., & dos Santos, R. G. (2009). *Ayahuasca religions: A comprehensive bibliography and critical essays*. Santa Cruz, CA: Multidisciplinary Association for Psychedelic Studies.

Loizaga-Velder, A., & Loizaga Pazzi, A. Therapist and patient perspectives on ayahuasca-assisted treatment for substance dependence. In this volume.

MacLean, K. A., Johnson, M. W., & Griffiths, R. R. (2011). Mystical experiences occasioned by the hallucinogen psilocybin lead to increases in the personality domain of openness. *Journal of Psychopharmacology, 25*(11), 1453–1461.

Melcher, T., Falkai, P., & Gruber, O. (2008). Functional brain abnormalities in psychiatric disorders: Neural mechanisms to detect and resolve cognitive conflict and interference. *Brain Research Reviews, 59*(1), 96–124.

Osório, F. L., de Macedo, L. R. H., de Sousa, J. P. M., Pinto, J. P., Quevedo, J., Crippa, J. A. S., & Hallak, J. E. C. (2011). The therapeutic potential of harmine and ayahuasca in depression: Evidence from exploratory animal and human studies. In R. G. dos Santos (Ed.), *The ethnopharmacology of ayahuasca* (pp. 75-85). Trivandrum, India: Transworld Research Network. Retrieved June 9, 2013 from: http://www.trnres.com/ebook/uploads/rafael/T_12998352185%20Rafael.pdf.

Palhano-Fontes, F. P., Oliveira, J. P. M., Alchieri, J. C., Soares, B. L., Coelho, N. G., & de Araujo, D. B. The therapeutic potentials of ayahuasca in the treatment of depression. In this volume.

Pedrero-Pérez, E. J., & Mota, G. R. (2008). Diferencias de personalidad entre adictos a sustancias y población general: Estudio con el TCI-R de casos clínicos con controles emparejados. *Adicciones, 20*(3), 251–261.

Verdejo-García, A., Lawrence, A. J., & Clark, L. (2008). Impulsivity as a vulnerability marker for substance-use disorders: Review of findings from high-risk research, problem gamblers and genetic association studies. *Neuroscience and Biobehavioral Reviews, 32*(4), 777–810.

Wechsler, D. (1997). *Wechsler Adult Intelligence Scale* (3rd ed.). San Antonio, TX: The Psychological Corporation.

Chapter 12
Healing with Yagé: An Interview with Taita Juan Bautista Agreda Chindoy

Brian T. Anderson, Beatriz Caiuby Labate and Celina M. De Leon

Abstract Taita Juan is a Cametsa traditional healer and yagecero from the Sibundoy Valley in Colombia. As a member of the new generation of Colombian taitas traveling the world, he has acquired clients and apprentices from throughout the Americas and Europe. He is perhaps best known internationally for having been detained by United States Customs officials and charged with possession with intent to distribute a Schedule 1 drug (ayahuasca) in 2010; he was subsequently released and deported. In this interview, we explore Taita Juan's views on how ayahuasca can be used to diagnose and heal illness. We address how clients are prepared for ceremonies (i.e., diet, sexual activity) as well as how he determines which patients can safely receive ayahuasca or other plant medicines (i.e., proscriptions based on health conditions or medication use). The interview also explores how the substance itself is ritually handled, including preparation, dosage, and its combination with other purgative plants and healing techniques such as *limpias* (cleansings), perfumes, and music. We discuss how Taita Juan's treatments are occasionally used in conjunction with conventional allopathic medicine. We also discuss his claims to have cured cases of heroin addiction, cancer, and AIDS, and address the drug addiction treatment clinic he and his assistants are

B. T. Anderson (✉)
Department of Anthropology, Stanford Univeristy, Main Quad, Bldg 40, Rm 42B, 450 Serra Mall, Stanford, CA 94305, USA
e-mail: bta5ht@gmail.com

B. T. Anderson · B. C. Labate
Núcleo de Estudos Interdisciplinares Sobre Psicoativos (NEIP), São Paulo, Brazil

B. C. Labate
Centro de Investigación y Docencia Economómicas—CIDE Región Centro, Aguascalientes, Ags, Mexico
e-mail: blabate@bialabate.net
URL: http://www.bialabate.net; http://www.neip.info

C. M. De Leon
Psychology and Interdisciplinary Inquiry, Independent Researcher, Oakland, USA
e-mail: celinadeleona@gmail.com

B. C. Labate and C. Cavnar (eds.), *The Therapeutic Use of Ayahuasca*,
DOI: 10.1007/978-3-642-40426-9_12,

founding in Central America. Finally, the interview explores not only Taita Juan's experience of being detained and released by the United States government, but also the legal ramifications this has had for the traditional use of ayahuasca in Colombia and elsewhere.

Introduction

As the use of ayahuasca for therapeutic and spiritual purposes has spread from the Amazon to urban areas of South America and beyond, the most widely known forms of the beverage's use have been based on Peruvian vegetalista and Brazilian syncretic religious traditions. Meanwhile, relatively little popular and academic attention has been paid to the Colombian traditions of drinking ayahuasca, or *yagé*, as it referred to there. This text (Caicedo 2014) serves as an introduction to the therapeutic uses of yagé originating in Colombia by means of an interview with one Cametsa traditional healer from the Sibundoy Valley, Taita Juan Agreda Chindoy.

In the 1990s, yagé use in urban areas of Colombia became an established phenomenon consisting of ritual "sessions" led by indigenous taitas and their apprentices, who were frequently either of mestizo or European descent (Caicedo 2014). The acceptance of yagé use in Colombia in the form of "traditional medicine" has also aided the diffusion of knowledge and practices of yagé consumption via mass media and popular culture (Uribe 2008). Over the years Taita Juan has assumed a strong presence in this expansion, having learned his healing craft from his father—Taita Martin (Guerrero 1991)—from his patients, and directly from the plants he uses. In his role as a taita, he has become the godfather to over 80 children, has served as an elected representative of the Cametsa people, and has a robust clientele from his local community as well as from as far away as North America, Europe, and Asia; some who have now become his apprentices. Having observed his yagé rituals in Colombia and abroad, we interviewed him in order to understand how he sees his work as a healer, and how he embodies his position as a taita through his knowledge, humor, and humility. His interactions with legal and medical authorities in the United States and Colombia are emblematic of the regulatory challenges and potentials that ayahuasca healing in shamanic and related emerging contexts—which are neither strictly "therapeutic" nor "religious"—will undoubtedly face as it continues to spread the world over.

In February 2013, two interviews were conducted in Spanish over Skype, 10 days apart, with Taita Juan answering from his home in Tamabioy, Colombia. Follow-up and clarification of Taita Juan's responses were done over email and telephone, and then added to the transcript that was subsequently translated to English. An appendix has been included which lists some of the medicinal plants grown in Taita Juan's garden in Tamabioy.

Interviewer: "Taita, can you please tell me your full name?"

Taita Juan: "Yes, my name is Juan Bautista Agreda Chindoy."

I: "Where were you born and in what year?"

T: "I was born in the municipality of Sibundoy in the Putumayo of Colombia on April 6, 1968."

I: "Can you please tell me about your community?"

T: "I belong to a community called the Cametsa. We are organized under a cabildo, and we have our own autonomy. We are made up of 6,000 indigenous people. In the municipality of Sibundoy, there exists two communitites: The Inga and the Cametsa. We belong to the Cametsa. Sibundoy is a small valley located in the department or the state of Putumayo."

I: "Your father also lived and grew up in this community?"

T: "Yes, he was native of the Sibundoy Valley and lived here his entire life."

I: "What did your father do for work?"

T: "In the beginning he had various trades, such as cultivating the traditional foods and taking care of the traditional field, and he was also dedicated to carpentry, woodcarving, and to traditional medicine."

I: "Was your father also a Taita?"

T: "Yes, I learned traditional medicine with my father, who died just 1 year ago."

I: "He taught you to be a Taita?"

T: "Yes, we are six brothers and sisters, and of the six of us, myself and my brother Floro are practicing traditional medicine."

I: "What does it mean to be a Taita?"

T: "Here the community classifies us in two ways: Someone is called a Taita if they lend service to the cabildo as a traditional authority, and then there are also those of us that practice traditional medicine."

I: "Can you explain the elected positions that you have held with the cabildo?"

T: "I had the opportunity to give service to the cabildo twice. The positions are for 1 year and there is no financial reward. The first time was in 2002 and I was elected *alguacil* mayor [mayor's assistant]. In this position, I was in charge of justice issues within the community. Sometimes I had to incarcerate people in the cabildo's jail and this was very difficult for me. Also, I was responsible for administering the sentences dictated by the governor.

In the year 2012, I was elected *alcalde mayor* [head mayor]. I was in charge of social and economic issues. Many times I was the governor in charge as well. This was more difficult because I had to resolve all different types of community problems. Also, in this position I was in charge of creating and implementing projects, and in this way I did a lot of work with the taitas and mamitas of the community. We succeeded in achieving recognition of traditional medicine on a local level and also within the state. Also, a group of taitas and mamitas unified to continue working together as an association."

I: "When was the first time that you drank yagé?"

T: "I don't remember because I always drank it since I was a kid."

I: "How was it to start drinking yagé as a boy and then to eventually become a Taita? How was this path of learning?"

T: "My father was always preparing us since we were little, although it's difficult for a child to understand the interest in drinking yagé. And then, after one is 15, one begins understanding a little more the importance of drinking the medicine because one understands what the remedy is showing us so that we can heal. Since I was young, on each full moon my father did rituals with crystals, animal skins, and bones, but I never understood it. Only now do I understand that this was a very special preparation he was doing for us to dedicate ourselves to the medicine."

I: "Did you decide to dedicate yourself to studying the medicine or was it something that you accepted because your father or your family told you that you would be a Taita someday?"

T: "My father was always encouraging us to drink the medicine because drinking medicine is a little difficult. Now we have changed a little how we prepare the medicine, but in those times with my father, what we were drinking was very bitter, and on top of that we had to drink a lot. When we were cooking with my father, he was cooking it very liquidy—totally liquid—and because of this, it was necessary to drink a lot. One had to drink as much as one full cup, more or less like a cup of coffee; 300–400 cm of yagé. So, it was very strong, and more than anything the taste was strong. But now we have changed this and we concentrate it more. Now we drink 5–10 cm and it's much easier to drink it."[1]

I: "And why is the yagé more concentrated now?"

T: "For the purpose of traveling with the medicine to other cities or out of the country; it's much easier to carry a small amount, as opposed to before when we had to carry a lot. Imagine one cup of medicine for each person. When my father was carrying yagé to Bogota, he was carrying 20 liters, more or less. If the group was big, we drank all of the 20 liters in just one night—a large quantity. It is because of this that it is more concentrated, and the most that I carry is 5 liters for 200–300 people. The amount that we give now may be about two to three teaspoons per person, depending on the person; but the effect is the same."

I: "Do you remember when the transition happened for you, from being the son of a Taita that was forced to drink yagé, to being someone who wanted to learn and dedicate himself to the medicine?"

T: "It was after I was 18 years old. I was aware that it was important to continue drinking yagé and also to continue practicing."

I: "Was there something in your life that helped you come to this realization?"

T: "In the beginning, I did not have visions, but then there was a moment in which the visions were revealed and I had the opportunity to make a painting of my first vision; a very simple painting. I showed it to the people and it had a big impact on them because it was very beautiful. These people, in addition to buying it, gave me a whole painting kit: oils, watercolors, acrylics, pastels, and all different types of pencils and erasers. They wanted me to continue painting my visions because it was easy to make copies. This is what motivated me to return to

---

[1] 1 cup = 8 oz; and 5–10 cm = 1–2 oz.

drink yagé, and to continue with more dedication, because I had to continue painting."

I: "In addition to painting, you also work with other forms of traditional art?"

T: "Yes, we started 10 years ago to work with traditional art, and it is interesting because the yagé has also helped influence this, especially with colors and designs. We work with weaving beadwork, weaving industrial fiber, and with natural fiber. We also do wood carvings, masks, stools, spoons, tables, chairs: a little bit of everything (Fig. 12.1)."

I: "Are the visions that show you what to paint part of the healing?"

T: "No. There are different reasons why someone drinks yagé. For someone who is continuously drinking, the interest is that the remedy shows him more and more, like how to treat people, how to cure people, and how to decode diseases. On the other hand, he who drinks to heal himself will be dedicated only to the disease that he has."

I: "Is there a difference between yagé and ayahuasca?"

T: "No, there is no difference. It's the same, but in each region they give it a different name. In the Putumayo it is called yagé, in the Amazon it is called ayahuasca, especially in Ecuador and in Peru. And in the part of the eastern Amazon, around the borders of Colombia and Venezuela, it is called caapi. These are the most well known names, but it is the same yagé.

There are many varieties; the most noticeable and distinct kinds are, for example, *Tigrehuasca*, which is the variety that has marks of a tiger on the bark of

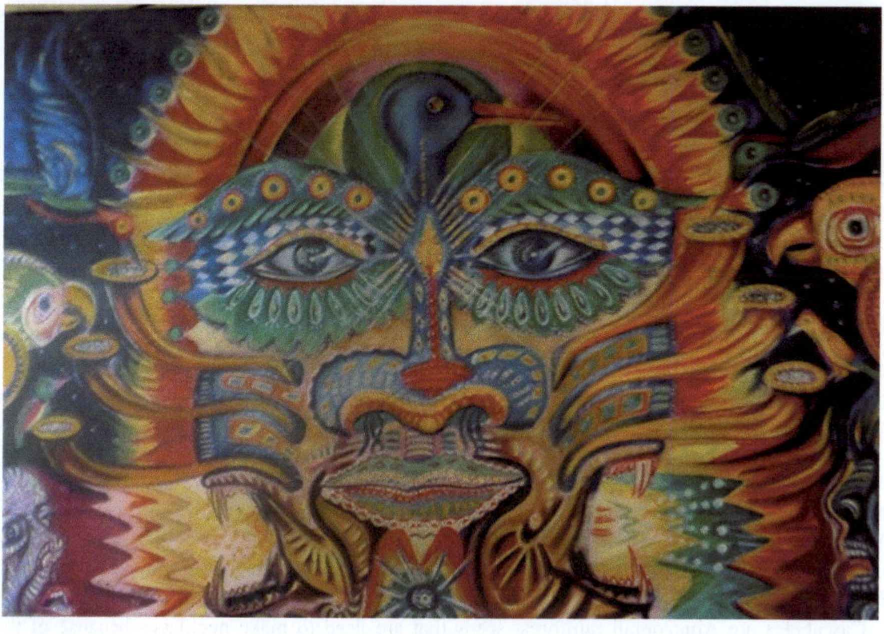

Fig. 12.1 Painting by Taita Juan Agreda Chindoy. Credit: Taita Juan Agreda Chindoy

the vine itself. And sometimes white moss grows on it in patches like the shapes of a tiger skin. There is also the *culebrahuasca*, which is distinguished because it has many knots. And the other is *intihuasca*, which translates as 'yagé of the sun.' It's a normal vine but it's differentiated by its thickness.[2] There are other varieties, but they are not as distinct as the ones I named.

The objective, more than anything, for tigrehuasca and intihuasca is to heal, as much spiritually as in the physical body. For this reason, each person that is going to drink has to be conscious that they are seeking healing. One must not drink just for the sake of drinking; rather, one must know what one is doing. Here in the indigenous community, when someone feels sick, they know that they should drink yagé to get well; not just for curiosity, because it doesn't work that way."

I: "What are the plants that are used to prepare yagé?"

T: "There are only two plants that create the effect of yagé. Yagé in itself is a vine, a crawler. The other plant, chagropanga [*Diplopterys cabrerana*], has the leaves. The two of them together create the effect of the purge and the visions. It's like a light bulb: There are two cables that create the connection for the light bulb to work. This is how the yagé functions, there are two plants; the connection between them is what causes the effect. Because if you only cook the yagé vine, you will only purge, and if you only drink the chagropanga nothing will happen. The connection of the two is what creates the effect."

I: "But you also know people that use other plants like *borrachera*?"[3]

T: "Yes, here we have 12 varieties of *borrachera,* and one of these is for consuming, but I do not use it. It's very strong. I have tried it, and the effect lasts 12 hours before you are conscious again. You do not remember anything you do, and it takes 3 days in order to fully return to consciousness. There are many plants that are added to the medicine, but I am saying that we only use yagé and chagropanga. We do not use others."

I: "How is the yagé ritual?"

T: "Well, at first when someone is explaining this, it may be difficult to understand in its totality; but you all have had the experience, and you all felt and should feel why it's important to do the ceremony. Because, first off, we are explaining the way that the yagé grows, where it comes from, what you receive, and what the intention is. All of this is explained to a person: This is how the prayer is done through the song, through the harmonization of music, with the necklaces, the cascabeles[4] that make music, the harmonica, and all of this. We are always calling to our ancestors who preserved this tradition, and we also pray a lot, because each plant has its elemental energy, its spirit. First, you have to thank it for

---

[2] All of the varieties listed are *Banisteriopsis caapi*; the way that they grow and how they are harvested is what distinguishes the different types. See Appendix for more information.

[3] *Borrachera* mostly refers to a variety of species in the *Brugmansia* family that are sometimes mixed with yagé; the Camseta also refer to some plants as borracheras that are not of the *Brugmansia* family.

[4] Cascabeles are Amazonian rainforest seeds that are used to make necklaces because of the rattling sound that is created when the seeds hit each other.

the privilege to work with it, and then you have to ask that the intentions of each person be blessed."

I: "How is the experience of using ayahuasca to decode a disease and to diagnose?"

T: "When there are complicated diseases, many times patients arrive as a last resort because the doctors do not know what they have. Sometimes we are able to diagnose without yagé, by just looking, because we have worked according to what the medicine teaches us and we have understood a particular aspect of the disease that clearly will not appear in any of the doctor's exams, no matter how advanced the exam; but we can see that it is an energetic illness. If the illness persists, we drink more yagé with the objective to see what the problem is; what disease we are dealing with. Also, the medicine shows us in what manner it will heal. It shows us what medicine we are going to apply and in what way we should use the different therapies."

I: "When you say that you are able 'to see which disease the person has,' are there things that you can see, in the sense of your eyes being open?"

T: "Yes of course, you can see them. Though sometimes, if you are not paying attention, or if you haven't learned how, then you will not be able to decode why some energies are there. It could be an animal, a plant, or a person that is totally different or strange. One deciphers why these spirits are present in the sick person. Or sometimes we simply ask, or we drink the remedy, so that we may receive guidance on how to heal. The remedy teaches what is missing for a patient with a complicated disease."

I: "The yagé is able to give suggestions for other remedies. But, sometimes, the yagé is also able to cure on its own?"

T: "In many cases, yes, but in others, no. That is why I always tell you that yagé is an essential foundation but it won't heal all diseases. Other plants are needed according to the disease."

I: "What are the differences between Western medicine and the medicine of yagé?"

T: "That is why I am explaining that when an energetic disease is present, it will not show up in any exams. We can decode the energetic disease with the plants that we have."

I: "Can both medicines be used in a complementary manner?"

T: "Yes, of course, because there are some very complex diseases that, in some cases, require surgery that we are not able to perform. And, in the same way, when there is an energetic disease, it is not going to appear in any type of exams, no matter how good they are. But, because of our training, we are able to cure the energetic disease because you cannot see it, but you can feel it."

I: "Or do they conflict?"

T: "No, to this day we have worked well together because we have to work being realistic about what is happening with the disease. Because sometimes, for instance, there is a tumor and we can't do anything. The patient will need surgery. We are not completely responsible for the disease. For this reason, we have to diagnose it. One could also end up saying, 'I am not able to heal you'; not everything can be cured and sometimes we have to send people to the hospital."

I: "Do you have experience working alongside Western doctors?"

T: "Yes, I have the assistance of two clinics in the city of Medellin. In one, I work with a female doctor, and in the other with a male doctor. Both groups are always sending patients to see me when they see that drinking yagé could be beneficial, as well as to do treatments with other types of plants."

I: "Are there many doctors that drink yagé with you?"

T: "Yes, from all over. Yesterday morning we drank yagé and there was a Chilean doctor and he was watching the analysis: how a person that came in with arthritic leg pain was responding. We made an assessment of how he has improved up until today. The doctor was surprised; he wanted to keep working with the plants. There are doctors like this everywhere I go. And there are crazy doctors, too [Laughter]" (Fig. 12.2).[5]

I: "And how do the doctors view your work?"

T: "Until now, I have been doing my work, and every time they are more accepting of collaborating with traditional medicine. Again, remember that we do not only use yagé for different illnesses, we use other plants, too. Sometimes we give yagé to patients and then their Western doctors come to understand why we do this. Those who disagree the most are the psychiatrists, and also the toxicologists. They are oriented by a basic level of understanding, by the chemistry of yagé, but they do not understand its ancestral healing power.

So, when we really work together with the Western doctors, they have seen how the patients react in a really good way and for that reason there is a lot of acceptance of traditional medicine; so much so that they themselves have agreed to drink yagé."

I: "Why do you think that the psychiatrists are the ones that are the most against it?"

T: "Because the psychiatrist is always trying to control madness. The toxicologist always says that it is toxic. So they are never going to be in agreement. They don't understand the ancestral power of yagé."

I: "How would you define 'health,' 'to be healthy'?"

T: "If we drink yagé and we are not sick, it is very helpful in purifying and preventing diseases, because we are able to detoxify ourselves from certain foods that we eat that make us sick. In this way, we can prevent and alleviate a little bit some pains, especially in the young. But also we are aware that sometimes there are things that we have to experience and for this reason, despite the best medicines that there are, we will not be able to cure."

I: "Is there a difference between how you use the medicine to treat people in your community as opposed to people from the city or foreigners?"

---

5 Taita Juan is poking fun at Brian Anderson here because he knows that Brian is a medical student.

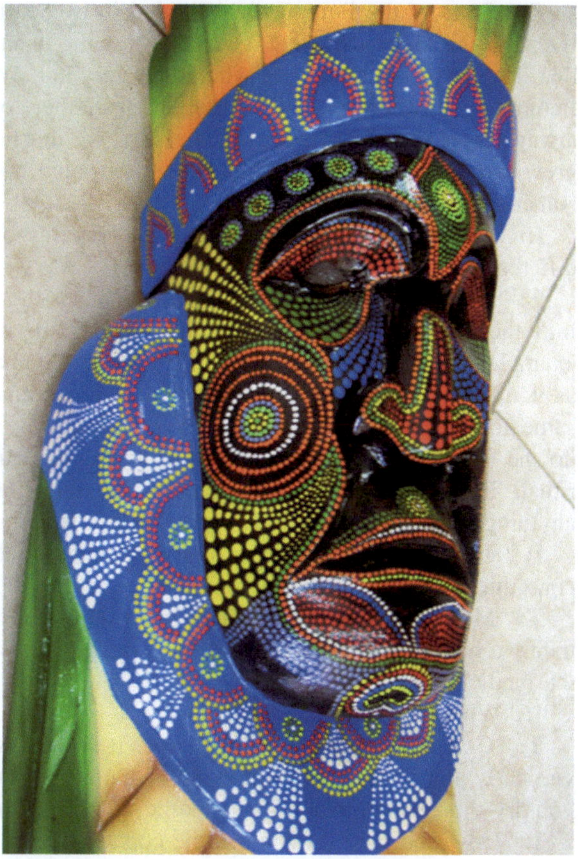

Fig. 12.2 Mask by Taita Juan Agreda Chindoy. Credit: Taita Juan Agreda Chindoy

T: "Sometimes, when it is not explained correctly, the whole world wants to drink just for the experience. Here in the community, they are very conscious that they need to drink it when there is a sickness, or for a clear purpose, not just for an experiment just to know what yagé is about. Really, it is used when there is a need. To the people of the city, and from all over the world, this is what we explain so that they become aware of what the yagé ritual is about."

I: "So then the way of treating people does not vary much if someone is from your community or from the city?"

T: "No, it's the same. Illness is the same. For instance, a cancer for someone from the city is the same as a cancer for someone from the community."

I: "And where does the yagé come from that you use?"

T: "The yagé mostly grows in warm climates, more or less at 25–30 °C. Here in the Sibundoy Valley, we live in a variable temperate climate of 10–20 °C. It's a little cold. It's difficult to grow yagé here. Nonetheless, I have some planted. I have plants that are 14 years old and that are very mature, but I still haven't tried them yet to see what result they give. That's why we bring yagé from the lower Putumayo.

The State of the Putumayo is divided in two parts: The upper part, where we live, and the lower part; that is more or less the Amazon Basin, the forested zone; that is close to sea level, and where it is very hot. We are very close to the lower Putumayo, between 3 and 4 h away, and from there on the yagé grows, so we have always brought it from there. In the past, we did not cultivate this remedy as it grew naturally; but now that it is being used more, we have to cultivate it, because sometimes it is scarce."

I: "Depending on how someone prepares the remedy, will there be differences?"

T: "Yes, a lot. This is a medicine that carries the intention of how it was made into the ceremony. That's where the ability to really heal comes from. For example, you have to make a ritual to plant it. You have to plant the yagé as much as you have to plant the intention of it being a remedy for it to be healing. The same goes for when you harvest it: You do the same thing. When you cook it, you do the same, and when you drink it, again, the same. Everything is done with ritual. That's why when some people take the vine and cook it without doing anything, it really doesn't have a good effect. It is through the ritual that it heals."

I: "Have you drunk a preparation of a medicine that was made poorly and that consequently affected your ceremony?"

T: "Many times. When this happens we use copal. If the ritual isn't going well, then we harmonize ourselves with the copal. We also sing different songs so that the medicine flows well."

I: "What is copal?"

T: "Copal [*Protium copal*] is a tree. It is the resin of a tree that you can cut vertically and from there it drips out. What comes out is the resin of the tree, and you dry this. Sometimes it looks like a rock. With this, we make the *saumedio*."[6]

I: "How and why do you use the copal in the ritual?"

T: "If there are certain types of bad energies, when you can perceive that something is not right: In these moments we can burn copal, and this helps to maintain the harmony in the people and in the ritual. Also, we use a combination of different essences when people are nervous, if they are feeling a lot of fear, if there is unrest, or, well, if something happens and it's necessary to do different therapies. Depending on the state of the person, we use these types of therapies.

This was born out of an idea of mine because I saw that people have to be very conscious in order to receive the complete message of the medicine. If we go to some parts of the lower Putumayo, there, they don't do anything for people having a hard time. Maybe they sing and do a cleansing with branches, and they also do *sopladas* with *chonduro*[7] if the person is in a bad place. If they can't control the person, they just tie the person up with a rope and that's it. I don't believe that is good because that person is going to suffer a trauma. I think it's better to use these

---

[6] *Saumedio* is a local term for incense.

[7] The root of the chonduro is used to make an infusion with water and alcohol that is then utilized for the *sopla*, i.e., the blowing of a fine mist on a patient.

little tricks that have worked very well in the past. This is the reason why people wake up in the morning after the ritual very happy to have received the message of the medicine so well."

I: "How do you prepare yourself for the yagé ceremonies?"

T: "I am always prepared, with the clear intention to heal and to cure with the necklaces, the *waira*,[8] a good little remedy, and with a strong prayer guided by the patients' needs. However, this varies a lot with each ceremony."

I: "Is this part of being a taita, always being ready to go do a ritual?"

T: "Yes, from the point that one starts the path, you must always be ready. Imagine that sometimes groups of 10, 15 people arrive, and you are not thinking about anything besides getting to your house, and sometimes you have to give them yagé: It's because you are prepared. Sometimes patients arrive—it has happened to me—that they arrive when I am already sleeping. A group arrives and you have to wake up and serve them. It's not necessary to prepare for months, and much less for years, in order to do a ceremony; you always have to be ready."

I: "Do you have to get dressed in a certain way or say a special prayer before you start a session?"

T: "Yes, like our father taught us, and as I learned from all the time we shared with other taitas, the medicine has an elemental energy that sometimes manifests in the vision in the form of what you should wear and how you should do the ceremony. When I started and I was practicing, I only had a waira and a *cascabel*, which makes a rattling sound. But, little by little, the items started arriving in the way that things happen when someone drinks yagé. And now I have necklaces of teeth, the cascabeles, and the crown of feathers. These are important for doing yagé ceremonies; they distinguish the person who can heal" (Fig. 12.3).

I: "Are there certain recommendations that you give to your patients before they drink yagé?"

T: "We try to evaluate a person regarding their state of health; if they have an illness, if they are taking a drug or medication for an illness, or if they just want to clean themselves out. Many are not prepared, and for this reason I explain why one should drink."

I: "Have you worked in the past with a patient that you thought should not drink yagé for health reasons?"

T: "Yes, of course. Above all, people older than 80 or 90 years will have difficulty being able to drink yagé because at that age they are often in a difficult condition with various illnesses. Sometimes they arrive thinking that yagé will help with pain or some other circumstances, but in these cases it is very difficult, so I don't give it to them."

I: "Are there some medicines that a patient should not take if they are going to drink yagé?"

[8] A waira is a collection of leaves tied together to form a ceremonial tool.

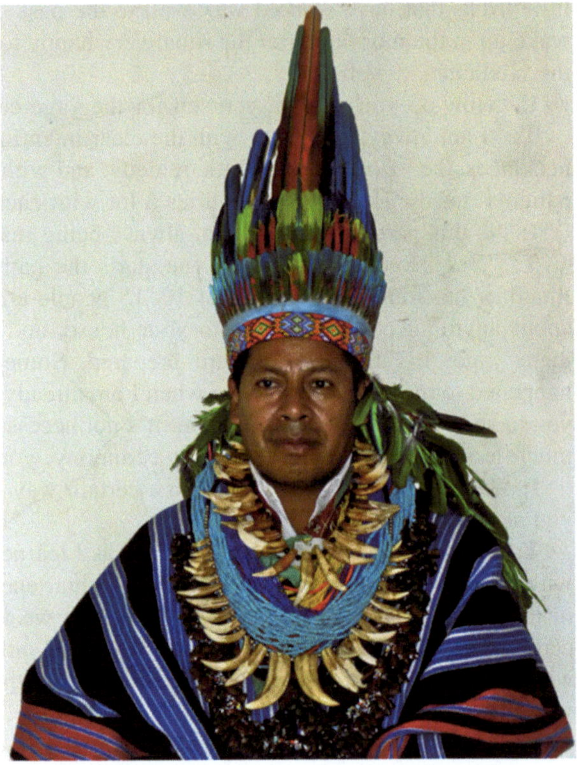

Fig. 12.3 Taita Juan Agreda Chindoy in ceremonial regalia. Credit: Brandon Hirzel

T: "Yes, generally the psychiatric drugs are the ones that don't mix well. When the patient's case is very complicated, we give other natural medicines that don't require yagé being given too."

I: "So, yagé can be dangerous to some types of people?"

T: "If you don't use it well, yes it is dangerous. It is always taken with a guide, with the taita, with the shaman because he or she knows how to manage energies. If the illness is something strong, there are going to be complications, and if there is not someone that understands it or can help, sometimes the patient can suffer some kind of trauma. This is why it is important to do it in a ceremony and with a guide because whatever happens, one can work with different therapies, using different plants, essences, and massages. Before, we used to do an evaluation, and sometimes a person in a very critical position would arrive. Understanding this, we are able to help with different therapies and we are able to work very well."

I: "Recently, in Colombia and in other countries, there have been deaths related to drinking yagé, either during the session or afterward. Can you explain why this happened?"

T: "Yes, there have been several deaths. The people involved need to speak up to clarify what happened, because before you know it someone will take the body for an autopsy to know what caused the death. Sometimes we cannot fight against the destiny of our final hour. Many people arrive at that moment. I have seen a woman who, 3 hours before the ceremony, preparing herself to drink yagé, died in the bathroom. It has also been the case that many people have not been able to use the autopsy to blame yagé, because the yagé has not been shown to be the cause of death.

But in other cases, yes, the taita had been irresponsible. A little while ago in one part of Colombia two people died in a ceremony. But, according to what the press reported, the taita gave the medicine to the people during the day and left them alone without staying there to guide them. The people were looking for help in the critical moments and, because no one was there to help them, these two people died; on top of that, several others went to the hospital. There was a lack of responsibility. For this reason we always recommend that when people do the ceremony, they do it with someone with sufficient experience."

I: "Is it possible to use yagé for the purpose of doing something bad to another person?"

T: "Yes, yes, that could certainly happen. Just as there are good people, there are also bad people in all places. Also there are people who do not have sufficient experience and they begin to distribute medicine, and this is a complicated situation. Sometimes they don't manage to really understand the message of the medicine, and there is confusion, and for this reason it does not go well for many people."

I: "How do you decide the quantity of yagé to give each person?"

T: "It is like Western medicine: There is a dose for kids and one for adults. Because when you buy a Western drug they ask, "Is this for a kid or for an adult?" If it is a kid, you are not going to take a dose for adults, right? Likewise, we are not going to give the same amount to drink to a kid as to an adult. Or also if the adult is in a weak state.... according to how the person is doing, they might not get the same dose. You have to see their physique and their illness. All of this is a question of analysis, in order to determine the dose."

I: "What is the objective of giving yagé to a kid? Is it different to give it to an adult?"

T: "Yes, especially the part related to the vision is very different because kids are very innocent. But it has worked very well to open the appetite, because kids generally don't have a good appetite, they don't want to eat and they are picky about food. Yagé helps them a lot to eat well and not be picky with food; moreover, they can expel their parasites. But they have a dose that is not for having a journey; rather it's to develop the mind, to maintain health, and to expel parasites. Also, it helps them a lot with studying, it opens their mind."

I: "Can you tell us a little more about how yagé can help kids with their studies?"

T: "It really facilitates their understanding of what they are taught in school. They can understand much more easily. That's why when they are doing poorly in grade school or high school, we resort to giving them yagé, so that they can understand and do well."

I: "Is this is a common practice in the community?"

T: "Not just in the community, also with the mestizos."

I: "Is the dose to develop the mind smaller?"

T: "Of course, yes, especially for little kids. It depends on their age, because we have given yagé to infants just a few hours after their birth."

I: "Are there other reasons why you'd give yagé to kids?"

T: "There are some kids that are children of taitas who begin to prepare since they are children to learn how to heal. This was the case for me. I was prepared through yagé and other plants so that I would follow the apprenticeship in traditional medicine, as I said before."

I: "Are there also cases of adults who you'd give yagé to so that they can learn better?"

T: "Yes, yes of course."

I: "And do you do this frequently?"

T: "When it is for learning, you do it frequently. But it is very different if it's for a student in grade school, in high school or in university. For a student of the medicine, it is possible to drink every day, but for a student in grade school, high school or university, every month is good. When the drinking is only for medical purposes, you only drink when you are sick."

I: "Can you give us examples of other treatments that you use apart from yagé?"

T: "I use treatments for all classes of illnesses, depending on what the person has. It is a complicated issue. You know how many illnesses there are; there are thousands. Because of this, we have to see in what way we are going to heal. Yagé is the foundation, the guide of many illnesses, but yagé does not heal all. We have to resort to many other plants."

I: "What is another common plant that you use in healings?"

T: "There are many purgative plants, so many. Here there are planted around 80 medicinal plants. When I see them I remember them: The name and what it is used for. Or when the patient is here also I know which plant in the garden I am going to go get to do the treatment. If I begin to talk about each plant, I think we will still be here explaining it all when the sun comes up."

I: "What is a limpia?"

T: "We do a limpia [cleansing] to complement the yagé ritual because sometimes we wake up with certain energies that come from our past experiences and we need to expel these energies. It is an energetic illness that one feels but does not see. That's why an illness like this will simply never appear in an x-ray. Hence the doctors say, 'No, there is no illness, all is good' when they do the exam, but the patient continues in pain.

In the same way we do a limpia for certain people that have what we call 'bad air' or 'bad wind' in which they have vomiting, diarrhea, and fever. They caught it when they were feeling good and then, all of a sudden, they have this type of symptoms. So we also do the limpia with certain branches that are called a waira, and an extraction of a plant that is called chonduro. With these we do a *soplo* and it goes away. In the ceremonies, I do a limpia, especially when there are new people. So, it's not always; it depends on how the people are doing. There are people that don't need it. But for the majority of occasions, yes, they need it."

I: "What does it mean to make a soplo?"

T: "All traditional healers work with the soplo, preparing coco chonduro mixed with water, sometimes, when you can, you make it with blessed holy water. Depending on the diagnosis of the malady that the patient has, you do a ritual invoking the ancestral power, so that, through the soplo, you can get rid of the bad spirits that provoke pains. You do the soplo by drinking a little bit of the chonduro remedy in the mouth and then blowing a mist on the body of the sick person. You also blow looking at the parts that are most painful. It heals with the soplo; the patient reacts instantaneously and gets better."

I: "Can you give me an example of a serious illness that you have treated through yagé? For example, cancer or AIDS?"

T: "Yes, I have lost count of the number of cancers I've cured, but I have cured many. Also, you have to see what type of cancer it is because there are a lot of types of cancer, and you need to check if it is progressing rapidly. When the cancer has already spread through the body it is very difficult to cure. Either way, I'll return to confirm that in these cases of difficult illness, one cannot cure with yagé; you can help a lot with yagé, but you cannot cure with yagé.

As of today, I have also had two cases of AIDS that were cured. They are two women, one from here in Colombia and another from Holland. I made them treatments, with yagé of course, and at the same time they were taking different medicines, but all natural, with plants. I believe they were in treatment for 3 months. We know that they were cured because I sent them to have a laboratory test and they did not have it anymore.

This is not to say that the whole world is going to get cured because some people that have these illnesses assimilate the medicine we give them here, and others do not. For this reason, some people have not been able to heal. There are also those that I have cured of difficult cases of drug addiction by using yagé complemented by other plants. To this day, I have the stories of two people that have left heroin, a complicated disease. But I have already cured so many people of addictions to *basuco* [coca paste], marijuana, alcohol, and cigarettes that I've lost count."

I: "How long did it take for the people that you treated to be cured of their heroin addiction?"

T: "One month."

I: "Is it true that you have thought about creating a clinic in Central America to treat addictions?"

T: "Yes, we are working to create a center in Costa Rica, and we shall see how that goes. We are trying to set things up to see how it could work. We see some difficulties because it is hard for people to arrive at the place. We have thought about creating a centralized location that people could easily access. The same goes for here [in Colombia]; things are going well, though not totally, but we are working on this."

I: "Is it true that you were detained in the United States a few years ago for bringing in yagé?"

T: "Yes, approximately, two and a half years ago."

I: "Can you tell us a little about it?"

T: "Yes. I was detained in the Houston airport. It is a pretty long story. But what is certain is that when I arrived, they confiscated the yagé, and sent it to a laboratory and found DMT. That was when I learned that yagé has a substance called DMT. DMT is what is what activates the vision and, for them, anything that provokes visions is a drug, a hallucinogenic drug. So they think like this: All that produces visions is going to be a drug that causes madness in people and is toxic. They do not understand the spiritual part or how we handle this. They will never understand that yagé is a very special kind of DMT. They think like this and that's why they arrested me."

I: "How many days were you detained?"

T: "I was there 1 month."

I: "And what did you do during this month?"

T: "I don't know if you want to hear the story of what I did for a whole month [laughter]. What I can say is that I studied a little about the DMT that is in yagé to understand it. I studied what DMT really is. I realized that many plants have DMT. Here there is a plant that is a crawler. They use it in the garden because it has beautiful flowers, and this has the same DMT. But reading into this more, for example, in one part of a book it says that it is very strong, and that it can cause a cerebral shock and could even lead to death. I was able to appreciate the different types of plants that have DMT; there is a variety, and there are some that really are very poisonous.

These poisonings do not happen with yagé because it has an ancestral power. It comes, being guided since ancient times, worked with by our ancestors. There have been legends and myths, but they don't know exactly what time it came from nor who discovered it. Since I have known my father—who died at 93—he would say that when he was a boy, his grandparents also spoke a lot about yagé. So, there are many, many, many years in which it has been worked with. They are not going to understand that there is an ancestral power in the plant, and furthermore, for this reason, one makes a ritual. One makes a very special prayer in order to be connected with the ancestors, as well as with the elemental energy of the plants.

We have never classified the yagé as dangerous, so even though it has the DMT, our elders have worked with it so that it is entirely healthy. Because they focus on the substance, on what it contains, they put me in jail and I was never able to justify myself to them. Only the lawyers were able to really justify that we use it as medicine, supported by the more or less 400 people that testified that it is medicinal.[9] They also understood that if I had not been indigenous, it would have been very difficult to get me out of prison."

I: "During this time you did not have yagé, but did you continue healing people in the prison while you were there?"

[9] He is referring to the signatures obtained during his US incarceration from people in Colombia and internationally that vouched for the "medicinal" quality of yagé and, specifically, their experiences with him.

T: "Yes, the yagé is a guide that teaches one through apprenticeship, but one does not need to be under the effect of yagé to be able to heal. I had the opportunity to heal, more than anything, a person with a fracture, and he got better."

I: "In the end, the government of the United States said that you had to leave the country?"

T: "Well, they dropped the charges, because of what the lawyers did, but I had a visa that they took away. I have the right to return after 5 years."

I: "Did this event change your work in Colombia in some way?"

T: "Not at all. Now, I have more clients. I had a lot of support; people have been more interested after this, wanting to have more contact with me."

I: "And how is the issue of legalization in your country?"

T: "The traditional healers of the municipality of Sibundoy have been coming together because of the issue of legalization. We formed an association of traditional healers so that we may be recognized, as well as the medicines that we use. We got a resolution from the cabildo. We are recognized in principle in the municipality of Sibundoy; as much in the cabildo as in the municipality. With this we will go to the Department, or State, within Colombia. Now we are trying to bring this to the Ministry of Health so that we are recognized as traditional healers as well as our medicines. We want to legalize not only yagé, but also all of the medicinal plants.

I: "In which countries have you worked in, as of today?"

T: "I have been, more than anywhere, in Argentina, Uruguay, Chile, and Ecuador. Also I have been in Panama, Costa Rica, Mexico, and the United States."

I: "How many people do you think have drunk yagé with you?"

T: "Here, I am not able to say. I started at 20 years old and now I have 24 years working at this. It's innumerable. We have sometimes, approximately, 100 people a month. Depending on the place, sometimes more."

I: "Do you have apprentices, people that are learning to be taitas?"

T: "Yes. A little while ago I had 17. Of the 17, 10 are men and the rest are women, also from other countries. And the medicine women are not called taitas, rather *mamas*."

I: "People that are not from your community, who are from the big cities of the world, can they become taitas?"

T: "Yes, of course, as long as they have the willingness in the apprenticeship they will achieve it. Although there are very few who truly learn to do good work at healing."

I: "Thank you Taita, we wish you much success."

T: Thank you.

Acknowledgments We would like to thank Pamela Ruiz Flores López for the transcription of the original interview with Taita Juan, Gustavo Caldarelli for his assistance with the translation of the interview to English, and Clancy Cavnar for the revision of the text. Finally, we would like to thank the Taita for his time and patience in doing this interview and for his willingness to share so openly his knowledge of Cametsa healing practices—both those he was taught and those he himself has developed over his years of caring for patients hailing from near and far. We also thank him for sharing his artwork here with us.

Appendix: Select Medicinal Plants in Taita Juan's Garden

[In the preparation of this text, not all English-language names and scientific names were available to the authors]

Ajenjo—Wormwood—*Artemisia absinthium*
Amansaguapo
Anamu
Arnica—Arnica
Borrachera Amarillo—Trumpet Flower—*Brugmansia aurea*
Borrachera Blanco—Trumpet Flower—*Brugmansia arborea*
Borrachera Rosada—Trumpet Flower—*Brugmansia insignis*
Borrachera Rosada—Trumpet Flower—*Brugmansia suaveolens*
Botoncillo de Mar
Calendula—Calendula—*Calendula officinalis*
Canelon
Casco de Vaca
Cauco
Cedron—*Aloysia triphylla*
Chonduro Rojo
Chontambe
Coco Chonduro
Cuiyangillo
Diente de Leon—Dandelion—*Taraxacum officinale*
Eneldo
Escobilla
Escorsonera
Euculyptus—Euculyptus—*Eucalyptus globulus*
Euculyptus—Euculyptus—*Eucalyptus leucoxylon*
Gente Chonduro
Hoja Santa
Insulina
Limoncillo—Lemongrass—*Cympopogon citratus*
Manzanilla—Chamomile—*Matricaria recutita*
Menta—Mint—*Mentha spicata*
Millonaria
Oregano—Oregano—*Origanum Vulgare*
Ortiga—Nettles
Paico—Wormseed—*Dysphania ambrosioides*
Pajakan
Poeleo
Quererme
Romasa
Romero—Rosemary—*Rosmarinus officinalis*
Sabila—Aloe Vera—*Aloe barbadensis*

Sangre de Drago—*Croton lechleri*
Sauco- Elderberry—*Sambucus nigra*
Seguidora
Sidra
Tarta
Tigre Chonduro
Tomillo—Thyme—*Thymus vulgaris*
Toronjil—Lemon Balm—*Melissa officinalis*
Valerana—Valerian—*Valeriana officinalis*
Violeta—Violet—*Viola odorata*
Vira Vira
Waira Chonduro
Yagé—*Banisteriopsis caapi*
Yerba Buena—Peppermint—*Mentha arvensis*
Yerba Dulce

References

Caicedo, A. (2014). Yage related neo-shamanism in Colombian urban contexts. In B. C. Labate & C. Cavnar (Eds.), *Ayahuasca shamanism in the Amazon and beyond*. New York, NY: Oxford University Press. (in press).

Guerrero, H. (1991). Pinta, pinta, cura, cura, gente. In E. Amodio & J. Juncoso (Eds.), *Espíritus Aliados: Chamanismo y curación en los pueblos indios de Sudamérica* (pp. 209–253). Quito: ABYA-YALA.

Uribe, C. A. (2008). El yajé, el purgatorio y la farándula. *Antípoa, 6*, 113–131.

Chapter 13
Postscript—Psychedelics in Unlocking the Unconscious: From Cancer to Addiction

Gabor Maté

Abstract Complex unconscious psychological stresses underlie and contribute to all chronic medical conditions, from cancer to addiction, from depression to multiple sclerosis. Therapy that is assisted by psychedelics, in the right context and with the right support, can bring these dynamics to the surface and thus help a person liberate themselves from their influence. Special focus will be given to the writers' experience in treating addictions and other stress-related conditions, both with aboriginal people and in non-indigenous contemporary healing circles. This work has been done under the guidance of indigenous Peruvian shamans and their Western apprentices.

Elsewhere in this book, worthy colleagues-experts-have discussed the science and theory of ayahuasca. Here, in this postscript, I have the more modest task of providing an account of what I have personally learned and witnessed, and of offering a perspective on why the plant and its effects call to me as a physician interested in healing.

Until 5 years ago—I write this in 2013—I knew nothing about ayahuasca, having only vaguely heard about it. As a practitioner trained in the orthodox Western allopathic model, I have long been aware not only of the astonishing achievements of modern medicine, but also of its limitations. What we, as medical doctors, cannot cut out, poison or burn, we can only alleviate, at best. We are mesmerized by cure and know nothing about healing. We can mend broken bones, transplant hearts and livers, but can do little for fractured souls or help transform traumatized minds. Above all, we do not get that people's illnesses, mental or physical, are not isolated, accidental, and unfortunate events, but manifestations of lives in a psychological and social context, the results of experiences and beliefs and lifelong patterns of relating to the world. Hence, we can suppress manifestations but rarely get at causes. We separate the mind from the body and the

G. Maté (✉)
941 West 22nd Avenue, Vancouver, BC V5Z 2A2, Canada
e-mail: gabor@drgabormate.com
URL: http://www.drgabomate.com

B. C. Labate and C. Cavnar (eds.), *The Therapeutic Use of Ayahuasca*,
DOI: 10.1007/978-3-642-40426-9_13,

individual from the environment. And we are arrogant, not in the sense that we think we know everything, but in our conviction that what we do not know is not worth knowing; what we have not studied is not worth investigating, that frameworks of awareness parallel to ours have no validity, are not worth exploring.

I have worked in family practice, palliative care with the terminally ill, and with addictions in Vancouver's Downtown Eastside, notorious as North America's most concentrated area of drug use. Both from personal observation and from the study of the new science of psychoneuroimmunology, I knew that cancer, and most chronic illness, represented lifelong emotional patterns of self-suppression, based on early childhood emotional loss or suffering. Too, I saw that addiction—whether to drugs or to any ultimately self-harming habit, be it sexual roving, gambling, compulsive working, internet surfing, or shopping—is always an attempt to escape pain, to shed, if only temporarily, an unbearable unease with the self. It was after my book on addiction (Maté 2010) was published, in which is demonstrated the relationship between childhood trauma and adult substance dependency, that I began to receive inquiries about what I knew regarding ayahuasca and the healing of addiction. I knew nothing, and after a while found the inquiries importunate and bothersome. Keen as I was to investigate ways of healing beyond the narrow medical model, I, too, did not want to have to learn about something new. I could not imagine how a psychedelic substance would help anyone overcome addiction or help heal PTSD or ingrained patterns of self-neglect that contribute to illness.

The universe had other ideas. I have since worked with ayahuasca, and such work, while a small part of what I do, has become the most exciting among my healing activities, the one in which I see the most transformative potential. In the healing retreats we have conducted (we: my friends, ayahuasqueros—more about them below—and I), we have worked with people struggling with drug use and sexual addiction, people facing cancer and degenerative neurological illness, depression, post-traumatic stress disorder, anxiety, and chronic fatigue, and just people seeking wholeness, meaning, an experience of their true selves rather than their ingrained but inauthentic habitual patterns. We have worked with people looking for themselves, for their parents, for love, for God, for truth, for their child selves, for community, for nature. I cannot say that everyone found everything they were looking for, far from it. I can say that most people took major steps forward on their path toward authenticity and found significant liberation from stultifying, limiting mind patterns, and behaviors. Some have transformed their lives. Some are no longer addicted. Many are no longer content to be other than who they are.

"Since the end of February, my first ayahuasca experience, I am daily experiencing a shift in my consciousness, my presence within and with others including animals. I see everything I've done from a completely new perspective and live it. Daily." So writes a man his 30s, himself with a history of trauma, who works with traumatized people in British Columbia, Canada.

> I am able to see the difference I make to ease pain in others, help them see themselves in a different light and give them a bit of brilliance and sparkle even as they are rolled out in ambulances, while both of us are aware that we will not see each other anymore in this form.

A similar chord is stuck by a man from the opposite shore of North America and with a different life path, a real estate broker from New York: "In my day-to-day capitalistic pursuits I often meditate on ways that I might help other people in a deeper way." And, from a woman whose life had been blighted by chronic pain and addiction, the template for which had been a history of childhood sexual abuse:

> Today I stand in awe of life's blessings and the sacred and precious nature of life. No wonder it is a miracle. I never understood until now that life continues in its miraculous nature from the point of conception until we draw our last breath.

Anyone who has worked with the ayahuasca as a facilitator, healer, guide, or shaman will be familiar with such testimonials to the power of the plant and the potential blessings it confers. But wherein resides that power, and what in the experience with it grants such benefits? And what might be some the risks?

My own first experience with the plant was in a ceremony led by a Peruvian shaman, in Canada. There were a few words of introduction, some silent meditation, but little else by way of preparation. We drank, about forty of us in a large tent, and sat in silence. And then the music began, and some icaros in native Peruvian languages, but mostly Spanish-sung cantos and some songs in English, to the accompaniment of guitars and percussion. I do not recall after what period of time, but I found tears flowing from my eyes, tears of joy, tears of love, and tears of gratitude. Love for whom? Love. Gratitude toward what or for what? Gratitude. And I saw and felt how I had myself fled from love so much of my life, failed to recognize it, feared to embrace it, betrayed it. I understood how so many—all—of my habits, including my addictive behaviors, were an escape from pain I had not wanted to feel, from a deep fear I had not wanted to experience. And with the presence of love I also knew that there was nothing to escape from, no reason to run.

I was able to grasp why so many people had written to me suggesting ayahuasca as a modality in the treatment of addiction: If we can allow ourselves to experience the pain, we don't need to run away from it, we do not need to seek oblivion in the temporary release substances or behaviors can grant us. And, of course, if we touch the core of love, we see there is nothing to run from any more. There never was, if we but knew it.

I experienced the plant twice more within a week, and by that week's end I was committed to incorporating it, somehow, into my work. The opportunity arose almost immediately, as I met Canadian ayahuasqueros who had studied in Peru under the guidance of a Shipibo shaman. They were humble and dedicated servants of the plant. They had participated in many ceremonies, some held in isolated jungle venues, in solitude, alone for days, following diets (*dietas*) without many of the condiments and comforts of "Western" food: Not for the faint hearted.

In the Amazon Basin, where they had learned and honed their craft, the ceremonies are led by traditional shamans in villages where the culture supports and holds the experience; where the community provides the ongoing context for the learning, healing, and transformation that may result. Our dilemma was: how to adapt the work in the urbanized, fragmented, materialistic society of North America? And, further, how to provide a healing experience for people with complex psychological patterns engendered by an alienated, denatured, non-spiritual culture that celebrates individualism but discourages individuality that promotes conformism without offering real community? How to create a safe, supportive environment for this work?

Our first thought was that in the North American setting the challenge is to provide a context that somehow approximates, or at least substitutes for, the original environment in which the plant has been used, even if only transiently. Having a group of strangers gather for a ceremony one evening and disperse in morning would not suffice. We have to create a temporary village, bring together a group of people who are committed to their own and to one another's growth, and we have to keep them together long enough for the process to unfold. Second, the event needed to occur away from the noise- and activity-pollution of the city, close to nature, enfolded by the sounds and sights, and smells of nature. Hence, the concept of a week-long retreat in a rural setting where people would live together, if only for a few days, share meals, and get to know one another very intimately in a short space of time.

But the deeper problem is rooted in the very nature of the ayahuasca experience itself. The plant teaches what we need to learn, but not always in a language immediately accessible to us. In a culture whose symbols are largely artificial, would the symbols conjured by the plant be understood by participants? Often they are not. The visions the plant brings to people can be beautiful, magnificent, and inspiring and engender the purest joy and gratitude; they can also be threatening, incomprehensible to the mind, and arouse terror. The emotions evoked can be gentle and soothing and suffused with peace and happiness; they can also be excruciatingly painful, frightful, and induce experiences of profound loss. The felt sense can be of ineffable freedom or of dark imprisonment. People can see and be their divine selves or be identified with the most diabolical elements of their personalities. Without preparation, processing and integration, the ayahuasca experience can be confusing and, for many, incomplete.

It has long been understood that the transaction between the plant and the human is never just one of a chemical effect. According to my ayahuasquero friends, the plant has a spirit; *is* a spirit. As a scientifically trained physician, I have no idea what they are talking about. Yet, on some level, I know they are right. It is certainly not a matter of "here, drink this tea and call me in the morning." The ceremony, the setting, the chanting, the relationship of shaman, and guide to participant are as least as important as the brew. That is why I was so amused to read a well-known Canadian writer publicly explain that he drank the tea in some friend's living room, without any ceremonial support, and experienced "nothing." He was fortunate, I think.

For reasons discussed above, in the North American, or more generally, in the Northern hemispheric setting, even the ceremony may not be enough. It is, for some, but may leave others bewildered. The deep psychological and spiritual dynamics potentially brought to our awareness during ceremony require guidance, both before and after, for their full integration. Even participants who have lovely experiences may not derive the complete benefit without some guidance and help with interpretation.

As one who offers such guidance, I am unconcerned with the subjective nature of a person's process, whether or not he saw beauty or monstrosity, whether or not she felt relief or intense discomfort, joyousness or horror. What matters is the teaching in each person's experience, and that teaching arises from their lives, their formative influences, their present situation, and their present needs.

"We ordinarily believe that we know who we are, what we are, what we are going to do, what life is about, what should happen," writes the great spiritual master A. H. Almaas. "Inquiry means challenging all these things. Do we really know?" Almaas was teaching about inquiry in a different context, but whether or not he would endorse such a view, I see the ayahuasca experience as primarily one of inquiry. Everything that occurs, or does not occur, is the subject of curiosity, of exploration. The question is simply, what is the meaning of the experience I am having? How does it relate to where I have been and to where I may be going? Who is having the experience, or whom do I believe is having the experience? From such a perspective it really does not matter that this person visualized beauty while another beheld trauma. We are not seeking this or that experience; we are seeking the truth in any experience. There are no "bad trips," only opportunities to learn. It is never the painful or frightening visions or emotional states that make an ayahuasca journey bewildering or disturbing—only the lack of meaning a person may be left with, for lack of proper guidance and support. Ayahuasca, in the right setting, helps to reveal meaning.

That addictions or illnesses like cancer or rheumatoid arthritis or multiple sclerosis are related to trauma is a novel idea to doctors trained in the biological and genetic determinism characterizing modern medical practice, but it is hardly news to anyone who has interviewed addicted human beings or who is familiar with the research literature on the relationship between childhood adversity and adult disease.

Childhood trauma—either the direct trauma of abuse or the indirect trauma of emotional loss—engenders addiction for three main reasons. First, it ingrains profound pain in the mind and body of the child, pain that the person will later seek to escape. In my 12 years of work in Vancouver's Downtown Eastside, for example, I did not meet a single female client who had not been sexually abused as a child; not a single person, male or female, who had not experienced some form of trauma, neglect or abandonment. The question in addiction, my mantra is, is not why the addiction, but why the pain. And that, of course, is what the research shows: For each adverse childhood experience, the risk of addiction increases exponentially. Second, traumatic experiences shape the neurological circuits of the developing child in such ways as to potentiate the appeal of substances. In short, the microarchitecture and neurochemistry of the brain reflect our formative influences, and chief among these are our relationships with our caregiving environment. Third, our self-view and our view of the world are also created by our early interactions. As the Buddha taught, we create the world with our minds. What modern psychology has contributed is the understanding that before we create the world with our minds, the world creates our minds.

As stated above, cancer, autoimmune conditions of the joints or the intestines, and neurodegenerative diseases may also be traced to negative early experiences. The latter can trigger lifelong a tendency towards inflammation, undermine the immune system, and impair or excessively activate the body's stress response mechanisms. Further, they result in the child's adapting coping mechanisms of emotional self-suppression that can significantly disable the immune system. Many studies have shown the relationship between emotional repression and disease. A recent Canadian study found that people abused in childhood have a nearly 50 % risk of having cancer as adults.

Ayahuasca can evoke direct but long-suppressed memories of trauma. It can also trigger emotional states and visions of horror and pain that are not direct recollections, but emotional imprints of trauma. There is nothing wrong with that—so long as the person can stay present to their experience, and can accompany themselves through the pain and grief and fear that may arise. As Peter Levine teaches us, trauma is not simply in what happens; it is in our inability or lack of opportunity to move through the process of trauma. For a child to move through his or her painful experience, he or she needs the presence of a supportive adult. Children become traumatized not only because terrible things happen to them, but also because they must endure that terror alone, without support. In fact, they must suppress even their conscious awareness of what occurs to them, simply in order to survive. Suppressed, deeply ingrained, sublimated, diverted, and compensated for in many completely inauthentic ways, the trauma becomes the source of addictive patterns and of coping mechanisms that lead to many illnesses of body and mind. The healing capacity of the ayahuasca experience resides significantly in the plant's ability to evoke the painful experiences of childhood self *while* having those experiences witnessed by the empathic curiosity of the adult self. "I went to all the sad places of my childhood," one participant shared, "but I accompanied myself there with understanding and love."

The ayahuasca ceremony can take us beneath the false world-view we developed and have lived since childhood, and can reveal the pain underneath he coping mechanisms of the false self. It is when that pain emerges that we see clearly what we have been running and hiding from, either by means of addictions or by other means that have protected us from feeling the hurt: being "nice," for example, taking on the needs of others while ignoring our own, manipulating our environment, and seeking approval or success or the acceptance of our peers or of our families. It is that pain that can manifest in disturbing visions or feelings during ceremony.

We may experience love and gratitude, as I was fortunate to during my first ayahuasca journey. Or, as many have, we may be visited by spirit healers in human, divine, or animal form. We may see jungle creatures and jungle plants, and these may talk to us, invite us, and guide us (I have never had such visions, though many I have worked with have). These experiences of love or guidance is our experience of truth, of the universal love that underlies all experience but is often, in our mundane lives, clouded and obscured by experience. This is how we learn that there is no reason to run.

Our retreat begins on the evening of arrival with introductions and with people sharing their goals for the retreat: what problem they wish to resolve, what they wish to learn, where they perceive the need for completion in their lives. There is no agenda other than what each individual brings. Our goal, the goal of the team leading the retreat, is to assist each person to find their truth. We trust that truth. We believe, as Jesus said, "You shall know the truth, and the truth will set you free."

The first day is spent in group process. People are assisted to explore their issues, their emotions, their beliefs, to relate all that to their formative experiences, to see how their past influences and, in many cases, rules their present. The ultimate intent is to enter and experience the present moment, to be free of beliefs and coping patterns that represent the past.

The first ceremony occurs that night. Beforehand, intentions are set—not as fixed and limiting goals, but as points of inquiry, as anchors to help people stay grounded in their purpose during ceremony. "I intend to experience my childhood," someone will say. Or, "I want to see what keeps me from love," or "I want to see my fear," or "my power," or "my clarity."

My role as guide/therapist effectively stops once the candles are extinguished and the brew is ingested, although I remain available to anyone who might need support. The ayahuasqueros chant—not generically, not to the group only, not according to some predetermined playlist, but sensitively to the unfolding group experience, mindful of the energies being generated and released, and responsive to the needs of individuals for their intervention. They work hands-on with people to release energetic or emotional blockages, to identify and unlock resistances. And throughout, they chant, though we all hear it, to specific people at specific times.

After sleep and meals, the next afternoon and the following day are full-immersion and detailed processing of each person's experience during ceremony. Now the teaching deepens and power grows, the coming of insight accelerates, the bonds among participants are strengthened, the opening to inquiry widens. Two more ceremonies follow, preceded and followed by the group work already described, with some participants requesting or needing some individual attention or counseling throughout.

It is astonishing and gratifying to witness the power, wisdom, mutual support, and love inherent in each group, no matter what the specific problems or intentions or concerns the participants individually may bring. And, need I say, to witness the power of the plant to catalyze people's growth, to empower their determination to be themselves, to experience their true selves, and to teach them the path they need to follow.

We have successfully applied this model not just to middle-class participants well experienced in psychological work, but also in an aboriginal community in British Columbia, heavily traumatized by oppression and abuse. The results, here too, have been gratifying and we have been invited to return repeatedly.

Ayahuasca is not for everyone, and even for the ones it calls, it is, once more, no panacea. The egoic personality, supported and threatened and egged on by the materialistic culture we live in, will seek to assert itself even in the face of new knowledge and new insight. Today's cathartic realization may, by next week, become just a vague memory. Unless ongoing work is done to integrate the learning, what the Buddha calls our "habit energies" soon re-establish their dominance. And the world, we may be sure, will—because it is largely unconscious—seek to invalidate and suppress our consciousness. We can go back to sleep. No matter how profound our insights, how lovely our connections to our fellow travellers, how fervent our intentions; we can continue to generate suffering for ourselves and for others in our lives. But the beauty of it is, we do not need to fall back asleep. We now have choice.

For some, the plant is contraindicated. People with a history of psychosis or mania are best to avoid it, and I would not accept them at a retreat; not for fear of what would emerge, but for the impossibility of providing long-term care and follow-up in a safe context. Nor can active drug users participate, as the issues of craving and withdrawal would vitiate their experience. But recent users, no longer in withdrawal, have benefited greatly, for reasons I hope I have explained above. People have overcome cocaine addiction, sex addiction, and alcoholism.

Even when cure is not possible, healing happens. A man with late-stage ALS—amyotrophic lateral sclerosis, known in North America as Lou Gehrig's disease, in England as motor neuron disease—attended one of our retreats. After his first ayahuasca ceremony he said, "I came here because I wanted to live. Now I understand that wanting to live is not the same as living longer. It means being fully alive while my life lasts." His last year was peaceful, full of much wisdom, joy, and shared bliss with his family and friends.

"I have always believed no one wanted me here on this Earth," one participant wrote a few months after her retreat:

> This has drastically colored most all of my experiences. However, during the ayahuasca ceremony, I listened to a voice saying "I don't want you to go away, I don't want you to go away," over and over and over. Also during the ceremony, I cried and remembered the innumerable times in my life I had disappeared when I had listened to the voice that said no one wants me here. Now, providing that basic building block of attention to myself, I find that when I remember I want me here, I have a very different experience of myself and the world. I feel solid in a new way. I do exist. I am here. All of the times I was convinced that no one wanted me here, I was bringing that belief to the situation. It wasn't actually happening anywhere except in my mind. I have always thought people didn't like me. Now I know I'm loveable.

That connection to our true selves, hard to achieve or regain in the face of trauma or loss, is what is most precious in this life. Fundamentally, what the plant offers is no magic. It is only the reality and the love: our birthright. And that, I believe, sums up the science, theory, and practice of ayahuasca, as of all true healing modalities: reality and love.

References

Maté, G. (2010). *In the realm of hungry ghosts: Close encounters with addiction*. Berkeley, CA: North Atlantic Books.

Correction to: Ayahuasca as a Candidate Therapy for PTSD

Jessica L. Nielson and Julie D. Megler

Correction to:
Chapter 3 in: B. Caiuby Labate and C. Cavnar (eds.), *The Therapeutic Use of Ayahuasca*, https://doi.org/10.1007/978-3-642-40426-9_3

In the original version of this book, the following correction has been incorporated: In Chapter 3, the name citation of "John Pasquina" has been removed. The book and the chapter have been updated with the change.

The updated version of this chapter can be found at
https://doi.org/10.1007/978-3-642-40426-9_3

B. Caiuby Labate and C. Cavnar (eds.), *The Therapeutic Use of Ayahuasca*,
https://doi.org/10.1007/978-3-642-40426-9_14,

Index

B. C. Labate and C. Cavnar (eds.), *The Therapeutic Use of Ayahuasca*,
DOI: 10.1007/978-3-642-40426-9, © Springer-Verlag Berlin Heidelberg 2014

MIX
Papier aus verantwortungsvollen Quellen
Paper from responsible sources
FSC® C105338

If you have any concerns about our products,
you can contact us on
ProductSafety@springernature.com

In case Publisher is established outside the EU,
the EU authorized representative is:
Springer Nature Customer Service Center GmbH
Europaplatz 3, 69115 Heidelberg, Germany

Printed by Libri Plureos GmbH
in Hamburg, Germany